Auricular Acupuncture Diagnosis

Dedication

To my teachers Yoshio Manaka and Johannes Bischko

For Elsevier:

Commissioning Editor: Mary Law/Karen Morley
Development Editor: Fiona Conn
Project Manager: Kerrie-Anne McKinlay
Senior Designer: Judith Wright
Illustration Manager: Merlyn Harvey
Illustrator: Graeme Chambers

Auricular Acupuncture Diagnosis

Marco Romoli
General Practitioner, Prato, Italy

With contributions by
Pierre Rabischong MD
Honorary Dean of the Faculty of Medicine, University of Montpellier, France

Filadelfio Puglisi
Bioengineer, Lecturer of Biomechanics for the Department of Motor Sciences, University of Florence, Italy

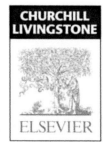

CHURCHILL LIVINGSTONE

ELSEVIER

Edinburgh London New York Oxford Philadelphia St Louis Sydney Toronto 2010

CHURCHILL
LIVINGSTONE
ELSEVIER

ISBN 978-0-443-06866-9

British Library Cataloguing in Publication Data
A catalogue record for this book is available from the British Library

Library of Congress Cataloging in Publication Data
A catalog record for this book is available from the Library of Congress

Notice
Neither the Publisher nor the Authors assume any responsibility for any loss or injury and/or damage to persons or property arising out of or related to any use of the material contained in this book. It is the responsibility of the treating practitioner, relying on independent expertise and knowledge of the patient, to determine the best treatment and method of application for the patient.

The Publisher

The
Publisher's
policy is to use
paper manufactured
from sustainable forests

Printed in the United States of America
Transferred to Digital Printing, 2011

Preface

Nowadays, with so many sophisticated diagnostic tools at our disposal (ultrasonography, CT, MRI, PET and so on), it may seem unrealistic to rely on simple procedures such as the inspection and palpation of the auricle for diagnosis.

However, despite great progress made in medical technologies, all practitioners need to make physical and psychological contact with patients. The ear lends itself well to this: through this small appendage of the body we can gain an overview of functional and psychosomatic disorders which cannot be investigated with conventional techniques. This diagnostic approach, however, calls for sufficient medical knowledge to interpret and correlate the information coming from the auricle with the symptoms of our patients.

This book is based on about 5000 observations made in both healthy subjects and patients affected by a large variety of diseases. My intention is to provide physicians and therapists with an innovative diagnostic model, giving them the possibility of a fuller understanding of their patients.

Given the increased interest in ear acupuncture over the past 50 years, it is my hope that this book will encourage readers throughout the world to add their personal experience to this constantly developing field.

MR 2009

Acknowledgements

I would like to express my gratitude to all my patients and colleagues who throughout time have made this work possible.

Special thanks go also to Marco De Vincenzi for his tireless processing of data; Andrea Giommi and Francesco Profili for their statistical expertise; Simone Fantoni and Stefano Bandinelli for their professional photographic consultancy; Giovanni Zagli for his precious help in searching out literature and Susan Seeley for her linguistic assistance.

Contents

Chapter 1

The history of the method

INTRODUCTION

In order to explain how such an interesting and innovative diagnostic and therapeutic system as that involving the outer ear remained unknown until about 50 years ago, we need to take a few steps back through the history of medicine, first to ancient times when a wide variety of animal and human ailments were cured using iron and fire. Cauterization was well known to Hippocrates (460–380 BC), who wrote in his last aphorism (section VII, no. 87), '*quaecunque medicamentis non curantur, ferrum curat, quae ferro non curantur, ignis curat, quae igne non curantur, ea incurabilia sunt*' ('those diseases which are not cured by medicines are cured by the scalpel; those which are not cured by the scalpel are cured by fire; those which are not cured by fire can be considered incurable').

The great surgeons Avicenna (980–1037) and Abū al-Qāsim, also known as Albucasis (d. c.1013), were particularly skilled in cauterization, and in selecting the appropriate instruments and techniques. Albucasis stated in the first book of his work,[1] dedicated entirely to cauterization: 'the cautery excels the drug by the rapidity of its success, the strength of its action, and the potency of its powers'. However, he admonished his pupils:

no one should attempt this operation unless he has had long training and practice in the use of the cautery, and is fully acquainted with the various human temperaments, and the character of the complaints in themselves; their causes, symptoms, and duration.

He removed some prejudices which still existed in this period:

> the Ancients disagreed also as to the fit time for cautery, affirming that spring was the best. Myself, I say that the cautery is suitable at all times; for whatever harm may arise from the season of the operation is utterly outdone by the benefit deriving from the cauterization itself; especially if the cautery is applied to pains that are severe, grievous, and swift, brooking no delay, because of the fear that the consequences may be more grave than the slight harm from the season.

His opinion was that:

> the actual cautery and its superiority over cauterization with chemical caustics is one of the secrets of medicine. For fire is a simple substance having no action except upon the actual part cauterized; nor does it do more than slightly harm any adjacent part. But the effect of cauterization with caustic may spread to parts at a distance from that burnt; and also in the part cauterized it may give rise to a disease difficult to cure or even fatal.

In the centuries to follow, the methods used were termed 'actual cautery' and 'potential cautery'. These indicated, respectively, treatment with red-hot iron and local application of caustics.

In Albucasis's time many parts of the body and several diseases were treated with cauterization, for example pleurisy, chest complaints, liver abscesses, diseases of the spleen, dropsy, piles and anal fistula, painful menstruation and infertility, toothache, migraine, sciatic pain, etc. In Chapter 5 of his book Albucasis described the following treatment for earache:

> when the ear gets a pain from the cold and is treated with laxatives and other medicine as mentioned in its section and the pain nevertheless persists, heat the cautery termed punctate. Then after it has been heated prick with it in a circle right round the ear, or around both if there is pain in both, after the place has been marked with ink; the cauterizations being a little away from the ear. Let the cauterization be of ten punctures or thereabouts round. Then dress the places till healed.

Albucasis at work is depicted in a series of miniatures accompanying the Latin translation of his text (Fig. 1.1).

The method of cauterization spread throughout Europe, and many physicians applied the actual

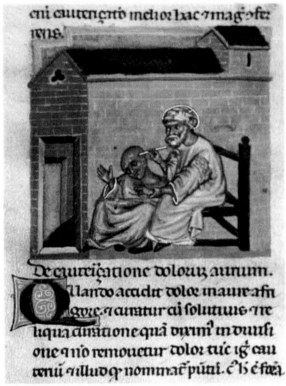

Fig. 1.1   Albucasis applying the cautery in a case of earache. Miniature from Abu'l Qasim Halaf Ibn Abbas al-Zahrawi, *Chirurgia*, second half of 14th century. *(Reproduced with the permission of the Wellcome Institute for the History of Medicine, London.)*

cautery until well into the 19th century. In France, the country in which the practice of cauterization had most support and was most widespread, it was used in the hospitals of all the principal towns, and the person who in 1811 best summarized the history of the actual cautery and best described the technique was a Frenchman, Pierre-François Percy (1754–1825), a surgeon at the court of Napoleon, who had had considerable experience on the battlefield. Percy[2] ordered at least 10 instruments of different dimensions and shapes to be forged for various uses. The heated instruments were inserted into a special wooden handle (Fig. 1.2).

The instruments were classified into three groups:

1. *cautères objectifs* – brought close to the part to be treated but not into contact with it (used, for example, for bleeding piles or nosebleeds)
2. *cautères transcurrens* – touched the affected part rapidly and superficially (used, for example,

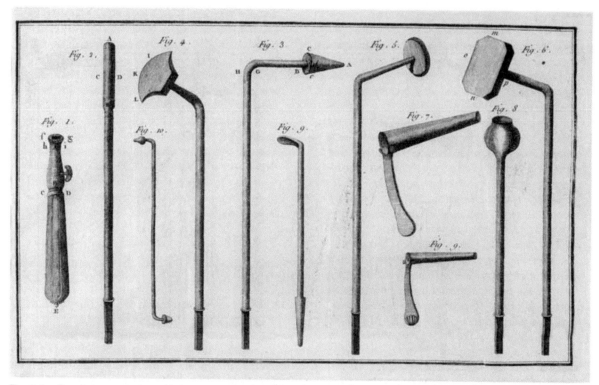

Fig. 1.2 Percy's ten cauteries with handle on the left. *(Reproduced with the permission of the Wellcome Institute for the History of Medicine, London.)*

for delicate tissues such as the lips and eyelids but also for rheumatism and sciatica)
3. *cautères inherens* – applied and held in place for more or less time, to act deeper.

In England the practice of ironing the painful part with a laundress's iron (the skin being protected by being covered with a piece of thin flannel or brown paper) had long been in vogue for various types of pain. However, it was only after 1830 that physicians such as Henry William Fuller[3] and James Syme[4] proposed the use of the actual cautery for lumbago, stiff neck and other forms of 'muscular rheumatism', which at that time included sciatica.

An exceptional case report comes from one of the great surgeons of the history of medicine, Joseph Lister. Having qualified in London, Lister went to Scotland, where in 1854 he became Syme's house-surgeon at the Edinburgh hospital. During his stay he probably witnessed patients being treated with the actual cautery, as in the following case:[5]

Case IV. – Disease between the Atlas and Axis: Actual Cautery applied with great benefit.

Thomas Smith, aet. 27, admitted the 20th of June, 1854. Generally enjoyed good health till eighteen months ago, when a stiffness of the neck came on without any assignable cause, with pain when he turned round his head on the pillow; the pain increased greatly, and deprived him altogether of sleep for seven weeks, during which time he lost three stone in weight. There was severe pain in the head as well as in the neck, aggravated to an extreme degree by either nodding or turning of the head, particularly the latter, which, indeed, he at last never did without turning the rest of the body also. He applied to numerous medical men in Birmingham, where he lives; and blisters and caustic issues were repeatedly applied to the back of the neck, but never gave more than very slight and very transient relief, and he says that from the commencement of his complaint he never had one minute's freedom from pain, except during sleep, till he came here.

At this time he was, according to his own account, about as bad as he had been at all. His countenance wore a peculiar expression of mingled suffering and apprehension, as Mr. Syme expressed it. He complained of severe pain in the neck and head, aggravated by any sudden movement, so that there was a great constraint about all his actions. He always kept his head bolt upright except when in bed, and could neither lie down nor get up without supporting his head with his hands; he never turned his head without the rest of the body, but gentle nodding was not very painful. There was great swelling of the upper part of the neck, and he could only open his mouth a little way; deglutition was extremely difficult, and a remarkable prominence of the bodies of the upper cervical vertebrae was to be felt in the pharynx.

On the day after the admission, Mr. Syme applied the actual cautery over the spinous processes of the upper cervical vertebrae; the man was not under chloroform, and said he hardly knew whether the pain was greater even at the moment than what he had experienced from caustic issues, and immediately afterwards he told us that he did not feel the pain of the burn at all. Next day he found less pain in moving the head, and in two or three days his countenance assumed a cheerful aspect. A steady daily improvement has since taken place in his symptoms, and at the present time (the 15th of July) he has no pain whatever when he sits at rest, and can also use strong and active exertion without uneasiness, and no longer requires to support his head in lying down or rising; he can turn his head round pretty freely and look up to the ceiling, and it is only in sudden movements of the neck that he feels any pain at all. The swelling of the neck has greatly subsided, and he can open his jaws wide, and swallow with comparative facility. The sore on the neck is almost healed, and he talks of leaving the hospital in a few days as cured.

Remarks. – The above cases speak for themselves; and I might add several others, that exemplify in an equally striking manner the beneficial effects of the actual cautery in certain forms of articular disease. It will be observed that is by no means so painful a remedy as is generally supposed, and also that its good effects are more than can be attributed to the mere discharge of pus from the sore which it produces, seeing that a great improvement commonly occurs within a few hours of its application, and long before suppuration is established.

It is now many years since the use of this means of counter-irritation was introduced into Great Britain by Mr. Syme; but although a constant series of successful cases have since continued to demonstrate its value to those who have witnessed his practice, yet I am satisfied that it has not hitherto been sufficiently generally appreciated. Case IV is an example of its efficacy against a most formidable disease, where caustic issues had been long tried in vain. I believe many limbs and lives have been sacrificed that might have been saved by the actual cautery, and by it alone; and having been myself very strongly impressed with the importance of the subject, I should be truly glad if any surgeon who may have hitherto overlooked it, should be induced by the above report to inquire more closely into its merits.

CAUTERIZATION OF THE EAR

It is not easy, even approximately, to identify exactly when cautery was first applied to the external parts of the ear (auricle) for therapeutic purposes.

If we limit our research to ancient Europe, there are traces in folk medicine which indicate that the external ear also had some significance in the prevention of disease. One noteworthy folk tradition is the custom of wearing earrings to improve sight or to prevent eye disease. Sailors of the European coasts and mountaineers of the central Alps shared this tradition, even though contact between these two populations was exceedingly rare in previous centuries. The custom, passing from one generation to the next, was popular in the valleys of Switzerland, Austria and northern Italy, and a common saying there, even in recent times, was 'gold fits good sight', referring of course to the wearing of a gold earring.

Among the more reliable pieces of information on cauterization of the ear in ancient literature, the quotations from the work of Johannes Scultetus or Schultheiss (1595–1645) reported in Percy's book[2] are remarkable. The physician was the pupil of the famous anatomist Adrian van der Spieghel of Brussels (1578–1625), also known as Spigel. The pupil observed the teacher cauterizing the antitragus of patients with toothache on the same side as the pain. This was a technique which he had applied also on himself: 'hac nova chirurgia dolor non amplius revertitur...ejusque virtutem in se primum expertus est auctor; post modum, me praesente, in non paucis aliis' ('with this new surgery the pain does not relapse so intensely...the value of which the author appreciated first on himself; afterwards, in my presence, also on not a small number of other patients').

Another excellent witness, not so many decades later, was the anatomist Antonio Valsalva (1666–1723), who performed the first rigorous and documented differentiation between outer, middle and inner ear. In his book,[6] based, according to his biographers, on 16 years of tireless work dissecting more than 1000 human skulls, particular mention is made of cauterizations carried out by healers on the posterior part of the lobe with the aim of treating toothache. Valsalva wrote:

the surgeon must apply a red-hot iron of four lines length [about 1 cm – author's note] *transversally on the back of the antitragus, because the nerve will certainly be included. For the rest a slight thickness is sufficient and there is no need to cauterize deeper than the cartilage.*

Figure 1.3 shows the location of the site which was most frequently cauterized.

The experiences from the 17th century reported above hold particular significance for practitioners in the 21st century and the following remarks may be made:

1. a topographic correlation was unexpectedly found between the symptom to treat (toothache) and the specific area to cauterize (the antitragus,

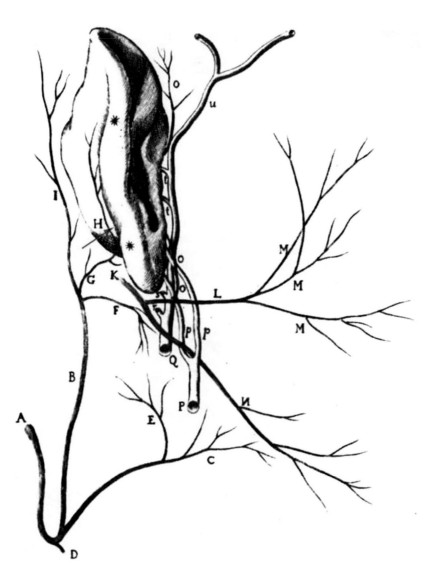

Fig. 1.3 The site (arrow) of cauterization for toothache according to Valsalva.[6] '*H = Locus, ubi ramus cujus ustio à quibusdam practicis ad tollendam odontalgiam proponitur, certius uretur*' ('H = The site where the branch was more certainly burned by some healers for treating toothache').

whether on the lateral side or the medial surface of the auricle)

2. cauterization had to be performed on the side corresponding to the pain
3. it had to include a neural branch to be effective
4. there was no need to apply the red-hot iron too deeply.

Transferring this knowledge to the present day, and adding our current knowledge of the neurophysiology of ear acupuncture, it may be said that in order to succeed with stimulation: one must first be very familiar with the somatotopic representation of the human body on the auricle; in the case of a painful syndrome it is best to select the points on the same side as the pain; one should be aware that the most effective auricular points are often located close to the nerve endings; and to be effective it is not necessary to practice invasive stimulation, as for example with needles, but an even more superficial stimulation such as massage, electric stimulation, magnet pearls, *Vaccaria* seeds, etc. may be applied.

Without any doubt, the most crucial year for the development of contemporary ear acupuncture was 1850. In that year the French *Journal des Connaissances Médico-Chirurgicales*, in its issue of 1 May, published an article on the cauterization of the ear as a radical treatment for sciatica. The report by Dr Lucciana of Bastia, Corsica, described a female patient who had been suffering with disabling sciatica for between 8 and 10 months. She was treated with opium and moxa by the physician himself and admitted to hospital for 25 days, during which she underwent several treatments, including, for example, cupping and blisters, without result. When she was discharged the pain was still quite severe and she chose to be treated by a blacksmith who applied a red-hot iron to her outer ear to 'cut her sciatic nerve' which was the explanation given at that time. She recovered and after 20 days she was pain-free without relapse. The physician was so impressed by this and other similar cases that he urged observation of the Corsican blacksmiths at work. They simply used a red-hot iron with a firm hand if they were experienced, or alternatively applied a thin metal plate, no thicker than 1 mm, to the ear. The plate had a small opening to permit entry of the tip of the cautery, designed with a stop, to a maximum depth of 0.5 cm (Fig. 1.4). The operation was simple and it was sufficient to cover the burn with fresh butter or olive oil shaken in water. The effect of cauterization generally took place after 8–10 days, though in some cases it was instantaneous.

Dr Lucciana's drawings, clearly illustrating the site for treatment on the root of the helix, triggered a series of reports throughout the following months in the whole geographical area. It is essential to cite two physicians living about 600 km apart who read the same article. The parallels between their two stories are surprising: Joseph François Malgaigne (1806–1865) and Giambattista Borelli (1813–1891) were both head surgeons at their hospitals, in Paris

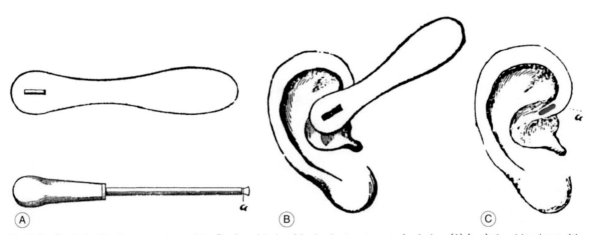

Fig. 1.4 Cauterization instruments used by Corsican blacksmiths in the treatment of sciatica: (A) (top) the thin plate with the small opening into which the tip of the cautery was introduced (bottom); (B) the thin plate applied on the root of the helix; (C) the site of cauterization.

and Turin, respectively; both were editors of a medical journal, the former of the *Journal de Chirurgie*, later known as the *Revue Médico-Chirurgicale*, the latter of the *Gazzetta Medica Italiana – Stati Sardi*. Both wrote reports of their own experiences soon after Lucciana's publication. Malgaigne made a first evaluation on 18 patients cauterized at Saint Louis hospital in Paris: one-third benefited by complete pain relief from the first day; one-third experienced complete or marked relief, but relapsed into pain after 2–24 hours; the last group of patients had no relief at all. He declared: 'It must be acknowledged that this is not a method of constant efficacy, however it is one of the most powerful methods, and when it works, the most rapid in its action'. The uncertain results of the operation probably led Malgaigne to seek out other areas in which to improve the percentage of success. The same thing occurred with Borelli who used to treat one or more areas with superficial cauterizations of 1–2 cm in length and 0.5 cm in width (Fig. 1.5). His conclusions were very interesting:[7]

> *Further research is now necessary to find an answer to some important questions regarding not only the disease but also the physiology concerned:*

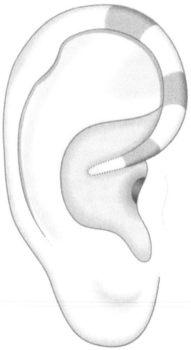

Fig. 1.5 The three areas used for cauterization by Giambattista Borelli.

> – *which is the exact point of the auricle to cauterize to obtain the best and most constant effect against sciatic pain?*
> – *does cauterization of the ear with caustic give the same result as actual cautery?*
> – *does cauterization performed under anesthesia have the same value as that performed with full consciousness of pain?*
> – *does intensity of pain felt during cauterization have some relation to its therapeutic effect?*
> – *which types of sciatica are more rapidly and constantly healed by cauterization?*
> – *finally, is the therapeutic effect of cauterization exclusive to sciatic pain or could it be extended to other kinds of very acute pain, especially to toothache, to facial, cervical-brachial, femoral neuralgias and iliac-scrotal pain?*

In England, cauterization of the auricle did not have the same popularity as it had in France. News from the continent was, however, reported in British journals. *The Lancet* of 19 October 1850 published a short comment about the treatment of sciatica (p. 451):

> So respectable an authority as Mr. Malgaigne, of Paris, has lately been publishing cases of sciatica, which were cured by cauterization of the lobe of the ear. From various accounts which have appeared in the medical periodicals of France, it would appear that this somewhat far-fetched counter-irritation or derivation is of old origin, and has been lately revived. It is confidently stated in the Revue Médico-Chirurgicale that a great proportion of cures has been obtained.

A few years later the same journal (*Lancet*, 14 June 1856, pp. 656–657) published an article by Dr Septimus Gibbon with the title 'Cases of sciatica, treated principally by cupping and tonics'. The physician wrote:

> We cannot refrain from adverting, while upon this subject, to the revival, a few years ago, by Mr. Malgaigne, of a remedy in popular use in Corsica – namely, the application of the actual cautery to the tip of the ear. Upon what principle the cure is effected here we are at a loss to determine, but several reported successful cases were given in the French journals at the time. We rather suspect the remedy had the effect of frightening away the pain.

The few physicians who in those years applied the method correctly on selected patients obtained

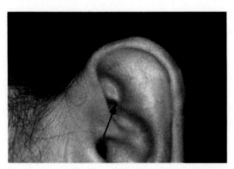

Fig. 1.6 An example of cauterization (site indicated by arrow) for sciatica made by an anonymous medical doctor (Tuscany, about 1950).

appreciable results. The majority, cauterizing instead the same area for several different pain disorders that were not sciatica, failed to achieve any positive results. The technique therefore declined rapidly as any knowledge or understanding of the underlying neurophysiological mechanisms was completely lacking. In 1855, Duchenne de Boulogne, who had always been firmly opposed to this technique, tackled the issue again, declaring that the therapeutic effect was only due to the acute and sudden pain of the cauterization itself. The auricle therefore played no role at all, and any cauterization performed in any part of the body could have been effective.

The method then sank into oblivion but, as with other treatments which have some intrinsic base of efficacy, it has survived among the population up to the present day, handed on by healers, monks and medical doctors (Fig. 1.6).

THE DISCOVERY OF AURICULOTHERAPY

A century later auricular cauterization was brought back to light and ear acupuncture had a new lease of scientific life. The years 1950–51 were important ones for the French physician Paul Nogier of Lyons (1908–1996). Nogier was impressed by the scar on the anthelix borne by some patients who had been treated for sciatica by healers in south-eastern France. The unanimous tale of these patients was that of a rapid recovery from pain within hours, or even minutes, after treatment. An evident connection between cauterization and the alleviation of pain could not be denied and Dr Nogier, without preconception, started treating patients in the same way. At first he applied cauterizations and later a less harmful method such as pins or acupuncture

needles. He gave much thought to the possibility that some unknown reflex areas might be located on the ear. At that time he was unaware that the site of the cauterization was different to the site which was popular in the 19th century. Nogier later commented:[8]

Have the traditions been distorted? Note that the former site on the helix, of which I now understand the efficacy, would never have allowed me to discover auriculotherapy.

Nogier tirelessly passed 'hundreds of hours' palpating and stimulating patients' auricles in order to relieve the different pain syndromes they presented. The result was a long series of failures and he wrote about that difficult time: 'the ear refused to yield its secret to my insufficient analytical method'. It was only in 1953, while he was studying manipulation techniques of the lumbosacral spine with another colleague, that he discovered the right key (Fig. 1.7):

I realized in a flash that the cauterized part of the anthelix could perhaps correspond to the lumbarsacral articulation and, in this case, the anthelix could entirely represent the spine, but with the head pointing down corresponding to the antitragus: the auricle could therefore appear as the image of an embryo in the uterus.[9]

Once he had discovered the correspondence between the anthelix and spine Nogier proceeded systematically with the identification of other zones, drawing inspiration from the segmental organization of the human body. The representation of the shoulder girdle was therefore to be found not far from the cervical spine, and the hip was close to the lumbosacral tract. Nogier soon understood that medical knowledge was necessary to treat diseases successfully. In his own words: 'It is essential to make a good diagnosis in order not to confuse the painful organ with its projection on the skin'. On this topic he reported the following case:

My children's tutor, aged 65, with high blood pressure around 180 mmHg, one evening this year told me she had had a pain in her right foot the whole afternoon. The pain was rather curious, short, intense, returning every two or three minutes. We were sitting down to dinner and I proposed relieving it immediately through acupuncture on her ear. I placed the first needle in the region corresponding to the foot without result; I applied

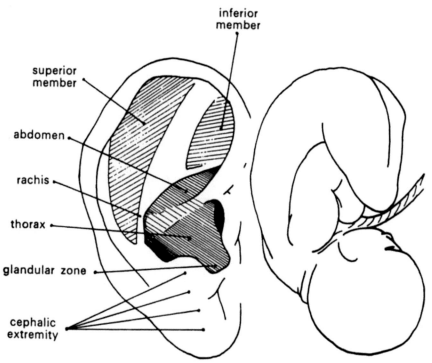

Fig. 1.7   The auricle and fetal image according to Paul Nogier *(reproduced with permission)*.

a second and probably a third but I was a little confused as she felt no relief at all. I suddenly realized her pain was not of gouty origin, but probably arterial pain originating in the lumbar-sacral sympathetic plexus. A puncture in this neural-vascular zone, which I have shown on the internal border of the anthelix, finally relieved what was only a reflex spasm.[10]

In February 1956 Nogier was invited by Dr Niboyet, a leading authority in acupuncture, to hold his first conference at the First Symposium of the Société Méditerranéenne d'Acupuncture in Marseille. In September of the same year he was invited by Dr Gerhard Bachmann (1895–1967), president of the German Association of Acupuncture, to give a similar speech in Wiesbaden. A few months later a report of his 6 years of research was published in three different issues of the journal *Deutsche Zeitschrift für Akupunktur (DZA)*.[10] The first detailed maps of the ear were officially born and Dr Bachmann himself made the drawings, as he was a skilled artist, having graduated in architecture before graduating in medicine (Figs 1.8, 1.9). As *DZA* was regularly read by Russian, Japanese and Chinese physicians among others, the

article and its maps rapidly spread all over the world. China was the first country to translate the article and validate the new diagnostic and therapeutic method. Just 1 year later, in the December 1958 issue of the *Shanghai Journal of Chinese Pharmaceutics and Medicine*, Yeh Hsiao-Lin published a summary of Nogier's three articles entitled 'Introduction to ear acupuncture therapy'.

It has to be remembered that every new discovery in the field of medicine is greeted not only with admiration but also with criticism, and sometimes with envy. The same thing happened to auriculotherapy, which was welcomed with enthusiasm by an increasing number of physicians but also had to face the comments of some incredulous colleagues.

In an article published in 1958 in *DZA* entitled 'Beware of fanciful acupuncture',[11] Dr De la Fuye of Paris challenged the hypothesis that a representation of the body permitting the physician to differentiate the knee, the elbow, the buttock, the abdomen, and even the individual vertebrae, could be identified on the outer ear. He concluded that 'this is childish and I propose to return to this issue in the next 200 years!' However, 50 years have already passed and ear acupuncture does not appear to have lost any of its vitality. The name of Nogier is

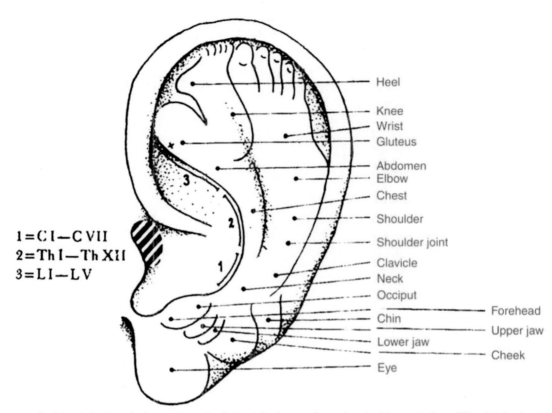

1 = CI—C VII
2 = Th I—Th XII
3 = LI—LV

Heel
Knee
Wrist
Gluteus
Abdomen
Elbow
Chest
Shoulder
Shoulder joint
Clavicle
Neck
Occiput
Forehead
Chin
Upper jaw
Lower jaw
Cheek
Eye

Fig. 1.8   Paul Nogier's 'historical' map drawn by Gerhard Bachmann *(reproduced with permission of Dietrich Bachmann and DZA).*

Fig. 1.9   Paul Nogier's 'historical' map drawn by Gerhard Bachmann *(reproduced with permission of Dietrich Bachmann and DZA).* 1 = bladder; 2 = kidney; 3 = pancreas; 3a = gallbladder; 4 = liver; 5a = esophagus; 5b = cardia; 5c = stomach; 5d = small intestine; 5e = large intestine; 6 = lung; 7 = heart; 8 = subcortex; 9 = internal nose; 10 = endocrine; 11 = spleen

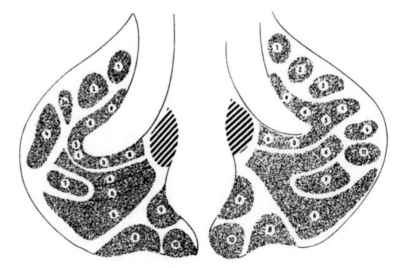

remembered everywhere in the world but, unfortunately for the author of this controversy, only few physicians remember the name of Dr De la Fuye!

THE CONTRIBUTION OF CHINA TO THE DEVELOPMENT OF EAR ACUPUNCTURE

Since the late 1950s, government institutions of the People's Republic of China have been in charge of restoring the reputation and promoting the practice of Chinese medicine. According to Hsu,[12] three 'innovations in acumoxa' (*zhenjiu*) were promulgated by the government during the Maoist periods of the Great Leap Forward (1958–61) and the Cultural Revolution (1966–76): analgesia (*zhenjiu mazui*), scalp acupuncture (*touzhen*) and ear acupuncture (*erzhen*).

The first, analgesia, became popular nationally and gained international recognition after delegations sent to China in the late 1960s and early 1970s visited hospitals in the big cities. They reported some impressive photographic documentation of surgical interventions performed with acupuncture analgesia.[13] The technique was applied during head, chest and abdominal surgery, stimulating acupuncture points on the body and on the auricle both manually and electrically. This application of acupuncture lost its popularity in the 1980s, both in China and in Europe, largely because the technique was time-consuming to apply and because the level of induced hypoalgesia was insufficiently predictable in different subjects and different types of intervention.

Scalp acupuncture was mainly practiced by highly skilled physicians in government hospitals and only for some specific diseases. This is perhaps the main reason why the technique did not spread so extensively among Chinese acupuncturists. Ear acupuncture, however, though imported from the West, has maintained its popularity outside government institutions up to the present day. Factors in its favor are probably that it can be easily applied, easily learnt and understood, and is extremely economical. But historical reasons have also been put forward to explain this great interest in the diagnostic and therapeutic value of the auricle. It has been said that in previous centuries the classical textbooks of Chinese medicine always attributed a great deal of importance to the ear. One example is *Ling Shu*, part of *Huangdi Nei Jing* (known also as the Canon of Medicine), compiled and rearranged by several authors over an extensive period of time (about

475 BC to AD 23). Chapter 28 reports: 'The ear is the place where all the channels meet', and Chapter 29 advises: 'By inspecting the condition of the ear, one knows whether the individual has an illness or not'.

Several techniques for treating disease were described in ancient times either as folk remedies or as specific treatments proposed by individual physicians. Among them are reported: the tradition of smearing, filling or blowing drugs into the ear; moxibustion of the apex for cataracts or acute conjunctivitis; massage of the helix to prevent deafness; needling of the helix, once more, to treat parotitis or to expel Wind for relieving backache, etc. According to Huang,[14] auricular therapy was long supposed to have the function of regulating the deficiency of *qi*, strengthening the senses, invigorating the function of Liver blood, nourishing *Yin* and regulating the function of the Kidney.

Despite this consideration for the ear there is no mention in ancient Chinese literature of a somatotopic arrangement of the auricle as proposed by Nogier. The only exception is probably the posterior or medial surface of the ear which was described in detail, mainly for diagnostic purposes, by Zhang Di-Shan of the Qing dynasty in 1888. His book 'Essential Techniques for Massage' contained what is perhaps the first Chinese auricular map to be drawn. The illustration reports five regions corresponding to the five *zang* organs (Heart, Kidney, Spleen, Liver and Lung) (Fig. 1.10A). This view has some analogies to the disposition of the five elements but also to the threefold division of the body into Upper, Middle and Lower Burner according to traditional Chinese medicine (TCM). Even the tongue, among the various systems which describe the correspondences between specific areas and individual organs, could present some analogy with Zhang's chart.[15] The document has been accepted as part of the historical heritage by all contemporary Chinese authors and included officially in the process of the standardization of nomenclature completed in 1993 (Fig. 1.10B).

In the story of the development of ear acupuncture we should also mention Dr Xu Zuo-Lin of Beijing who in 1959 performed what was probably the first clinical validation on 255 patients for the most different diseases.[14] Using Nogier's maps, Xu introduced a series of new points which were linked to TCM. One of them was *shen* (the point of vitality) which became universally popular among acupuncturists as Shen men and is included in several Western maps (Fig. 1.11).

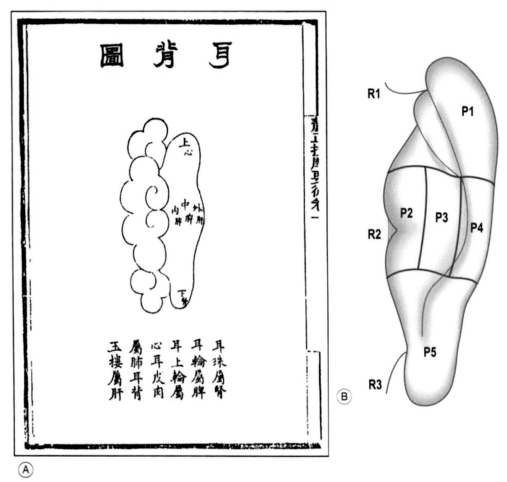

Fig. 1.10   (A) The 'historical' map of the posterior surface of the ear according to Zhang Di–Shan (1888) *(reproduced from* Modern Chinese Acupuncture *by Ping Chen, Paradigm Publications, 2004, with permission).* (B) The current Chinese standard location of ear points on the posterior surface. P1 *(erbeixin)* = heart; P2 *(erbeifei)* = lung; P3 *(erbeipi)* = spleen; P4 *(erbeigan)* = liver; P5 *(erbeishen)* = kidney; R1 *(shangergen)* = upper ear root; R2 *(ermigen)* = root of ear vagus; R3 *(xiaergen)* = lower ear root.

The discovery of an increasing number of new points was the result of a rapid development of auricular therapy in clinical practice and research. It is noteworthy that army doctors, especially those of the Nanjing garrison,[16] were among the first physicians to study the application of ear acupuncture on soldiers. They stated:

> *ear acupuncture neither needs equipment nor has any limitation of place and climatic condition; no matter where it is practiced: indoors or outdoors, in a laboratory, construction site, battlefield or classroom, this treatment can be applied.*

In the early years of the Cultural Revolution a campaign took place for a big increase in medical personnel in rural areas. Over a million 'barefoot doctors', also versed in the art of needling, took care of about four-fifths of the population. The first Chinese maps were probably conceived for them and showed a mosaic of illustrated anatomical parts which were easy to consult and use during practice. In the subsequent maps each part was further defined by a number, by the denomination in Chinese characters, and finally also by its translation to other languages.

In another important year for ear acupuncture, 1973, two physicians of the neurosurgical unit of Kwong Wah hospital in Hong Kong published an article about a new approach for relieving withdrawal symptoms and counteracting drug addiction.[17] They used only the Lung point, at the center of cavum conchae, and stimulated it electrically,

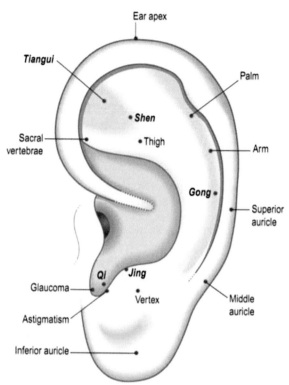

Fig. 1.11 Some new auricular points proposed by Xu Zuo-Lin.

One of the most relevant aspects in the recent history of ear acupuncture has been the effort on an international level to find a solution to the tendency to steadily increase the number of auricular points, thus creating confusion in the terminology used. The first attempt to provide a new system of nomenclature to describe the auricular points was proposed by Terry Oleson of the UCLA Pain Management Center of Los Angeles. In 1983 he developed an original 'auricular zone system', subdividing each major anatomical area and attributing a single letter and a number to each zone[19] (Fig. 1.12). His aim was to facilitate clinical understanding and research investigations into the accuracy of auriculotherapy.

bilaterally, for half an hour at a time with the frequency gradually increasing from 0 to 125 Hz. In the first days of treatment the patient received two or three stimulations per day followed by one per day for the next 4–5 days. Withdrawal symptoms ceased gradually 10–15 minutes after stimulation and 'a sense of general well-being was described by all patients undergoing treatment. They felt less drowsy, and much more interested in their surroundings than before, and they quickly gained an interest in conversation and reading'.

The success of this treatment convinced Dr Michael Smith of the Lincoln hospital in New York to form in 1974 the nonprofit association, the National Acupuncture Detoxification Association (NADA). The aim of NADA was to promote the training of acupuncture detoxification specialists in the USA and other parts of the world to treat all kinds of addiction. Acupuncture treatment without electrical stimulation of five auricular points (Sympathetic, Shen men, Kidney, Liver and Lung) was able to relieve withdrawal symptoms, prevent the craving for drugs and increase the rate of participation of patients in long-term treatment programs.[18]

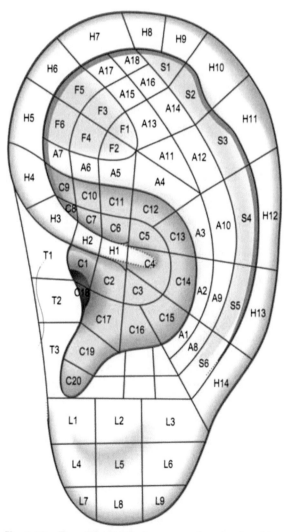

Fig. 1.12 The original auricular zone system developed by Oleson and colleagues (reproduced with permission).

The need for standardization of auricular points was felt urgently at that time and in 1982 Chinese researchers were entrusted by the World Health Organization's (WHO) Regional Office for the Western Pacific to establish the draft of a 'Standard Scheme of Auricular Points'. The scheme was presented after 5 years of discussion and revision in Seoul by Wang Deshen and Deng Liangyue[20,21] of the China Academy of Traditional Chinese Medicine of Beijing. A preliminary standardization of the anatomical areas of the outer ear was proposed. The subdivision into twelve different zones published in the report was, however, not definitive and a further 5 years of discussion were necessary before a final document emerged in which the number of the anatomical areas was reduced to eight.[22]

At the same WHO meeting of 1987 the following three inclusion criteria were proposed to standardize the different auricular points:

1. an international common name in use
2. a proven therapeutic value
3. a generally accepted location.

Points that fulfilled all three criteria were classified with an alphanumeric code (a two-letter abbreviation and one number), Pinyin, Han character and English name. For example, the 'wrist' was classified with the code SF2, with Pinyin *wan* and Han character 腕. Points that fulfilled the first and second criteria were not attributed a code, but only Pinyin, Han character and English nomenclature. Points that failed to fulfill all three of the criteria were excluded.

Of the 90 points proposed to the International Committee by Chinese researchers, 43 entered the first category, 36 the second and 11 the third. The standardization process, after a last WHO meeting in Lyon (1990), was then continued mainly by Chinese researchers, and in 1993 reached a total number of 68 points accepted at national level.[22]

The persistence of some disagreement regarding the standardization of auricular points and areas in the Western and Chinese charts calls for a systematic and rigorous clinical validation in the future, taking into account the different historical backgrounds when categorizing diseases and clinical syndromes.

References

[1] Albucasis. On surgery and instruments. London: Wellcome Institute of the History of Medicine; 1973.

[2] Percy M. Pyrotechnie chirurgicale-pratique. Metz: 1811.

[3] Fuller HW. On rheumatism, rheumatic gout, and sciatica. 2nd ed. London: John Churchill; 1856.

[4] Syme J. The principles of surgery. 4th ed. London: John Murray; 1856.

[5] Lister J. The collected papers of Joseph, Baron Lister. Vol. 2. Oxford: Clarendon Press; 1909.

[6] Valsalva A. De aure humana. Bologna: 1704.

[7] Borelli G. Riflessioni pratiche sulla cauterizzazione dell'orecchio nella cura dell'ischiade. Gazz Med Ita Stati Sardi. 1851;2:10–12;5:33–5;6:54–5.

[8] Nogier PFM. Handbook to auriculotherapy. 2nd ed. Brussels: SATAS; 1998.

[9] Nogier PFM. Traité d'auriculothérapie. Moulins-les-Metz: Maisonneuve; 1969.

[10] Nogier PFM. Über die Akupunktur der Ohrmuschel. DZA. 1957;3–4:25–33;5–6:58–63;7–8:87–93.

[11] De la Fuye R. Nehmt Euch in acht vor phantastischen Akupunkturen. DZA. 1958;1–2:22–3.

[12] Hsu E. Innovations in acumoxa: acupuncture analgesia, scalp and ear acupuncture in the People's Republic of China. Soc Sci Med. 1996;3:421–30.

[13] Niboyet JEH. L'anesthésie par l'acupuncture. Moulins-les-Metz: Maisonneuve; 1973.

[14] Huang Li-Chun. Auriculotherapy – diagnosis and treatment. Bellaire: Longevity Press; 1996.

[15] Maciocia G. Tongue diagnosis in Chinese medicine. Seattle: Eastland Press; 1994.

[16] Compiling Group of Nanjing Military Headquarters. Ear acupuncture. Shanghai: People's Publishing House; 1973.

[17] Wen HL, Cheung S. Treatment of drug addiction by acupuncture and electrical stimulation. Am J Acup. 1973;1:71–5.

[18] Smith MO, Khan I. An acupuncture programme for the treatment of drug-addicted persons. Bull Narc. 1988;1:35–41.

[19] Oleson TD, Kroening RJ. A new nomenclature for identifying Chinese and Nogier auricular acupuncture points. Am J Acup. 1983;4:325–44.

[20] WHO Regional Office for the Western Pacific. 3rd WHO regional working group on the standardization of acupuncture nomenclature. Seoul: 25–30 June 1987.

[21] Deshen W. The third WHO regional workshop on the standardization of acupuncture nomenclature. J Trad Chin Med. 1988;3:221–8.

[22] Technical Supervision Bureau of State. The nomenclature and location of ear acupuncture points. Beijing: Chinese Standard Publishing House; 1993.

Chapter 2

Anatomy, embryology and neurophysiology

Pierre Rabischong

GENERAL PRINCIPLES

MEN DID NOT BUILD MEN

We have the solution and not the problem.

Humans are the most recent species to appear on Earth and the only one able to understand the great complexity of all biological systems. The comprehensive approach that we advanced many years ago presupposes that the technical specifications of organs and functions correspond to a logic and intelligent program of construction. Therefore it is necessary to begin observation of a function by identifying the technical requirements necessary to achieve it, like an engineer investigating a machine that he did not design. After that, moving to the anatomical solution allows us to validate it and to appreciate the choice of biocomponents and the organization of command and control systems. In other words, this approach, going from function to morphology, can be compared to the inverse dynamics used in mechanics. In fact being obliged, after collecting scientific data from the observation of a biological problem, to formulate an explanatory theory, it is very important for us to keep in mind that a *logical plan of construction exists* and that this is no place for fantasy or personal feelings. At the present time we have measurement technology available for evaluating any kind of biological, physical or chemical phenomenon. In the clinical field, however, the situation can be a little bit different: sometimes a good clinical result indicated by a patient and partially validated by a physician may generate an interpretation lacking in precise scientific proof. The empirical practice of medicine is full of such interpretations which do not change the results but which can form the basis for a more or less convincing education program. Nevertheless, a hypothesis remains a hypothesis until it has been scientifically validated. This rigorous approach is mandatory when we are examining a clinical therapy such as auriculotherapy. We will try later to integrate the clinical data obtained for this technique within an acceptable functional scientific framework, leaving some doors open for future investigation.

EMBRYOLOGICAL DEVELOPMENT

The development of the embryo is guided by very precise instructions contained in the genetic code, with a specific reproducible timetable for every species. Starting from a small group of polyvalent cells, each organ and function is built and interconnected. The crucial role of the nervous system as control integrator explains its early identification in the ectoderm of the embryo as neural plate, neural groove and then neural tube induced by the notochord which also organizes the construction with the metameric segmented mesoblastic components of the spine and muscles. This initial overdevelopment of the neural tube is responsible, in all species, for the spiral shape of the embryo, rolled up around the vascular system, with the heart pump in the center pulsating very early in order to transport the required building and trophic material to all parts. At the end of the third month, each organ and function is in place. This complex growth program is perfectly regulated in its timing and everything is designed to minimize the influence of external factors, called epigenetic factors, by providing a physical and biochemical protective environment within the uterus, first for the embryo and later for the fetus. Some mistakes do occur, causing, fortunately, a low percentage of malformations.

THE NERVOUS SYSTEM

The nervous system is in general more complex than was thought. The more we know about it, the more we can appreciate its remarkable organization which can explain all biological and physiological phenomena. The incredible miniaturization of the components of neurons and the enormous capacity of their synaptic connections creates a very powerful, flexible and plastic neural network. It is no longer possible to discover new morphological structures within the brain, but the extremely complicated multimedia interconnections that we can increasingly better identify through revolutionary modern methods of imaging are still to be fully understood. A good example is the acupuncture point, which physically and structurally exists without any doubt, but which is difficult to integrate logically in the plan of human construction. The maps we make of neural pathways and centers, in our common tendency to represent them, are in fact very far from being a true representation of nervous organization; in reality it is increasingly difficult to envisage a 'holistic conception' of the nervous system. However, some very precise laws of functioning have been defined and accepted. This means that we cannot speculate on the role of a particular nervous structure without precise scientific arguments and evidence. This is, for example, the case with the reticular formation: for many teachers this is developing into a magical key but it lacks irrefutable neuroscientific proof for its use. Two other important points need to be considered: neural signal processing and the relationship between the cerebrospinal system and the vegetative or autonomic system.

TRANSMISSION AND PROCESSING OF NEURAL SIGNALS

Transmission and processing of neural signals occur in two conditions: first there is a *direct nervous conduction* along the fibers by a depolarization wave traveling from one node of Ranvier to another at a velocity that depends on the diameter of the myelin sheath. The maximum speed is in the order of 120 m/s corresponding to the largest sensory fibers of 25 μ diameter. Second, this neural conduction, neuron to neuron, is also regulated by the *synaptic doors* using neurotransmitters as keys for opening them and passing through. This technical originality, introducing a chemical code to facilitate or inhibit a signal, explains the clinical importance of neurochemistry as crucial to the understanding of nervous function. In addition there are some specific sites within the central nervous system responsible for the secretion of specific neurotransmitters, such as the monoaminergic centers (noradrenergic, serotoninergic and dopaminergic) in the brainstem and the cholinergic centers. The neuromodulation produced by all these neurotransmitters uses, like the endocrine glands, the circulation of the blood and also the cerebrospinal fluid. The action can be slower than direct nervous conduction and in most cases is more prolonged in time.

The cerebrospinal system has two parts: a *central part* located in the encephalon (brain, brainstem and cerebellum) and in the spinal cord, where in the gray matter the sensory inputs are separated from the motor outputs, and a *peripheral part* grouping all the sensory and motor nerves.

Regarding the general organization of the sensory inputs, it is important to remember that the different sensory fibers coming from different types of receptors with their different calibers are the dendritic expansions of the first neuron of the sensory pathway located in the spinal or cranial ganglion outside the central nervous system. There are more skin receptors than sensory fibers conveying the signal, which is the expression of a peripheral sensory convergence still not fully understood: is it the same type of receptor on the same fiber or different types? In addition, in their distribution, spinal and cranial nerves have a cutaneous and muscular territory and also, by sympathetic or parasympathetic fibers, a visceral territory, the main conscious expression of which is logically manifested on the skin by projected pain, according to its poor representation within the conscious somatosensory cortex. This central neural interference mechanism between different kinds of input has to be explained by the organization of the spinal and thalamic relays described later. This is therefore the neurophysiological justification for the dermatological metameric reflexes with an important sympathetic component provoked by pinching the skin in relation to visceral dysfunction, described after Head[1] by Jarricot,[2,3] which also exists at the level of the auricle. In addition, *reflex activity* needs to be defined from the physiological point of view. It is the result of the conjunction between a stimulus and a reaction.

A reflex can be *monosynaptic*, like the myotatic reflex due to the link of a Ia sensory fiber from a muscular spindle with an alpha motoneuron of the anterior horn of the spinal cord generating a muscular contraction, or *polysynaptic*, with a delayed reaction like the spinal withdrawal reflex of lower limbs after painful pinching of the skin, or the contraction of the iris after light stimulation. It can also concern *neural multicentric activity* such as general vegetative reactions (tachycardia, skin pallor, etc.) after mental induction (fright, anxiety, stress, etc.)

or, particularly, conditioning situations as demonstrated by Pavlov. In this context, it is possible to talk of *reflexotherapy* if certain well-defined stimuli result in pain relief or restore normal functioning. Neural architecture is composed of different interconnected levels creating a complex heterarchic control system which finally operates at the cortical level in conscious and unconscious mode. The commonly poor knowledge of the pilot of the human machine in biology or bioengineering was provided in the program, allowing him to decide and command difficult tasks executed by unconscious processes within the very complex and rich neural network. This can explain why, in order to understand any physiological problem, it is not enough to refer to the conscious part of nerve function, which represents only a small part of it. In fact, in order to have a clear view of a function it is mandatory to try to perceive all the parameters and interconnections acting in a completely unconscious manner.

The *vegetative* or *autonomic system* has two polarities controlled by the *sympathetic* and *parasympathetic* nervous systems. Their architecture is the same: first, specific centers within the central nervous system (brainstem and sacral spinal cord for the parasympathetic and C8/L2 spinal cord level in the intermediate gray matter for the sympathetic); second, ganglions connected by preganglionic myelinated fibers (white communicating ramus) with the centers and supplying vegetative organs by postganglionic unmyelinated fibers (gray communicating ramus). Those fibers are small in diameter (in the order of 3–6 µ) and therefore have a low conduction velocity. The differences between sympathetic and parasympathetic systems lie in the organization of the ganglions.

In the *sympathetic system*, the ganglions are located in a long interconnected chain on both sides of the spine with some plexus grouping of fibers along arterial vessels before distribution: cardiac, pulmonary, esophageal, coeliac, superior and inferior mesenteric, hypogastric plexuses. The superior cervical ganglion supplies the encephalic territory by fibers traveling along the vertebrobasilar artery and the internal and external carotid arteries.

In the *parasympathetic system* there is no chain but isolated ganglions appended commonly to the nerve, resulting in the innervation of a territory, as for the three branches of the trigeminal nerve with the ciliary, sphenopalatine and otic parasympathetic ganglions having their centers close to the IIIrd, VIIth and IXth cranial nerve (CN) nuclei.

The domain includes all the visceral organs located within the trunk, all the digestive glands and all the arterial vessels equipped with a contractile system allowing regulation of the blood flow. The best indicator of the equilibrium between the two opposite components of the vegetative nervous system is the iris in the anterior chamber of the eye, which has a smooth sphincter innervated by the parasympathetic system (myosis) and a dilatator radial muscle innervated by the sympathetic system (mydriasis). The intercommunication between the two big systems is made at the highest level in the brain, mainly by the hypothalamus. This center, which represents only 4 g of neural substance, plays a powerful role in the control of specific functions such as hunger, thirst, temperature, aggression, sexual behavior and the whole of the endocrine system through its rich vascular and nervous connections with the hypophysis (pituitary gland). Its influence on the cardiovascular and digestive systems and its connection with the central nucleus of the amygdala make it an important component of the limbic system, particularly the part concerning emotional expression. Finally, it will be necessary to associate these two cerebrospinal and vegetative systems when looking for the particular physiology of the ear pavilion. The vascular reaction perceived in the pulsations of the radial artery after its manipulation corresponds to a non-specific vegetative vascular reflex existing in all cutaneous territories.

MORPHOGENESIS OF THE HEAD

At the initial embryonic stage, three tubes are aligned longitudinally: the *neural tube*, the *notochord* and the *primitive digestive tube* closed at both its caudal and cranial extremities. Two major developments will occur, drastically changing the morphology. First of all, the rapid overgrowth of the neural tube, particularly in its cranial part, will generate the five encephalic vesicles with the cephalic and pontine flexures after closing the neural tube like a 'zipper model' during primary neurulation (2–4 weeks) and secondary neurulation (4–6 weeks). Isolated on its lateral border is the neural crest, responsible for the spinal and cranial sensory ganglions as well as postganglionic fibers, glial cells and the adrenal medulla. The construction of the primitive skull base has two parts: first, the posterior part built around the notochord, which plays a role in the genesis of the vertebral

bodies, ending in the clivus joining the occipital bone process and a part of the sphenoid at the level of the sella turcica; second, the anterior prechordal part built around the olfactory ethmoid bone and the orbital neurocranium with a typical human skull base angle (kyphotic skull base as opposed to the lordotic skull base of carnivores). The *calvarium*, the second part of the neurocranium, becomes osseous by a different osteogenesis than the cartilaginous matrix of the skull base, made by direct apposition of bone on the continuous dural membrane. Therefore the growth of the telencephalon is the 'motor' of the expansion of the skull vault which is possible because the cranial sutures are growth lines. The telencephalon initially has a smooth aspect and progressively makes folds called gyri to increase the surface of the cortex. When it finishes its growth, the sutures close, starting from the endocranial side. The anencephaly which is the malformative lack of telencephalon means the absence of a skull vault. The hydrocephalic deformation in young children with anomaly of the circulation of cerebrospinal fluid demonstrates the importance of intracranial pressure for the expansion of the skull. The suture drawing is linear on the endocranial side and sinuous on the exocranial side, due to the alternating tractions of the muscles during growth. However, after a certain age it is absolutely impossible to move the bones, and the explanation for the clinical success of *cranial osteopathy* has to be found in manipulation not of cranial bones but of the skin covering the skull.

The second major growth process takes place around the *primitive intestinal digestive tube* which will first be actively open, creating the primitive mouth at the cranial extremity, later dividing into nasal cavity and oral cavity, and the anal canal and its opening at the caudal extremity. The ectoblast and mesoblast of the area will generate some folds around the digestive tube that we must call 'visceral arches' and not branchial arches. In fact, this denomination originated in Ernst Haeckel's theory of recapitulation, which said the human embryo follows different stages as a phylogenetic recapitulation, which is nonsense. The four visceral arches, contributing by their growth to the setting up of the embryonic face, correspond to the segmentation of the mesoblast with ectodermal and endodermal fissures.

The important point is to remember that every visceral arch will have a skin cover from ectoblast, skeleton and muscles from mesoblast building the

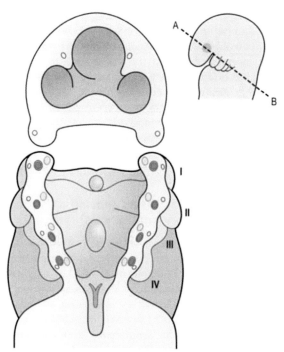

Fig. 2.1 Coronal section of the embryo's head showing the segmentation of the face isolating ectodermic and endodermic fissures and visceral arches.

splanchnocranium, and a specific cranial nerve from brainstem having motor, sensory and vegetative fibers innervating the territory (Fig. 2.1). Inside, the separation between the respiratory and digestive visceral tubes organizes the mandatory aero-digestive crossroads within the pharynx, allowing first the larynx to inject sounds into the mouth to be 'masticated' as phonemes and second, food to be injected into the esophagus without entering the respiratory tract, explaining the crucial role of the soft palate. The appropriate nomenclature is as follows:

- *First visceral arch*: 'mandibular arch', later developing the superior maxillary bone, the malar bone, the jaw with the temporomandibular joint (TMJ) and all the masticatory muscles (temporal, masseter, lateral and medial pterygoid, tensor tympani and tensor veli, the anterior part of the digastric, mylohyoid). The cranial nerve here is the *trigeminal nerve* (CN V) with its motor root and sensory root originating from the trigeminal ganglion with its three branches (ophthalmic, maxillary, mandibular) serving the three areas of the face (Plates IA, IB). A parasympathetic ganglion is appended to each trigeminal branch. The orbits contain the eyeballs which are diencephalic nervous expansions and have a roof of neural origin and a floor of visceral origin.

- *Second visceral arch*: 'hyoid arch'. This refers to the upper half of the hyoid bone with the muscles coming from the mandible (geniohyoid, mylohyoid) and the styloid process (stylohyoid, digastric). The cranial nerve which serves this area is the *facial nerve* (CN VII) with its motor root innervating all the muscles of facial expression, the stylohyoid, the posterior part of the digastric muscle and the stapedian muscle. The facial nerve during its trajectory on the face is a pure motor nerve because the facial muscles responsible for expression and language have no proprioceptive receptors and the goniometric control needed for movement coordination is given by CN V innervating the skin in which the muscles are included. The sensitive root of CN VII has a ganglion known as the geniculate ganglion from its location on the flexure of the facial nerve within the ear. It serves the anterior two-thirds of the tongue and a part of the auricle and external auditory meatus. The intermediate nerve (CN VII bis) or Wrisberg nerve should not be further mentioned as such, because it is really the sensory root of CN VII and not a correction of a mistake in counting the cranial nerves. The vegetative centers related to salivary glands (submaxillary and sublingual) are in the part of the brainstem related to the facial nucleus, but the distribution of the postganglionic fibers is made by CN V.

- *Third visceral arch*: 'hyothyroid arch'. This concerns the lower half of the hyoid bone and the upper part of the thyroid cartilage with the stylopharyngeal muscle, the upper and middle pharynx constrictor muscles and the levator veli. The cranial nerve in this area is the *glossopharyngeal nerve* (CN IX) with motor and sensory root for the posterior third of the lingual mucosa, the upper part of the pharynx and middle ear mucosa and vegetative salivary center for the parotid gland. However, the extrinsic laryngeal muscles (thyrohyoid, sternothyroid, sternocleidohyoid, omohyoid) are innervated by branches of the cervical plexus (C2, C3) which use the *hypoglossal nerve* (CN XII) as a tutor to make their distribution by forming a loop.

● *Fourth visceral arch*: 'thyrocricoid arch'. This concerns the lower part of the thyroid cartilage and cricoid cartilage with all the intrinsic laryngeal muscles (thyroarytenoid as vocal cord, posterior and lateral cricoarytenoid, interarytenoid). The cranial nerve here is the *vagus nerve* (CN X) which has three unequal territories. First, it has a sensory cranial distribution corresponding to its two sensory ganglions (upper jugular and lower plexiform) for mucosa of the pharynx, larynx by the superior laryngeal nerve, tuba auditiva and part of the external auditory meatus. Second, it supplies all the intrinsic laryngeal muscles by the recurrent inferior laryngeal nerve corresponding to the motor root of CN X visible on the lower part of the lateral aspect of the myelencephalon. This nerve has a recurrent trajectory to reach the lower part of the larynx, which represents the anatomical limit of the visceral portion of the head and neck. Third, CN X is the most important parasympathetic nerve, conveying vegetative fibers to all viscera of the trunk as far as the pelvis.

Particular mention has to be made of the so-called spinal accessory nerve or accessory nerve (CN XI). It derives from the cervical spinal cord (C1–C4) through fibers going out laterally and traveling up to the foramen magnum and then to the jugular foramen to reach two cranial muscles: the sternocleidomastoid (SCM) and the trapezius. It contains mainly motor fibers and needs for its proprioceptive part to carry out anastomosis with sensory fibers coming from the cervical plexus which it is possible to isolate by dissection before entering the SCM and the trapezius in the subclavicular space. It is important to understand that the same applies to all the purely motor cranial nerves: the oculomotor (CN III), trochlear (CN IV), abducens (CN VI) and hypoglossal (CN XII). These all innervate muscles of somitic origin: the six extraocular and the 17 tongue muscles. The mandatory sensory anastomosis is provided by the sensory nerve of the territory, the trigeminal nerve with its three branches.

As a consequence of this description, a new functional classification of cranial nerves can be adopted, with four groups:

1. The pseudocranial nerves

These are not cranial nerves which come from the brainstem with sensory and motor roots like the spinal nerves, but expansions of the encephalon of which they are a real part:

— the rhinencephalon coming from the telencephalon with the olfactory bulb receiving through the ethmoidal cribriform plate the nervous fibers of the olfactory mucosa and the olfactory tract, going to the olfactory cortex and orbitofrontal cortex
— the ophthalmencephalon corresponding to the retina which is a modified cortex with six layers coming from the diencephalon, the optic nerve being in reality an exteriorized central pathway surrounded by the three meningeal sheaths.

2. The pure motor nerves (having a mandatory sensory anastomosis) (Fig. 2.2)

— for the extraocular muscles: *oculomotor* (CN III) (superior, inferior, medial recti and inferior oblique), *trochlear* (CN IV) (superior oblique), *abducens* (CN VI) (lateral rectus)
— for the tongue muscles: *hypoglossal* (CN XII)
— for the SCM and trapezius muscles: *accessory* (CN XI), which is not really a cranial nerve but a cervical nerve with an intracranial trajectory in the posterior fossa.

3. The mixed nerves of the four visceral arches *(CN V, VII, IX, X)* as described above

4. The pure sensorial nerve *(CN VIII)*

The *vestibulocochlear nerve* (CN VIII) is concerned with two different functions (hearing and statodynamic stabilization of the head and body) with their own ganglions (Scarpa, vestibular) and nuclei within the brainstem (Fig. 2.3).

From the embryological point of view, the ear represents a convergent zone of different visceral arches explaining why the auricle is innervated by the four mixed nerves and the cervical plexus (Fig. 2.4). More specifically, the hyoid arch and the mandibular arch develop six buds along the first ectodermal fissure growing around the ectodermic invagination, which later will produce the external auditory meatus going to the neural placode and the mesoblastic components of the middle ear. Therefore the auricle is an original part of the body, made by skin and cartilage in which there are very rich neurovascular plexuses combining myelinated and unmyelinated vegetative fibers able to generate intense vascular reaction (red ear) in varying circumstances. *The auricle can in fact be considered as a neurovascular organ.*

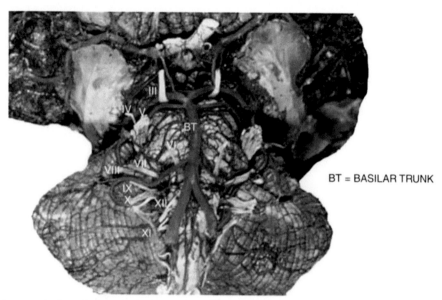

BT = BASILAR TRUNK

Fig. 2.2   Anterior aspect of cerebellum, brainstem and cranial nerves.

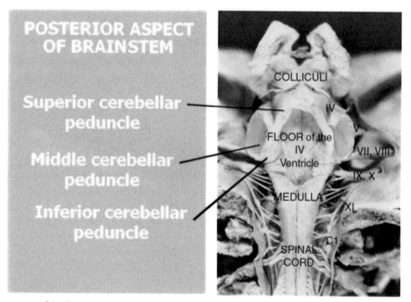

Fig. 2.3   Posterior aspect of brainstem.

THE NEUROPHYSIOLOGICAL BASIS OF AURICULOTHERAPY

In 1850 Dr Rülker from Cincinnati, Dr Lucciana from Bastia and Professor Malgaigne from Paris all noted, following an ancient Egyptian practice, that cauterizing the helix of the auricle can be effective in curing some sciatic pain. A century later,

Dr Paul Nogier[4] from Lyon started experimenting with this technique on patients and after many clinical observations he described the *cartography of the auricular points* with the now classic image of the inverted fetus projected on the auricle. His original contribution was progressively enriched by the research work of his pupils all over the world. Nogier[5] emphasizes *pain* as the main

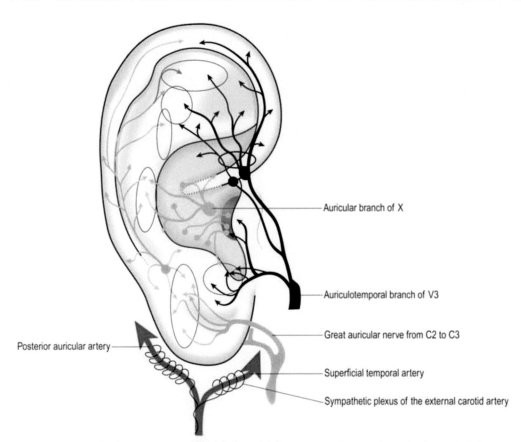

Auricular branch of X

Auriculotemporal branch of V3

Great auricular nerve from C2 to C3

Superficial temporal artery

Sympathetic plexus of the external carotid artery

Posterior auricular artery

Fig. 2.4 Innervation of the auricle coming from the four visceral arches and cervical plexus for cerebrospinal innervation and from the sympathetic perivascular plexus.

indication for auriculotherapy. But among all the results published it is important to identify those of scientifically unquestionable proof from those where the scientific basis is yet to be demonstrated.

THE IDENTIFICATION OF THE ACUPUNCTURE POINT

A major contribution was made by a group of clinicians from the Groupe Lyonnais d'Etudes Médicales (GLEM) and by researchers, particularly Claudie Terral[6,7,8] and Odile Auziech,[9] working in Unit 103 of the Institut National de la Santé et de la Recherche Médicale (French Institute of Health and Medical Research; INSERM) in Montpellier, France. The essence of the research program using physical, histological and physiological data collected between 1973 and 1983 can be summarized as follows:

- Following the demonstration by Niboyet[10,11] in 1963 that there was less electrical resistance in

Chinese acupuncture points, the most acceptable hypothesis was to consider either a skin surface effect related to the secretion of sweat glands, as pointed out by some researchers, or more consistently to consider the possibility of a specific subcutaneous structure, since cleaning the skin with ether/acetone did not change either the electrical properties or the detection of points on fresh cadaver skin (Fig. 2.5). More precise investigations were performed by Claudie Terral using both direct and sinusoidal (alternating) current. For this investigation, a curve plotter was built allowing recording of the instantaneous variability of intensity as a function of applied sinusoidal voltage of the electrical equivalent circuit changes. All those parameters were visualized on the oscilloscope with the output voltage in the X axis and the output current in the Y axis. A special exploratory electrode was designed, equipped with a strain gauge bridge measuring the pressure on the skin. It was able

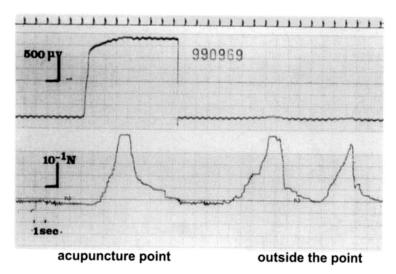

acupuncture point   **outside the point**

to identify 'stable low electrical resistance points' of the order of 10–560 kΩ with short latency detection and with a low level of mechanical pressure. These specific cutaneous points correspond to the traditional Chinese points and have a small surface area of around 1 mm². They can be surrounded by unstable points depending on the duration of the detection and the diffusion of the charge. With sinusoidal current it was possible by changing the metal of the electrode (pure magnesium, dural) and the duration of the point stimulation to describe a diode effect, thyristor effect as a marker of analgesia, and a tunneling effect as well as generator and supraconductive effects. This very interesting investigation clearly suggests a complex electrical activity at the level of the point.

- Logically suspecting a structural phenomenon to be accountable for this electrical behavior, a histological investigation was carried out in 1975 by Odile Auziech and Claudie Terral in the laboratory of René Senelar of the Faculty of Medicine of Montpellier. Black ink was injected at the level of the electrically detected point in rabbit and human skin in order to be sure to localize the right area precisely on serial histological sections. Using different staining methods such as Coujard-Champy or silver staining permits the description of the specific components of what we called 'neurovascular bundles': lax connective tissue with a shaft in the dermal layer/fibroblasts, fibrocytes, mastocytes, histocytes as well as mobile and fixed Langerhans cells and APUD

cells/neurovascular complex made by the intricate arrangement of myelinated and unmyelinated fibers within and around micro blood vessels (arterioles, veins and lymphatics)/ radiating matrix into the basal layer of the epidermis (Figs 2.6, 2.7, 2.8, 2.9). Observations made using an electron microscope revealed some local endocrine substance activity as well as some enzyme activity after electrical stimulation, particularly adrenaline secretion in the neural network. In 1984 Odile Auziech made special histological investigations on the auricle in vivo on rabbits and post mortem in human, with the outcome that three different types of neurovascular bundles located in three areas corresponding roughly to the three territories of innervation could be described: posterosuperior (½ the surface), anterosuperior (¼) and anteroinferior (¼). In 75 biopsies corresponding to 20 different points on the anterior aspect and three on the posterior, some typical features were described: medium size (80 μ) and horizontal shape within fatty connective tissue for *type I*; small size (60 μ) with many capillaries for *type II*; and large size (100 μ) and vertical shape in adipose tissue for *type III* (Fig. 2.10). Some holes through the cartilage in front of the point were observed in 2% of the cases and some typical aspect of glomus in 10%.

- The third approach was to build a physiological reproducible model to study analgesia[12] in the rabbit, which is particularly convenient for its type of symmetrical locomotion by simultaneous

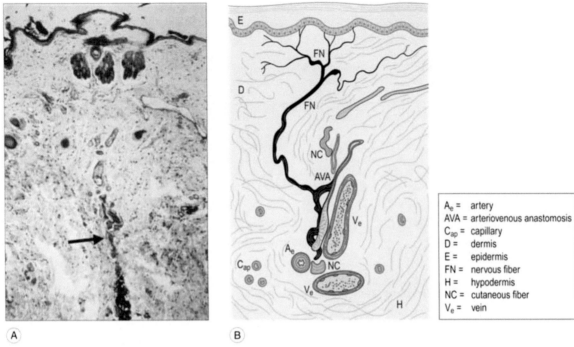

Fig. 2.6   Neurovascular bundle on rabbit skin showing the modification of the connective tissue and, deeper, the microvessel with myelinated and unmyelinated fibers: (A) histological section; (B) drawn representation.

Fig. 2.7   Magnification of the neurovascular bundle marked with arrow in Figure 2.6.

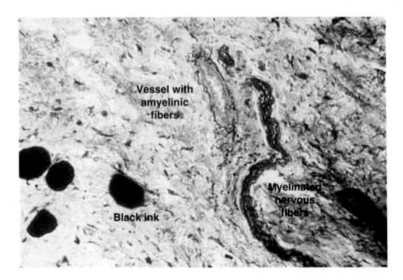

propulsion of the hind limbs. Therefore a pain test was done through painful mechanical skin prick with a force transducer in order to calibrate the stimulus which, applied to the hind limb, generates a bilateral withdrawal reflex. Two points, *Yishe* and *Tsusanli*, were electrically detected in one hind limb and needles implanted and connected with an electrical stimulator. The

interesting observation was that after 20 minutes of electrical stimulation a true analgesia of the stimulated limb was created, validated by the absence of the withdrawal reflex after mechanical painful puncture on this side and the persistence of the withdrawal reflex by puncture on the opposite side (Fig. 2.11). This demonstrates without doubt real skin analgesia on one side without

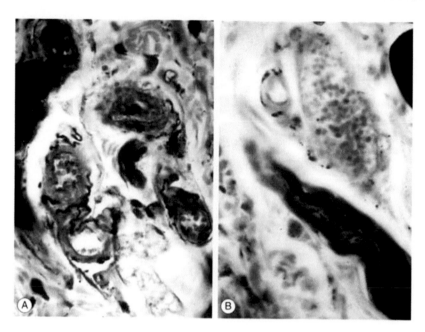

Fig. 2.8   Some details of (A) unmyelinated fibers on vessel and (B) myelinated fibers.

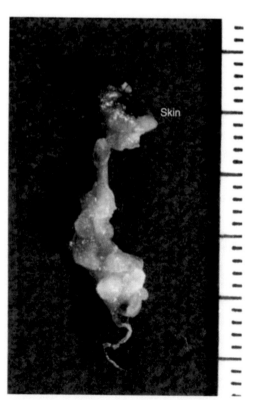

Skin

Fig. 2.9   Biological sample of the full neurovascular complex extracted from the skin of a human volunteer after electrical detection of the acupuncture point on the leg.

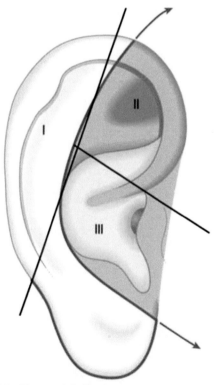

Fig. 2.10   The zonal distibution of the three histological types of neurovascular bundles within the auricle (from O. Auziech[9]). I = 'horizontal' type; II = 'compact' type; III = 'vertical' type.

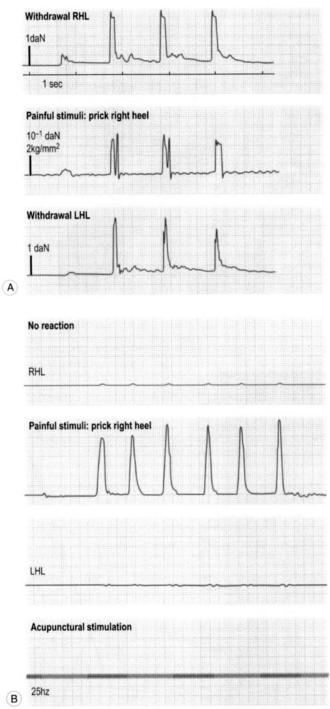

Fig. 2.11 Experimental demonstration of the analgesia induced by electrostimulation of needles placed in two neurovascular bundles of the posterior hind leg of a rabbit, validated by measuring the withdrawal reflexes (RHL = right hind limb; LHL = left hind limb) after painful skin stimulation (A) and by observing the lack of reflexes after 20 minutes of electrostimulation (B) (Unit 103, INSERM, Montpellier, France).

paralysis. A secretion of a neurotransmitter being suspected, 2 cm^3/kg of the serum of rabbits with induced analgesia was injected into naïve rabbits demonstrating a transfer of the analgesia into almost the same territory with diverse local variations. Opiate antagonists (nalorphine and naloxone) did not change the phenomenon and we suggested the possible action of an enkephaline neurotransmitter with a possible specific metameric action. Obviously more experimental investigations are needed and the reproducibility of the rabbit model will hopefully elicit new motivation for this work somewhere.

Finally, it is possible to summarize the results of these scientific researches as follows:

- the acupuncture point undoubtedly exists in view of the electrical, histological and physiological arguments presented above
- the auricle has a particular structural profile with a very rich vascular network and typical neurovascular bundles.

NEUROPHYSIOLOGY OF PAIN

The pain signal

Among the very rich scientific and medical literature on pain, it is possible to isolate some precise data:

- The pain signal integrated in nociception is a priority signal of unpleasant sensation traveling within specific pathways in the central nervous system (CNS) to the conscious cortex. It manifests as suffering through additional emotional components if prolonged in time, or by an alarm system inducing semi-automatic protective defense reactions (withdrawal reflex, running away). There is no unconscious pain. The level of suffering depends directly on the brain state and structure which means that every species has its own specific profile of suffering. Suffering is also possible without a physiological pain signal. Mechanisms of pain inhibition normally exist in certain neural circuits of the CNS.
- A pain signal can occur by stimulation of receptors over their normal range of function. For example, progressively increasing the temperature of a water flow on the skin causes pain to manifest with a semi-automatic withdrawal action. Pinching the skin can also cause a level of pain corresponding to an overstimulation of mechanical receptors. These two types of pain correspond to the progressive transition between

normal and painful sensation and have a very precise localization in the body. This means that it is necessary to find some neural system in the CNS able to recognize the painful character of a sensation and to transfer the signal to the somatosensory cortex for conscious identification.

- Different types of sensory fibers can be identified. First, myelinated fibers: Aα (Ia from muscular spindles and Ib from Golgi organs), Aβ and Aγ (II) from mechanoreceptors for tactile (Meissner, Pacini) and goniometric sensations (Ruffini), Aδ (III) of small diameter for pain and thermal sensations with a limited field of reception. Second, unmyelinated fibers: C (IV) with low conduction velocity and a wide field of reception for pain and thermal sensations from polymodal receptors.

The pain pathways

All the sensory pathways have their first neuron within the spinal ganglion for spinal nerves and within the cranial ganglion for cranial nerves.

A. Spinal cord level. The epicritic sensibility, concerning precise tactile discrimination and statokinesthetic sense given by the skin goniometric information coming from the Ruffini receptors, travels along the medial gracile (lower limb and abdomen) and lateral cuneate (upper limb and thorax) fasciculi in the dorsal column to the corresponding gracile and medial and lateral cuneate nuclei of the medulla. After synapses, the fibers cross the midline to form the medial lemniscus reaching the thalamic ventral posterolateral nucleus pars oralis (VPLo). They are then projected on to the primary somatosensory cortex located on the parietal postcentral gyrus with area 3 for precise tactile identification, areas 1 and 5 for stereognosia (body scheme) and area 2 for statokinetic perception. Note that the lateral cuneate nucleus is connected with the cerebellum in order to achieve the motor coordination which requires information first on stiffness of the muscles given by the muscular spindles (spinocerebellar tract), identifying the three possible states of the muscle: relaxed, contracted or stretched, and second on position and movement of body segment given by the skin via the lateral cuneate nucleus.

The protopathic sensibility, which concerns pain, temperature and crude touch by Aδ fibers articulated in the posterior horn with lamina I of Rexed as well as IV and V (nucleus proprius) and C fibers with II and III (substantia gelatinosa) and

VII and VIII, travels in the first conduction system of the dorsal and ventral spinothalamic tract representing the extralemniscal ways placed in the medulla and pons laterally to the medial lemniscus. They will later join to reach the thalamic ventral posterolateral nucleus (VPL) in the pars caudalis for the ventral and in the pars posterior for the dorsal spinothalamic tract (nucleus suprageniculatus). This protopathic system can be considered as an alarm system. A second conduction system is made by the spinoreticulothalamic tract conveying mainly C fibers more or less mixed with fibers of the ventral spinothalamic tract and going first to medullar and pontine reticular nuclei, second to periaqueductal gray matter and mesencephalic raphe nuclei and third to the reticular nuclei of the medial thalamus (intralaminar and parafascicular). They then reach the anterior cingulate cortex (area 24) and the close prefrontal cortex, adding to the precisely localized pure pain sensation, the emotional component characterizing suffering.

B. Brainstem level. This is directly related to the auricle. As in the spinal cord, the sensory fibers have their first neuron within the cranial ganglions (trigeminal, geniculate, superior and inferior of IX and X) sending fibers to the brainstem nuclei (Plate IC). Three of them are of particular importance:

First, the very long trigeminal nucleus divided into three different parts:

- The caudal part is the *spinal trigeminal nucleus* with its *pars caudalis* originating within the cervical spinal cord mainly at C2/C3 level, corresponding to the part of the cervical plexus which supplies a large territory of the auricle. C1 is linked with the supraspinal nucleus corresponding to the motor innervation of the muscles of the craniocervical Cardan joint moving the head along the two visual exploration axes: vertical and horizontal, and placed close to the tectospinal tract ending at the cervical level and connected with the visual superior colliculus for the mandatory visuomotor articulation integrated within the eye–head servomechanism. This pars caudalis is mainly devoted to the protopathic sensibility of the face and in fact of the entire auricle. Above, at medullary level, the pars interpolaris receives sensitive facial skin signals and is connected with the cerebellum for the goniometric information related to the deformation of the facial mask by the facial muscles (activated by the CN VII motor nucleus) corresponding to two different activities: first the

semi-automatic eyelid movement for corneal protection by lachrymal secretion and second the mouth movements for articulated language. The same problem invests the lateral cuneate nucleus sending goniometric information from trunk and limbs to the cerebellum. At the pontine level the pars oralis receives the epicritic sensations from the face. Some sensory fibers from CN IX and X innervating the middle ear, pharynx mucosa and external auditory meatus are also connected with the trigeminal nucleus, which is of particular interest for the understanding of the innervation of the auricle. After decussation, the fibers then go to the ventral posteromedial thalamic nucleus forming the ventral trigeminothalamic pathways. To simplify, one can bear in mind that the epicritic pathways join the medial lemniscus and the protopathic pathways, the spinothalamic system (Fig. 2.12A, B).

- The principal *sensory trigeminal nucleus* is isolated at the pontine level and located on the lateral border of the motor trigeminal nucleus which innervates all the masticatory muscles. Presumably it receives sensory fibers from the teeth and mouth and through sensory feedback allows control and regulation of the forces applied during mastication. Of course the commands for masticating come from the motor keyboard of the precentral gyrus but the force control has to use a closed loop regulation linking the sensory and motor trigeminal nuclei. Uncrossed fibers then go to the ventral posteromedial thalamic nucleus forming the dorsal trigeminothalamic pathway which is not so well known.

- The *mesencephalic trigeminal nucleus* is a long thin nuclear column leading to the upper part of the mesencephalon at the superior colliculus devoted to visuomotor articulation. It has a very original feature, collecting the proprioceptive inputs from Ia and Ib fibers (muscular spindles and Golgi organs) directly without synaptic relay in the trigeminal ganglion, not only from the striated masticatory muscles but also from the extraocular muscles, the nerves of which are purely motor and require a sensory anastomosis provided by the ophthalmic branch (CN VI) within the cavernous sinus. That explains the length of this nucleus and it is also conceivable that the 17 muscles of the tongue activated by the pure motor nerve CN XII send their proprioceptive information through the sensory anastomosis with branches of the lingual nerve

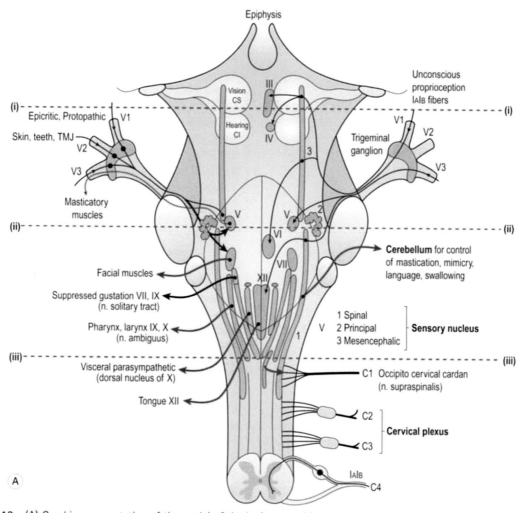

Epiphysis

Unconscious
proprioception
IaIB fibers

(i) ------- (i)
Epicritic, Protopathic V1
Skin, teeth, TMJ
V2
V3
Vision
CS
Hearing
CI
III
IV
3
V1
V2
Trigeminal
ganglion
V3

Masticatory
muscles

(ii) --- V V 2 --- (ii)
VI

Facial muscles
Suppressed gustation VII, IX
(n. solitary tract)
Pharynx, larynx IX, X
(n. ambiguus)
VII
XII

Cerebellum for control
of mastication, mimicry,
language, swallowing

1 Spinal
V 2 Principal   Sensory nucleus
3 Mesencephalic

(iii) --- (iii)
Visceral parasympathetic
(dorsal nucleus of X)
Tongue XII

C1 Occipito cervical cardan
(n. supraspinalis)
C2
C3
Cervical plexus

A
IaIB
C4

Fig. 2.12 (A) Graphic representation of the nuclei of the brainstem with particular emphasis on the trigeminal nucleus connections.

(V3) into the mesencephalic nucleus. This particular feature is exactly the same as that of the spinal cord where the Ia and Ib fibers go directly without relay to the alpha motoneurons of the anterior horn with a monosynaptic fast junction. This is not to be considered only in the myotatic reflex matter, but mainly in the fusorial servomechanism able to regulate from the periphery the correct level of force to apply for a particular motor task.

Second, the nucleus of the solitary tract. Its upper part (nucleus ovalis) is related to the gustatory sense through fibers from the sensory root of CN VII (anterior two-thirds of the tongue) and IX (posterior third). Its lower part receives sensory fibers of CN IX and X coming from the pharynx and

larynx which probably correspond to the superior laryngeal sensory nerve giving to the inferior laryngeal motor nerve a classic proprioceptive anastomosis called the 'anse de Galien' (Galen's anastomosis) along the lateral border of the cricoarytenoid muscle. In addition it is an important vegetative nucleus receiving input signals from vessel receptors and the digestive tract.

Third, the nucleus ambiguus which is a motor nucleus sending motor fibers to the pharynx (CN IX) and to the larynx by the inferior recurrent laryngeal nerve of CN X.

It is important anyway to know that some controversial opinions among neuroanatomists still remain regarding the exact location and functional role of some brainstem structures, but our proposed scheme is the most acceptable at the

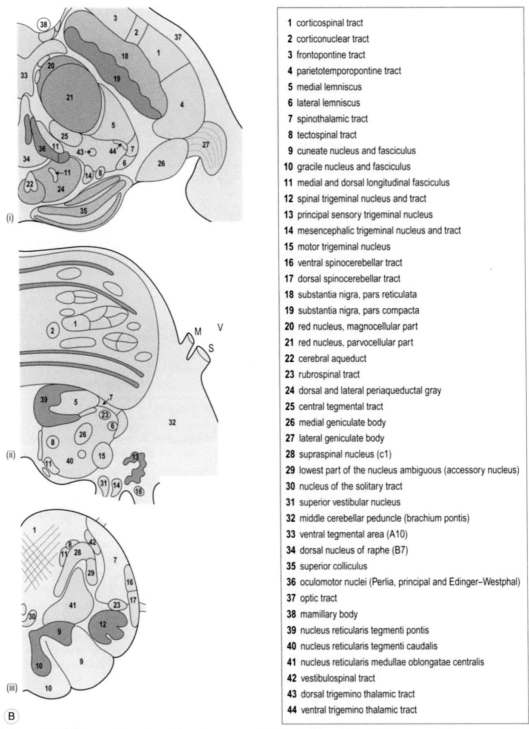

1 corticospinal tract
2 corticonuclear tract
3 frontopontine tract
4 parietotemporopontine tract
5 medial lemniscus
6 lateral lemniscus
7 spinothalamic tract
8 tectospinal tract
9 cuneate nucleus and fasciculus
10 gracile nucleus and fasciculus
11 medial and dorsal longitudinal fasciculus
12 spinal trigeminal nucleus and tract
13 principal sensory trigeminal nucleus
14 mesencephalic trigeminal nucleus and tract
15 motor trigeminal nucleus
16 ventral spinocerebellar tract
17 dorsal spinocerebellar tract
18 substantia nigra, pars reticulata
19 substantia nigra, pars compacta
20 red nucleus, magnocellular part
21 red nucleus, parvocellular part
22 cerebral aqueduct
23 rubrospinal tract
24 dorsal and lateral periaqueductal gray
25 central tegmental tract
26 medial geniculate body
27 lateral geniculate body
28 supraspinal nucleus (c1)
29 lowest part of the nucleus ambiguous (accessory nucleus)
30 nucleus of the solitary tract
31 superior vestibular nucleus
32 middle cerebellar peduncle (brachium pontis)
33 ventral tegmental area (A10)
34 dorsal nucleus of raphe (B7)
35 superior colliculus
36 oculomotor nuclei (Perlia, principal and Edinger–Westphal)
37 optic tract
38 mamillary body
39 nucleus reticularis tegmenti pontis
40 nucleus reticularis tegmenti caudalis
41 nucleus reticularis medullae oblongatae centralis
42 vestibulospinal tract
43 dorsal trigemino thalamic tract
44 ventral trigemino thalamic tract

Fig. 2.12, cont'd (B) Three axial sections: (i) at the mesencephalic level; (ii) at the level of the pons; (iii) at the medullary level, are represented with the identification of the different nuclei and pathways.

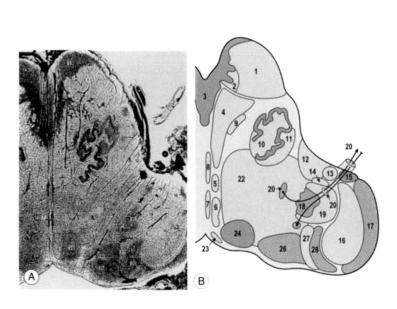

1 corticospinal tract
2 corticonuclear tract
3 arcuate nucleus
4 medial lemniscus
5 tectospinal tract
6 medial longitudinal fasciculus
7 nucleus raphe obscurus
8 nucleus raphe pallidus
9 ventral trigeminothalamic tract
10 inferior olivary nucleus
11 central tegmental tract
12 spinothalamic tract
13 ventral spinocerebellar tract
14 rubrospinal tract
15 corpus pontobulbare
16 inferior cerebellar peduncle
17 dorsal cochlear nucleus
18 spinal trigeminal nucleus
19 spinal trigeminal tract
20 nucleus ambiguus
21 fibers of the IX
22 nucleus reticularis gigantocellularis
23 dorsal longitudinal fasciculus
24 nucleus prepositus
25 nucleus of the solitary tract
26 medial vestibular nucleus
27 descending vestibular root
28 inferior vestibular nucleus

Fig. 2.13   An example of the possible identification and localization of nuclei and pathways: vessel microinjection with black ink (A); anatomical interpretation of the localization of nuclei and pathways (B) *(from Henri Duvernoy with permission)*.

moment, based on the data in the literature and the exceptional high-level research work carried out by Henri Duvernoy[13,14,15] from Besançon in France (Fig. 2.13).

The central pain control centers

In a didactic approach, it is possible to describe three main centers which explain the possible efficacy of auriculotherapy:

A. The spinal cord posterior horn selective gate. In 1965, Melzack and Wall[16] formulated the *gate control theory of pain*, suggesting that some inhibitory neurons of the substantia gelatinosa connected with Aδ and C pain fibers could be activated by sensory myelinated Aβ fibers closing the door to the spinothalamic tract conveying pain sensation. In fact, the posterior horn is divided into six lamina described by Rexed which contains many interneurons allowing connections between Aδ and C

fibers linked to lamina I, II, III and Aα and Aβ large myelinated fibers. The spinothalamic neurons are connected according to three modalities: high threshold (HT) for nociception connected with lamina I; low threshold (LT) for mechanical inputs connected to lamina IV/VI; and wide dynamic range (WDR) being the most numerous with three concentric zones: central, intermediate excitatory and peripheral inhibitory, giving priority to nociceptive stimulus (80% nociceptive neurons type II and type IV). M. Sindou[17] from Lyons, France, has done substantial work describing this organization in detail for its application in surgery. Some metameric interconnections are possible through the Lissauer tract. The role of *substance P* and *enkephaline neurotransmitters* suggesting local or regional metameric pain control should not be underestimated. Finally we have sufficient evidence to be able to ascribe to the posterior horn a further function than merely that of a selective gate, one more concerned with semi-automatic defense reflexes. It is also important to note that any external stimulation of the dorsal funiculus is very painful (C fibers), which is not the case with the anterolateral funiculus.

B. The brainstem reticular formation. This represents a very complex group of nuclei with an anatomical disposition in three columns all along the brainstem: the median, representing the six raphe nuclei, the central or medial reticular formation represented by five identified types of nucleus reticularis in the medulla, pons and mesencephalon, and the lateral reticular formation with six nuclei, among which is the medial parabrachial nucleus which, together with the nucleus coeruleus and subcoeruleus, forms the dorsolateral pontic tegmentum (Fig. 2.14). More than a precise description of all those nuclei, it is important to emphasize the great concentration of *neurotransmitter secretion centers* playing a crucial role within the regulation of spinal cord ascending and descending pathways. They can be classified into:

- *monoamine centers* with first noradrenaline (A1 to A7) with descending and ascending fibers (noradrenergic dorsal pathway from locus coeruleus A6 stimulating the cortex), second adrenaline and dopamine (A8 to A14) more concerned with the mesolimbic system and nucleus accumbens, third serotonin (5-HT) located only in the brainstem within the raphe nuclei (B1 to B9) with descending fibers (B1 to B3) inhibiting the sympathetic spinal centers and posterior horns for pain control, connected to the locus coeruleus (B3 to B6) and to the mesolimbic and mesocortical system (B7 and B8) to septal nucleus, hypothalamus and hippocampus

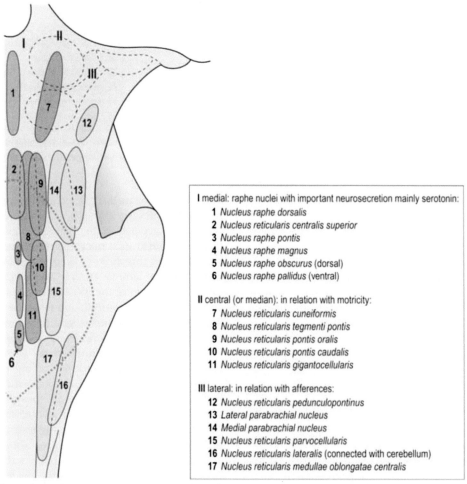

I medial: raphe nuclei with important neurosecretion mainly serotonin:
   1 *Nucleus raphe dorsalis*
   2 *Nucleus reticularis centralis superior*
   3 *Nucleus raphe pontis*
   4 *Nucleus raphe magnus*
   5 *Nucleus raphe obscurus* (dorsal)
   6 *Nucleus raphe pallidus* (ventral)

II central (or median): in relation with motricity:
   7 *Nucleus reticularis cuneiformis*
   8 *Nucleus reticularis tegmenti pontis*
   9 *Nucleus reticularis pontis oralis*
   10 *Nucleus reticularis pontis caudalis*
   11 *Nucleus reticularis gigantocellularis*

III lateral: in relation with afferences:
   12 *Nucleus reticularis pedunculopontinus*
   13 *Lateral parabrachial nucleus*
   14 *Medial parabrachial nucleus*
   15 *Nucleus reticularis parvocellularis*
   16 *Nucleus reticularis lateralis* (connected with cerebellum)
   17 *Nucleus reticularis medullae oblongatae centralis*

Fig. 2.14   The reticular formation of the brainstem *(from Henri Duvernoy with permission).*

- *acetylcholine centers* (ACh) in the basal forebrain (Ch1 to Ch4) and in brainstem (Ch5, 6, 8) with ascending fibers for the intralaminar and reticular nuclei of the thalamus and striatum and descending fibers to the brainstem.

Finally, the reticular formation of the brainstem has an important neurotransmitter secretion activity and a double system of connections: first *ascending from the spinal cord* (spinoreticulothalamic pathway with relay in the raphe nuclei and periaqueductal gray matter) and to the reticular thalamus (reticular nucleus surrounding the thalamus 'like a shield' with thalamocortical and corticothalamic fibers, intralaminar nuclei forming the median center, parafascicular nucleus, paracentral and centrolateral nuclei), and second *descending to the spinal cord* for inhibitory pain control. But obviously that is only a small part of the function of the reticular formation which is also related to all the management of visceral activities, servomechanisms and cortical ascending activation or deactivation during sleep.

C. The thalamic selective filter. As pointed out many years ago by Head and Holmes,[18] the pain control takes place mainly in the thalamus which is a large mass of gray matter located on the lateral wall of the third ventricle within the diencephalon. The classification of nuclei is still controversial, but it is possible to identify three groups of thalamic nuclei: *anterior* connected with the mamillary body and integrated within the Papez circuit of emotions; *medial* projecting to the frontal, prefrontal and orbitofrontal cortex and connected with amygdaloid nucleus, ventral pallidum and midbrain reticular formation; *ventrolateral* subdivided into ventral anterior (VA), lateral (VL) and posterior (VP) and in lateral dorsal (LD), lateral posterior (LP) and pulvinar. In addition there is the lateral geniculate nucleus as an integrator of the two retinal fiber flows and the medial geniculate nucleus as a relay on the auditory pathway going to the temporal lobe. The thalamus has a widespread reciprocal projection system with the entire cortex and roughly its caudal half is concerned with ascending sensory pathways including occipito-temporo-parietal cortex while the rostral half is foremost in relation to motor and limbic activities.

The VP is also called the ventrobasal complex. The medial lemniscus is projected to the VP lateral anterior (VPLa) for conscious statokinetic sense and to the posterior (VPLp) for tactile epicritic sensitivity. The spinothalamic fibers are also connected with the VPL mainly in its superior, lateral and posterior parts in a manner different to that of the lemniscal fibers. But the functional interaction of those two types of fibers is still controversial: do they really converge on the same thalamic relay neuron or are they projected in parallel with eventual interaction by interneurons? At any rate, it seems that 70% of the relay neurons of the VPL and VPM receive cutaneous inputs according to three functional modalities: 15–20% of nociceptive specific neurons; 20–30% of low threshold mechanical slow adapting (SA) or rapid adapting (RA) neurons; 50% of convergent WDR type neurons sensitive to noxious and non-noxious stimuli. The recognition by the cortex of the nociceptive nature of the signal in the 3b part of the post-central gyrus is largely dependant on the thalamic relay neurons and interneuron activity.

In addition, the importance of the trigeminal lemniscus (trigemino-thalamic pathway), also concerned in this activity and in which many sensory fibers from the auricle are traveling, could be an argument to validate the inhibitory action of a stimulation of the auricle on the pain projection of spinothalamic fibers from different body origin. This active thalamic inhibition of pain (ATIP) is a sort of competition between pain stimuli. Therefore it is plausible to consider the existence of oscillatory pain circuits in the thalamus as well as in the spinal cord in case of prolonged pain, reinforced by cortical actions (cingulate gyrus, limbic system, amygdala), which can be 'broken' by another pain stimulus: pinching, needling or electrostimulation of the skin on identified neurovascular bundles or auricular zones. In the experimental work we carried out in research Unit 103 at INSERM, we demonstrated the thalamic inhibition of painful stimuli on the hind limb of rabbit by recording evoked thalamic potentials within the parafascicular nucleus using a stereotactic frame and anatomical cross-sections for precise localization (Plate ID). Electrostimulation of the analgesic points lasting 20 minutes suppressed the thalamic potentials, but at 2 cm from the points it maintained them. This was also confirmed by G. Farnarier and colleagues[19] in Marseille and Chang Hsiang-Tung[20] in Shanghai. However, some hypotheses can be formulated: either the inhibition lies at the thalamic level or at the spinal level, or both.

CONCLUSIONS

The main objective of this chapter is to explain as clearly as possible the state of the art concerning the scientific basis of auriculotherapy. It is clear that some technical aspects remain to be understood, justifying a multidisciplinary research program on an international level. Some major points can be indicated:

1. Two facts explain the possible diagnostic and therapeutic effect of mechanical or physical stimuli applied on the auricle: first, the peripheral innervation of the auricle by three main nerves: the auriculotemporal nerve (CN V3); the auricular branch of CN X with fibers from CN VII and CN IX; the cervical plexus (C2/C3); and second, the possible central neural interference of different sensory fiber origins at the level of the brainstem and thalamus.

2. The somatotopy in the CNS is evidence of a preprogrammed ordering of inputs and outputs avoiding neural chaos. Therefore the sensory fibers coming from the lower limb are separated in the ascending pathways from those coming from the upper limb, trunk or head and it is logical to find such precise topographic organization within the spinal cord, the thalamus and mainly the cortex. When we touch our big toe, we have the feeling of a very precise local action, but the neural signal processing takes place more than 1 m or more away, within the brain cortex. That explains the very precise cutaneous projection on the post-central gyrus of the parietal lobe (sensory keyboard) with the body scheme, which is statodynamic according to the loop joining the motor keyboard of area 4 and the sensory keyboard of areas 3a and b, 1, 2 and 5. The classical homunculus described by Penfield is the anatomical expression of this irregular projection of all the muscles and all the cutaneous territories of the body. A visceral conscious body scheme does not exist which justifies their mandatory functional expression on skin. Regarding the somatotopy on the auricle, no scientific arguments can be found for the cartography proposed by different authors describing many points for brain structures such as the corpus callosum or anterior commissure, or for nervous plexuses or for visceral organs. It is necessary to avoid such intellectual constructions which are lacking real scientific basis and return to the description of 'zones' with some neurovascular bundles corresponding to a validated clinical action on pain or visceral dysfunction. In addition, time cannot change the structure of the nervous elements of the auricle, but only their functional behavior, possibly measured by their physical parameters. The same applies to the plantar part of the foot, largely used for reflexotherapies. Plantar skin is very rich in mechanoreceptors, particularly Pacini force transducers, because of its role as force plate in the regulation of the body's vertical posture. But it is no serious scientific argument to describe visceral somatotopic representations on it.

References

[1] Head H. Studies in neurology. London: P Keegar; 1920.

[2] Jarricot H. Sur certains phénomènes douloureux: viscéralgies, dermalgies réflexes, cellulites et quelques phénomènes réflexes d'origine thérapeutique. Essais cliniques et thérapeutiques. Lyon: Thèse de Médecine; 1932.

[3] Jarricot H, Wong M. De certaines relations viscéro-cutanées métamériques ou dermalgies réflexes en acupuncture. Méridiens. 1971;16:87–126.

[4] Nogier P. Traité d'Auriculothérapie. Moulins-les-Metz: Maisonneuve; 1969.

[5] Nogier P. Introduction pratique à l'auriculothérapie. Bruxelles: Satas; 1997.

[6] Terral C. L'acupuncture en France: douleur et acupuncture. Tempo Médical. 1976;34(2):43–63.

[7] Terral C. Induction du processus de régénération et de cicatrisation par stimulation électrique ou mécanique des points d'acupuncture. Méridiens. 1988;81:99–119.

[8] Terral C, Rabischong P. Scientific validation of acupuncture practice. J Altern Complement Med. 1997;3:55–65.

[9] Auziech O. Acupuncture et auriculothérapie: essai d'analyse histologique de quelques structures cutanées impliquées dans ces deux techniques. Montpellier: Sauramps; 1984.

[10] Niboyet JEH. Traité d'acupuncture. 3 vols. Moulins-les-Metz: Maisonneuve; 1970.

[11] Niboyet JEH. L'anesthésie par l'acupuncture. Moulins-les-Metz: Maisonneuve; 1973.

[12] Rabischong P, Niboyet JEH, Terral C et al. Bases expérimentales de l'analgésie acupuncturale. Nouv Presse Méd. 1975;28:2021–8.

[13] Duvernoy H. Human brain stem vessels. Berlin: Springer; 1978.

[14] Duvernoy H. The human brain, surface, three-dimensional anatomy and MRI. Wien: Springer; 1991.

[15] Duvernoy H. The human brain stem and cerebellum. Wien: Springer; 1995.

[16] Melzack R, Wall PD. Pain mechanism: a new theory. Science. 1965;150:971–9.

[17] Sindou M, Quoex C, Baleydier C. Fiber organization at the posterior spinal cord rootlet junction in man. J Comp Neurol. 1974;20:391–408.

[18] Head H, Holmes G. Sensory disturbances from cerebral lesions. Brain. 1911;34:102–254.

[19] Farnarier G, Planche D, Rohner JJ. Blocage des afférences nociceptives par stimulation périphérique percutanée chez le chat. Comptes Rendus Soc Biologie. 1978;171:1054–8.

[20] Chang Hsiang-Tung. Integrative action of thalamus in the process of acupuncture for analgesia. In: Kao F, Kao J, editors. Recent advances in acupuncture research. New York: Institute for Advanced Research in Asian Science and Medicine; 1979. 178–216.

Chapter 3

Morphology of the outer ear

CHAPTER CONTENTS

INTRODUCTION

The shape of the outer ear has long been a subject of interest to both artists and anthropologists. Artists have been impressed by the harmony of its lines and curves and much study was needed before they were able to reproduce it in paintings and drawings. For learners, a geometric scheme of the ear imagined to be inscribed in an ellipse was proposed in 1768.[1] The upper drawing in Figure 3.1 represents a major semi-axis divided into four parts and a minor semi-axis (half of the former) divided into three parts. The diagonal axis subdivides the upper left quarter into two approximately equal parts and this line is intended to indicate the prominent point of the helix at the junction between the first and second part. The lower left quarter is subdivided into three parts to localize the prominent point of the ear lobe at the junction between the second and third part (Fig. 3.1).

Anthropologists were more interested in the ridges and depressions of the pinna and dedicated themselves to systematically measuring and classifying the morphological signs of the ear in humans and primates.

THE ORGANIC EVOLUTION OF THE PINNA IN PRIMATES AND HUMANS

Charles Darwin (1809–1882), in his masterpiece *The Descent of Man, and Selection in Relation to Sex,*[2] wrote:

> The whole external shell of the ear may be considered a rudiment, together with the various folds

Fig. 3.1 How to draw the correct proportions of the outer ear (from a teaching text of 1768).

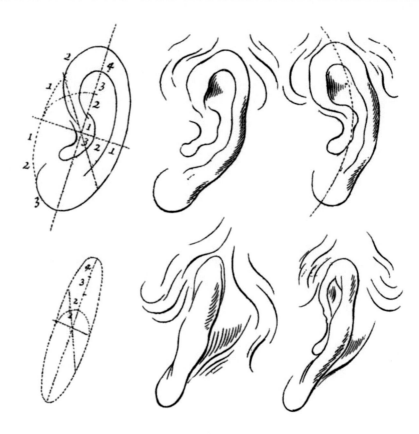

and prominences (helix and anti-helix, tragus and anti-tragus &c.) which in the lower animals strengthen and support the ear when erect, without adding much to its weight ...

Rudimentary organs are eminently variable; and this is partly intelligible, as they are useless or nearly useless, and consequently are no longer subjected to natural selection.

One of these 'rudiments' became famous as the 'tubercle of Darwin' but the true story of this distinguishing mark of the helix was told by the author himself:

The celebrated sculptor, Mr. Woolner, informs me of one little peculiarity in the external ear, which he has often observed both in men and women, and of which he perceived the full signification. The peculiarity consists in a little blunt point, projecting from the inwardly folded margin or helix. These points not only project inwards, but often a little outwards, so that they are visible when the head is viewed from directly in front or behind. They are variable in size and somewhat in position,

standing either a little higher or lower; and they sometimes occur on one ear and not on the other ... we may safely conclude that it is a similar structure – a vestige of formerly pointed ears – which occasionally reappears in man. (Fig. 3.2)

Darwin[2] made several comparative observations in primates and could not at his time understand the reason of the loss of mobility of the outer ear. He wrote:

The ears of the chimpanzee and orang are curiously like those of man, and I am assured by the keepers in the Zoological Gardens that these animals never move or erect them; so that they are in equally rudimentary condition, as far as function is concerned, as in man. Why these animals as well the progenitors of man, should have lost the power of erecting their ears we cannot say. It may be, though I am not quite satisfied with this view, that owing to their arboreal habits and great strength they were but little exposed to danger, and so during a lengthened period moved their ears but little, and thus gradually lost the power of moving them.

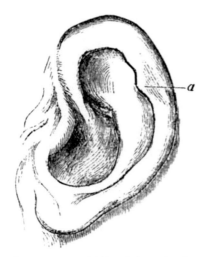

Fig. 3.2 Human ear, modeled and drawn by the sculptor Mr Woolner.[2] Point marked a = the 'projecting point' mentioned by Darwin.

Box 3.1   The Morphological Ear Index measured in different mammals: the higher scores belong to primates and humans, according to Schwalbe[3]

Hare	21.3	*Macacus rhesus*	93.0
Antelope	27.6	Chimpanzee	105–107
Pig	35.4	Orang-utan	122
Cat	58.8	Gorilla	125
Lemur macaco	76.0	Human	130
Cynocephalus baboon	84.0		

Darwin's observations influenced all following anthropologists who tried to find an answer to this query. Two famous researchers, the German Gustav Schwalbe (1844–1916) and Rudolf Martin (1864–1925) from Switzerland, demonstrated that the process of regression in primates and in man consisted essentially in a shortening of the tip of the ear, causing an inward curl of the helix and a rise of the upper branch of the anthelix. Schwalbe[3] measured the base of the ear (a–b in his study) and the so-called true length (d–c), from the tragus to Darwin's tubercle, and compared the morphological ear index (base × 100/true length) in various mammals and primates (Fig. 3.3; Box 3.1).

Humans had the highest score not only because length was reduced but also because the base of the ear was significantly larger. This increase was actually responsible for the progressive loss of mobility observed by Darwin. Nevertheless, the significance of the raised anthelix and the curled helix remained obscure and it was only several decades later that an explanation was found, thanks to modern technology.

The unanswered questions in recent times were fundamentally two:

- how could the human ear localize the direction of sound without moving the pinna?
- to what extent is the strange shape of the ear involved in the understanding of speech?

Several hypotheses were proposed on both subjects but the most interesting conclusions were probably those reached by the psychiatrist Johann Burchard[4–6] of Hamburg, who dedicated 30 years of his life to these issues. In a series of experiments

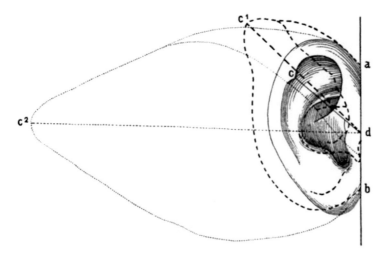

Fig. 3.3 The human outer ear compared with that of a baboon and that of a calf according to Schwalbe.[3] The human outer ear (represented by an unbroken line; a c b); the outer ear of a baboon (dashed line; a c[1] b) and the outer ear of a calf (dotted line; a c[2] b) were overlapped maintaining the same base length (a d b).

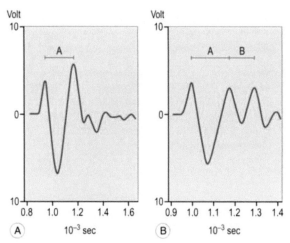

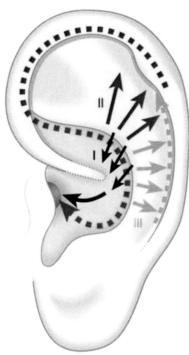

Fig. 3.4 (A) Specimen of 2-peak sound-wave transmission: in this case interval A was 0.22 ms = 7.2 cm. (B) Specimen of 3-peak sound-wave transmission: in this case interval A was 0.18 ms = 6.0 cm; interval B was 0.12 ms = 3.9 cm.) *(From Burchard.[6])*

Fig. 3.5 The three anatomical paths (I, II, III) of transmission of the sound wave to the external acoustic meatus according to Johann Burchard.

he noticed that a square-shaped click of 0.14 ms produced by the computer could be recorded with two or three peaks by a miniaturized microphone in the external acoustic meatus (Fig. 3.4A, B). Of 53 people (106 ears) placed in a noiseless room, 14% showed two peaks and 86% three peaks. In both groups interval A (between the first and second peak) and interval B (between the second and third peak) were significantly different when the direction of the sound was shifted from a perpendicular axis to the ear surface to points placed at 45° respectively in front, at the back and below ($P <0.01$) or up ($P <0.05$). These data confirmed the evidence that the human ear can actually localize sounds in space without moving the pinna.

Burchard's second hypothesis was that the three peaks could correspond to three different anatomical paths covered by the sound wave transmitted to the external meatus (Fig. 3.5). Calculating the average delays from one peak to the next, he obtained distances in cm which were significantly correlated with the length of the respective anatomical path measured with soft threads ($P <0.01$). He identified three possible paths: the first (I in Fig. 3.5) was the shortest way to reach the external meatus (about 0.1 ms corresponding to 3 cm) and could seemingly start from the lower concha and the wall of the anthelix; the second (II in Fig. 3.5) had a further average delay of 6.6 cm and could possibly start from the upper-middle portion of

the scapha and helix tunnel; the third (III in Fig. 3.5) had a further average delay of 3 cm and could possibly originate from the lower portion of the same anatomical parts. The incomplete consistency of peak 3 was explained by Burchard by the lack in these subjects of a sufficiently pronounced depression of this anatomical portion (as for example in Fig. 3.6 or in types 3 and 4 in Fig. 3.9A). Repeating the same experiment on chimpanzees and gorillas he found that these primates had only two peaks which were similar to peaks 1 and 2 in humans. The less curled helix and the distance between anthelix and helix make the third peak, typical in humans, impossible for primates. The author concluded that the triple signal and its variations of amplitude and interval were essential for the cortical recognition of sound which is fundamental in the analysis of speech.

ANTHROPOMETRY OF THE OUTER EAR

Anthropometrists, dealing with the measurement of size, weight and proportions of the human body, also introduced some anatomical landmarks for the

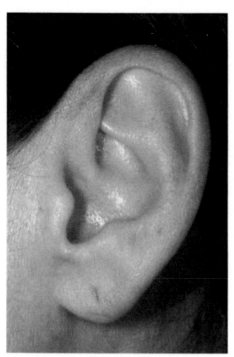

Fig. 3.6 Example of a pinna without the lower part of the scapha.

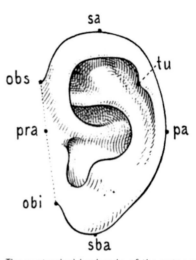

Fig. 3.7 The anatomical landmarks of the outer ear. obs = otobasion superius; obi = otobasion inferius; pra = preaurale; sa = superaurale; sba = subaurale; pa = postaurale; tu = Darwin's tubercle.

outer ear to be used for calculating its dimension. These are *otobasion superius* (obs), *otobasion inferius* (obi), which are the upper and lower points at which the pinna is attached to the scalp (Fig. 3.7). The line joining obs and obi is called the base of the ear. The other points are *superaurale* (sa) and *subaurale* (sba), which allow the measurement of the so-called 'physiognomic length', and *preaurale* (pra) and *postaurale* (pa), which are used to measure the 'physiognomic breadth' of the pinna. Both measurements are usually taken by the anthropologist using a special calliper.[3] Among the data gathered by different authors on large samples of the population are the average larger dimensions of the pinna in males compared to females. Another interesting phenomenon observed by various researchers is the constant increase of both measurements, particularly of length, during a subject's life.[3,7] Especially after the age of 50 there is a further increase which has to be correlated with various factors such as the flattening of the anthelix and the reduction of curling of the helix, but also the decrease of skin elasticity and the particular growth of the ear lobe. In addition the appearance of creases in the front of the tragus and the growth of hair on the external meatus are considered good parameters for judging a subject's age.

MORPHOLOGICAL VARIABLES

In the past anthropologists have studied the outer ear to make a reliable classification of the dominant and recessive trait of some recurrent morphological characteristics. Studies have been carried out on large groups of individuals of different racial and geographical origin. Another application of the inspection of the outer ear, nowadays superseded by genomic analysis, was sometimes proposed by forensic medicine as a control in the scientific clarification of paternity.[8,9]

The effort made by anthropologists to describe the morphological variables of the ear as exhaustively as possible is of great value and interest to us. The reader could actually be helped to differentiate some morphological characteristics with a more pronounced hereditary tendency than others acquired later in the patient's life (see the next section). Figure 3.8 reports the first which received particular consideration in the literature as a possible dominant or recessive trait.[7] In this description I have excluded any malformations associated with hereditary deafness, renal and vertebral anomalies and chromosome abnormalities such as trisomy 18 syndrome. The frequency of the illustrated characteristics is very variable: for example, according to Lange, in 908 subjects: the curled helix was visible in 60.1%; Darwin's tubercle in 59.8%; the

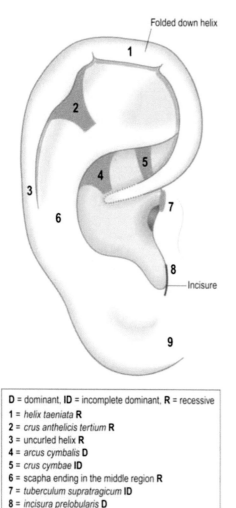

Folded down helix

1

2

5

4

3

6

7

8

Incisure

9

D = dominant, ID = incomplete dominant, R = recessive
1 = *helix taeniata* **R**
2 = *crus anthelicis tertium* **R**
3 = *uncurled helix* **R**
4 = *arcus cymbalis* **D**
5 = *crus cymbae* **ID**
6 = *scapha ending in the middle region* **R**
7 = *tuberculum supratragicum* **ID**
8 = *incisura prelobularis* **D**
9 = *ear lobe attached to cheek* **ID**

▨ = protuberances, raised areas

Fig. 3.8 Hereditary characteristics as having a possible dominant or recessive trait according to Lange.[7]

tuberculum supratragicum in 38%; the *helix taeniata* in 9%; the *crus cymbae* in 6.8%; the *incisura prelobularis* in 4.7%; the *crus anthelicis tertium* in 3.4%. Some significant sexual differences were observed, among them the higher frequency of Darwin's tubercle in males and the strikingly higher proportion of curled helix in females (76.8% in females compared with 44.2% in males)[3] (Fig. 3.9). These characteristics are seemingly correlated and Martin[3] gives us the following explanation to think about, and perhaps be amused by:

the regression process is more advanced in female ears, i.e. the shape of the female ear has reached a certain stability; instead the shape of the male ear is relatively more like that of the monkey and has less stability.

A further autosomal dominant familial trait, the *fistula auris congenita*, also known as pitted ear, has been observed in about 1% of Europeans and in 2.5% and 2.6% respectively in samples of the Chinese and Japanese populations (see Fig. 3.18).

Once the possible hereditary origin of the characteristics visible on inspection have been excluded, the practitioner should, however, recognize other signs possibly acquired later in the patient's life. These characteristics have been noted both by anatomists and by anthropologists[8–10] (Fig. 3.10). Some of them may be important in the diagnostic process based on inspection of the ear presented in this book (Ch. 4).

THE SHAPE OF THE OUTER EAR AS A POSSIBLE EXPRESSION OF DIFFERENT MODELING FACTORS

Two German anthropologists from Munich, Ludwig and Ilse Burkhardt, were fascinated by the peculiar shape of the outer ear and its great variability according to the individual constitution. In previous literature they found only the well known association between long and slim ears with a slightly curled helix and a leptosomic constitutional body type (Greek *leptos*, slender), and similarly between large and oval-shaped ears with a pronounced curled helix and a pyknic constitutional body type (Greek *pyknic*, thick). They may well have felt dissatisfied with this limited information when they started an observational study on 1206 deceased patients in the clinical departments at Schwabinger Hospital in Munich, observing them during autopsy.[11] Their aim was first to confirm the upper reported variability and at the same time to discover an innovative way to classify the different morphological types of ear. The parameters chosen were sex, age, profession, weight, height and other anthropometrical measurements such as the circumference of the head and of the thorax. The left ear of all subjects was photographed and the following measurements taken: length, width and angle of inclination of the pinna with respect to the scalp.

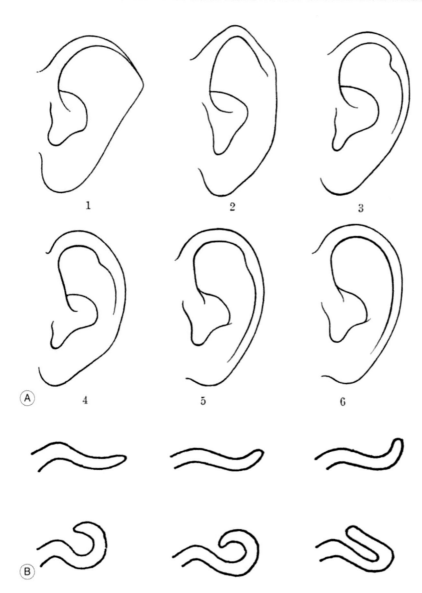

Fig. 3.9   (A) Classification of Darwin's tubercle according to Schwalbe.[3]
1 = *Macacus* shaped
2 = *Cercopithecus* shape
3 = clear tip
4 = rounded tip
5 = sketched tip
6 = not visible
(B) Different degrees of curling of the helix according to the same author.

For the purpose of classification a ranking was proposed for the following parameters:

1. aspect of the pinna as a whole (less developed, fleshy, slim, protruding)
2. length of the ear (short: up to 60 mm in males, 58 mm in females; medium size: 61–68 mm in males, 59–66 mm in females; long: >68 mm in males, >66 mm in females)
3. aspect of the helix (more or less curled)
4. tragus (hairy or not)
5. aspect of the ear lobe (small, fleshy, close to the skull)
6. angle of inclination of the pinna (up to 95°, >95°)
7. index of thoracic circumference × 100 ÷ height (small: up to 48 mm; medium: 49–55 mm; large: >55 mm).

The authors classified the data on 1132 subjects, excluding those of children, who were studied separately. From the beginning they were aware of the difficulty in defining clearly a series of morphological types of the ear. Nevertheless they identified at least five types: two of these had the most marked opposite characteristics and were

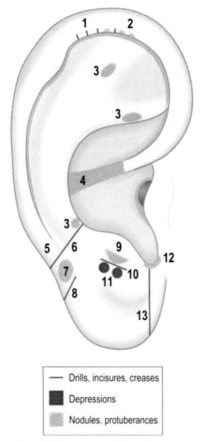

- — Drills, incisures, creases
- ■ Depressions
- ▨ Nodules, protuberances

Fig. 3.10 Descriptive non-hereditary characters reported in the literature by anatomists and anthropologists.
1, 2 = indentation or nodules of the helix border
3 = protuberances of the anthelix
4 = *processus cruris helicis ad anthelicum*
5 = deepening of the scaphoid groove
6 = *sulcus obliquus*
7 = *tuberculum retrolobulare*
8 = *sulcus retrolobularis*
9 = *eminentia anonyma*
10 = *sulcus supralobularis*
11 = depressed areas of the upper ear lobe
12 = *torus trago-antitragus*
13 = *sulcus lobuli verticalis*

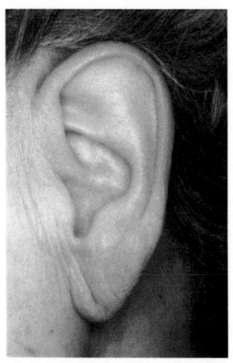

Fig. 3.11 Example of the 'cranial' type of ear: when the picture was taken the female patient was aged 66, her weight was 65 kg and her height was 165 cm (BMI = 24). Now she is 78 years old and the only disorders developed during the intervening time are a gastro-esophageal reflux syndrome and a mild cognitive impairment.

named 'cranial' and 'caudal', making up 23.5% and 26.1% of the total, respectively. A third group, for the type with intermediate characteristics, was named 'indifferent' and made up 41% of the total. Two more groups were added: the 'dorsal' and 'sickle-shaped' types, totaling only 5.3% and 4.1%

respectively. Examples of caudal and cranial types are shown in Figures 3.11 and 3.12. The recurrent characteristics in these groups are listed in Table 3.1.

The second part of the research is probably the most interesting for this book. The authors searched for an association between the morphological type of the ear and the main pathological findings at autopsy. Among the most frequent diseases they found were cardiovascular disorders, luetic (syphilitic) aortitis, tuberculosis, carcinomas, gallstones, prostate hypertrophy, pneumonia, endocarditis and sepsis. As shown in Table 3.2, a higher number of cases with cardiovascular diseases, gallstones, prostate hypertrophy and endocarditis were associated with the caudal type; lung tuberculosis, lung and stomach carcinomas, on the other hand, were more

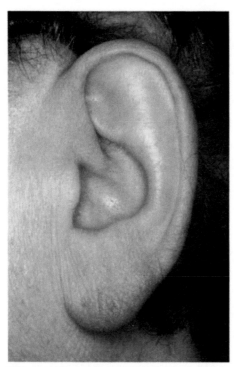

Fig. 3.12 Example of the 'caudal' type of ear: when the picture was taken the female patient was 67 years old, her weight was 130 kg and her height was 175 cm (BMI = 42). The patient had diabetes and hypertension and died 3 years later with acute congestive heart failure.

Table 3.1 The opposite characteristics of the cranial and caudal type of ear according to the Burkhardts

Cranial ear	Caudal ear
Tendency to proportionally higher dimensions of the upper (cranial) part of the ear	Tendency to proportionally higher dimensions of the lower (caudal) part of the ear
On the whole a slimmer aspect; the pinna is closer to the skull	On the whole a fleshy aspect; the pinna protrudes more from the skull
Tendency to a leptosomic constitution (see text)	Tendency to a pyknic constitution (see text)
The helix is less curled	The helix is more curled
The tragus is less hairy	The tragus is hairier
The lobe is smaller, thinner and closer to the skull	The lobe is larger, fleshier and protrudes more from the skull

frequently associated with the cranial type (see Table 3.2). As no statistical analysis was carried out by the authors themselves, we tried to identify a possible association between the morphological type and the disease using the χ^2 test. The hypothesis of independence could be discarded both for males and females ($P<0.005$). It was therefore possible to measure an association with the Kramer index (range 0 to 1), which yielded only 0.20 for males and 0.16 for females. The association therefore did not seem relevant but, limiting the analysis only to caudal and cranial groups, the χ^2 test was still significant for males and females ($P<0.025$) and the level of association increased to 0.5 and 0.4 respectively. The effort made to separate two morphological types with opposite characteristics did indeed produce a better understanding of the connections between the shape of the ear and the tendency toward specific groups of health disorders. The authors wrote:

we have to consider the possibility that life conditions and diseases can modify the constitution of a subject including the shape of his auricle.

Moreover, a third interesting observation was made on the population examined with regard to the possible association between ear type and profession. Excluding the negligible number of people with dorsal and sickle-shaped ears, the authors found some curious associations in 500 male subjects aged over 18. The cranial type was more frequent among farmers and blue-collar workers; the caudal type was more often found among dealers, white-collar workers and those occupying positions calling for brainwork, or leaders (Table 3.3). The Burkhardts concluded their extensive study hypothesizing that besides the other already reported factors, lifestyle linked to a profession representing it could possibly act as a modeling factor of the outer ear.[11]

This study was published in 1949, several years before Nogier's discovery and at least 20 years before Chinese acupuncturists reported their experiences concerning the diagnostic value of auricular inspection.

Table 3.2   The association in 1132 subjects (581 male and 551 female) between ear type and principal pathology; according to the Burkhardts[11]

				Male				
Ear type	Cardiovascular	Luetic aortitis	Tuberculosis	Carcinomas	Gallstones	Prostatic hypertrophy	Pneumonia	Endocarditis
Indiff.	59	13	32	57	17	18	10	21
Caudal	66	8	4	11	21	11	3	11
Cranial	36	6	37	54	12	4	6	4
Dorsal	11	0	9	11	6	4	1	2
Sickle-shaped	4	1	3	3	1	3	0	1
Total	176	28	85	136	57	40	20	39

				Female				
Ear type	Cardiovascular	Luetic aortitis	Tuberculosis	Carcinomas	Gallstones	Prostatic hypertrophy	Pneumonia	Endocarditis
Indiff.	73	8	36	40	53	–	10	17
Caudal	62	8	4	22	43	–	4	17
Cranial	27	1	22	32	15	–	1	10
Dorsal	4	1	4	4	1	–	0	2
Sickle-shaped	7	0	7	6	7	–	1	2
Total	173	18	73	104	119	–	16	48

Table 3.3   The association in 500 male subjects aged over 18 between ear type and profession, according to the Burkhardts[11]

	Ear type		
Profession	Indifferent (%)	Caudal (%)	Cranial (%)
Farmer	2.7	1.7	5.7
Blue-collar worker	27.8	13.4	29.1
Labourer	6.7	5.1	12.7
Baker	0.9	1.7	0
Tailor	2.2	3.4	0.6
Trader	7.2	15.9	7.6
White-collar worker	22.4	25.2	15.2
Leader-manager	4.5	7.6	4.4
Regular soldier	6.7	9.2	5.7
Artist, medical doctor, intellectual	4.1	6.7	4.4
Other profession	13.5	8.4	13.9
Unemployed	1.3	1.7	0.7
Total	100 (223 subjects)	100 (119 subjects)	100 (158 subjects)

THE SHAPE OF THE EAR AND THE PROBLEM OF THE TRANSCRIPTION OF POINTS

The research work carried out by the anthropologists Ludwig and Ilse Burkhardt and reported in the previous section is enlightening for an exhaustive appreciation of the great variability in the shape and dimension of the outer ear.

This section deals with a problem which I have long felt crucial, namely the correct transcription and recording of the points mapped on the auricle. Keeping clear records of the location of points and skin alterations helps to give a complete overview of a subject's past and current health. The adoption of a reliable system of transcription is also essential in the follow-up for a better understanding of the subject's syndrome. If, for example, a certain symptom is going to improve or disappear spontaneously we will no longer find the point or the area which was previously identified. On the other hand, persisting sensitivity despite treatment indicates that the corresponding district of the body is still affected.

The various methods of transcription of the auricular points are different but have the same intrinsic limits:

1. they are based on a bi-dimensional representation of the outer ear; the auricle, however, is tri-dimensional with its ridges and depressions
2. they do not take into account the variability of shape and dimension related to sex, age and constitution of each subject as explained in the preceding sections.

These combined factors are not easy to manage, even if a computed tri-dimensional representation of the outer ear were available, as in plastic surgery, for the reconstruction of parts of the face. While waiting for future techniques of this type we must be content with bi-dimensional maps and select the one which is simpler to use and which offers the fewest errors in transcription. It is understandable that every author considers his own graphic system to be more valuable than others. I need therefore to make a short review of this topic.

Probably the easiest way to illustrate a specific point to students is to insert a needle on a rubber model of the ear, as the Chinese and other practitioners do in the West. This method is very useful for teaching small groups, but not so useful if there are more than 8–10 students in a class and if it is necessary to record data during a course of therapeutic sessions.

Among the graphic systems which have been proposed we have to remember the following:

- The first one, known as 'Nogier's buffer'. This is still on the market (made by Sedatelec). It is an ink stamp easily used for reproducing the graph of the ear on the patient's record at every session. Each graph can be used to record points on the lateral and medial surface of the ear, updating the patient's situation. Its major inadequacy is its reduced dimensions (it is only 40 mm long and 24 mm wide on the lateral surface) which absolutely does not allow for a reliable transcription (Fig. 3.13).
- The various grids proposed by different authors which show squares coded by one letter and one number[12,13] (Fig. 3.14). This system is interesting for teaching and makes it easy to show students the coordinates of a given point or area. Its major defect is that the grid is superimposed on a model which may or may not correspond to the ear of the actual patient to be examined. Thus it is necessary to adjust the coordinates of the point to be transcribed. This system is therefore of limited interest in the case of clinical research on larger groups of patients.
- Oleson's graphic system. This has the advantage of precisely classifying the hidden and depressed areas of the ear[14] (Fig. 3.15). His solutions are useful for teaching and transmitting data among international acupuncturists and have undoubtedly influenced the standardization process of

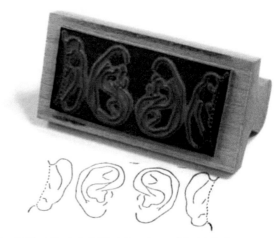

Fig. 3.13 'Nogier's buffer' *(courtesy of Sedatelec).*

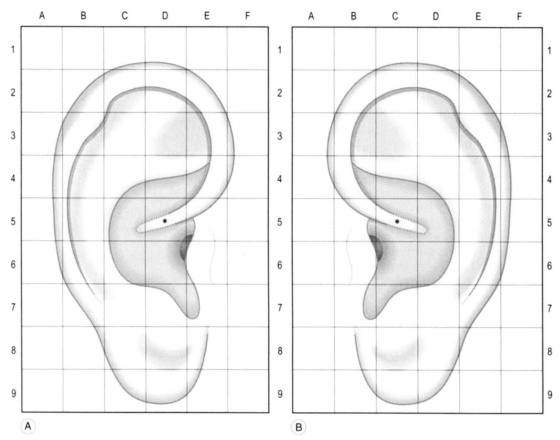

Fig. 3.14 Example of an auricular grid.

the Chinese school. However, even if the system adequately fits the ridges and depressions of the ear, it is possible that the clusters of points that are going to be transcribed from the patient's ear, or from a group of patients with a given syndrome, do not coincide with a particular subdivision of the ear.

- Some other graphic systems which use anatomical landmarks of the outer ear and a general reference point on the root of the helix that Nogier called point 0 (zero) (see next section).

On this subject, two authors, the Russian R. A. Durinyan and myself, have developed a grid with a variable number of sectors centered on point 0.[15,16] This system, which I officially presented in 1981, was recently named a 'sectogramme' (SG, Sectogram) by the French and is a satisfactory diagnostic and therapeutic tool. The SG is obtained by subdividing the auricle by three semi-axis lines,

A, B and C, going respectively through the visual intersection point of the posterior edge of the raising branch of the helix with the lower branch of the anthelix (A); through the antitragus–anthelix groove (*sulcus auriculae posterior*) (B); and tangent to the posterior edge of the tragus (C). The resulting main sectors, A–B, A–C and B–C, were themselves subdivided, into 16 sectors in the case of the first two and into eight sectors in the case of the third (Fig. 3.16). This arbitrary subdivision did not aim to produce sectors of equal angles (actually they vary between 8 and 11°) but was rather intended to offer to the practitioner a graphic instrument which could be suitable for auricles of different shapes and different dimensions. The SG is not therefore intended to replace existing methods such as, for example, the Chinese standardized areas; moreover, it could be probably improved in the future. (A copy of the Sectogram is provided at the end of the book for your use.)

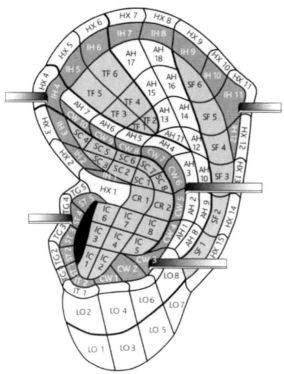

Fig. 3.15 Oleson's[14] chart *(with permission).*

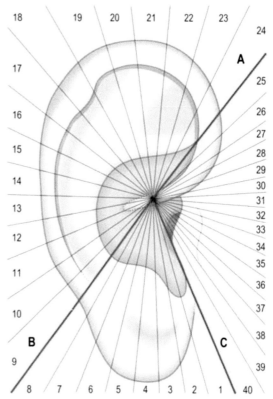

Fig. 3.16 Romoli's Sectogram, centered on Nogier's point zero, with the three half-lines A, B and C subdividing the auricle.

The SG does allow, however, several operations. The practitioner is able to:

1. follow the evolution of a syndrome in a patient receiving no treatment or undergoing therapies of different types (drugs, physiotherapy, surgery, body acupuncture, etc.)
2. facilitate the topographical diagnostic process, typical of the ear, for identifying the segmental origin (muscular, skeletal, visceral, etc.) of a current symptom
3. identify, in a subject or in a series of patients with the same disease, the sector/s showing a higher concentration of points. The spatial cluster analysis adopted in this book may be useful for identifying statistically significant clusters of sectors of high or low values (i.e. with a significant higher or lower concentration of points compared to the average number per sector).

I evaluated the reliability of the SG in 385 medical doctors attending theoretical–practical seminars of ear acupuncture between 2004 and 2007. After 16–18 hours of teaching they were asked to

participate in the following transcription exercise: two sets of points, I and II, were projected onto a screen one after the other. Each set was composed of three points located on three different parts of the pinna (helix, anthelix and ear lobe) (Fig. 3.17). The doctors were asked to transcribe the points of sets I and II in random order on the SG or on a map of the auricle without subdivision into sectors. These two modalities were compared for total average number of correct transcriptions as well as for their relative proportions on the different parts of the ear. The same procedure was adopted with the average total number of correctly identified sectors and their proportions. The results were that the total average number of correctly transcribed points was significantly higher using the SG ($P<0.001$) compared to an auricular map without subdivision in sectors (Table 3.4). Also the proportions of points correctly transcribed on the different parts of the ear (helix, anthelix and ear lobe) were significantly different (Table 3.5).

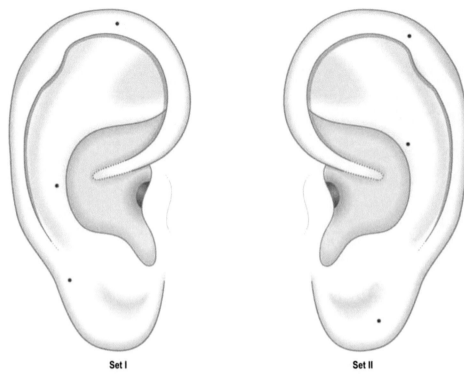

Set I   Set II

Fig. 3.17   The transcription exercise: set I of points on the left; set II on the right.

Table 3.4   Comparison in 385 students of the total average number of correctly transcribed points

	Sectogram Yes	Sectogram No	Z	P-value
A+B+C	1.84 (61%)	1.34 (45%)	10.17	<0.001

Table 3.5   Comparison in 385 students of the proportions of correctly transcribed points on three different parts of the ear (A = helix, B = anthelix, C = ear lobe)

	Sectogram Yes	Sectogram No	Z	P-value
A	0.73	0.49	6.93	<0.001
B	0.64	0.53	3.16	<0.005
C	0.47	0.32	4.17	<0.001

The same results were found comparing the total number of correctly identified sectors ($P < 0.001$) and their proportions on the three different parts of the ear.

The conclusions of the above evaluation (submitted for publication) are as follows:

The regular use of the sectogram allows practitioners to transcribe the site of auricular points and areas more precisely. By recording these locations from one session to the next it is possible to identify the clusters of points in one or more sectors which are relevant in every patient for diagnostic and therapeutic purposes.[17]

POINT ZERO AND THE 'PRINCIPLE OF ALIGNMENT' ACCORDING TO PAUL NOGIER

The SG is based on point 0 which was considered by Nogier to be the geometrical center of the ear. It is located on a distinct notch where the horizontal concha ridge meets the vertically rising helix root (see Fig. 5.10). It is noteworthy that the Chinese standardized map has the same denomination (center of the ear) for the root of the helix.

Paul Nogier was principally a clinician but he was also an expert painter and could therefore probably capture both aspects: the geometrical alignment of some points detected on the pinna and also the effect of their stimulation on the patient's symptoms. To find these alignments he invited students to examine the outer ear carefully, without any preconception, with a spring-loaded probe held vertically, passing gradually from one point to the next and applying the same pressure. When four or five points had been identified, he said, the student would be surprised to find some other tender points on the helix as an extension of the former. Nogier noticed that several alignments crossed the root of the helix in the notch described above, easily identified using the nail of the index finger.[18]

From the anatomical point of view this notch does not seem to have any particular meaning, except that it is placed in a zone which seems to be subjected to several transformations at the embryogenic stage. It is, for example, interesting that the root of the helix and its ascending branch correspond substantially to the zones which more frequently show the curious *fistula auris congenita* or 'pitted ear' cited in 'Morphological variables', above.

Perhaps the largest statistical study worldwide on this subject was performed in Japan. In a healthy population of 15 114 elementary and high school students this characteristic was observed in 396 subjects (2.6%). In 74% of the cases the fistula was unilateral and there was a slightly higher incidence in females. The total number of fistulae observed on both ears was 503, and 98.2% of them were located in the area comprehending the preauricular region, the prehelix and the crus helix[19] (Fig. 3.18). Several authors suppose the fistula to be caused by imperfect fusion of the tubercles derived from the first two branchial arches which could lead to entrapment of the epithelium to form preauricular cysts and preauricular sinuses or fistulae. Another interesting hypothesis is reported by Pearson who considered the pit to be caused by a partial retention of the primitive external auditory meatus.[20] Nevertheless, besides this bold association with the pits in the ear, anything reasonable may be said about the true sense of point 0.

In his untiring work Nogier was particularly impressed by the anthelix placed on an arch of circumference around this point. Actually the system of radii starting from the center of the ear and traversing the entire pinna helped him greatly in discovering what he called the 'segmental projections' or 'somatotopic organization' of the body. His clinical experience permitted him to say that:

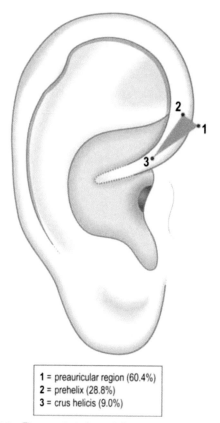

1 = preauricular region (60.4%)
2 = prehelix (28.8%)
3 = crus helicis (9.0%)

Fig. 3.18 The opening sites of *fistula auris congenita* and their percentages according to Dr Iida.

all the points on each of these radii are connected in such a way that any therapeutic action performed at the level of the border point and at point Zero (the extreme points of the radius) is transmitted to all points of that radius.

In this way Nogier was able to identify precisely the radii related to some specific vertebrae. He asked students to be very cautious and, for example, not to consider the line RTH8 passing through the vertebral point TH8 as in any way pertaining to the 8th or 9th thoracic nerve[18] (Fig. 3.19). But if we look at the case with herpes zoster of the 8th thoracic root reported in Figures 3.20 and 3.21, we can see that the lines proposed by Nogier actually have a meaning and are important for diagnosis and therapy. Through his explanation he perhaps intended stressing the importance of not confusing other structures located on the same line, the innervation of which could in no way be accepted as coincident. For example, in Figure 3.19, the location on the line RTH9 of the somatotopic representation

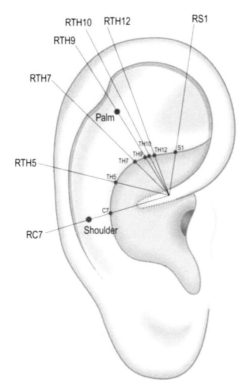

Fig. 3.19 Reconstruction of some radii according to Nogier's principle of alignment.

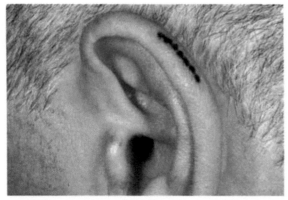

Fig. 3.20 Example of alignment on the helix in a case of herpes zoster located on the 8th thoracic root. The points which are tender to pressure are marked with non-toxic ink.

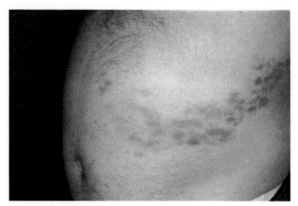

Fig. 3.21 Skin rash in the same patient.

of the palm of the hand, proposed by Nogier himself, seems unacceptable as its innervation stems from the plexus brachialis (originating from the ventral branches of the last four cervical spinal nerves and most of the ventral branch of the first thoracic spinal nerve). Nevertheless, if we look at the body acupuncture points which are in topographic correspondence to the auricular point TH9 and the palm of the hand, we find respectively point *Ganshu* (BL18), and point *Laogong* (PC 8). The former is located 1.5 *cun* laterally to the border of the spinous process of TH9; the latter is located between the second and third metacarpal bones where the middle finger touches the palm, closing the hand. Beyond the interpretation of these points according to traditional Chinese medicine (TCM), we can limit ourselves to considering only the different groups of therapeutic indications which are reported in the most important acupuncture textbooks. The reader may well be surprised to notice that the two points share overlapping indications, for example of cough, nosebleed and chest pain but also of deep anger and manic-depressive syndrome.[21] Therefore, even keeping both feet on the ground and attempting to maintain a scientific approach to auricular diagnosis and therapy, we should nevertheless be prepared to encounter several surprises during our work. The outer ear still holds secrets to be unveiled and no clinical observation, however strange and out of place it might appear, should be rejected.

References

[1] Anfangsgründe zur Zeichnungskunst fur Anfänger in XX Kupferrissen bestehend. Nuremberg: 1768.

[2] Darwin C. The descent of man, and selection in relation to sex. Vol. 2. London: John Murray; 1871.

[3] Martin R. Lehrbuch der Anthropologie. 1st vol. Jena: Gustav Fischer; 1928.

[4] Burchard JM, Irrgang B, Andresen B. Das äussere Ohr des Menschen als schallverdoppelndes Organ. Sprache-Stimme-Gehör. 1985;9:100–3.

[5] Burchard JM, Irrgang E, Andresen B. Die Funktion der menschlichen Ohrmuschel. Spektrum der Wissenschaft. 1987;6:66–74.

[6] Burchard JM. Über die Funktion der Ohrmuschel. Hamburger Ärzteblatt. 2001;6–7:301–2.

[7] Lange G. Familienuntersuchungen über die Erblichkeit metrischer und morphologischer Merkmale des äusseren Ohres. Z Morph Anthrop. 1966;2:111–67.

[8] Tillner I. Seltene morphologische Merkmale an der menschlichen Ohrmuschel und ihr praktischer Wert für die Vaterschaftsbegutachtung. Anthrop Anz. 1963;4:294–307.

[9] Mullis ML. Zur Frage der Kontrollfunktion der anthropologisch-erbbiologischen Expertise in der Vaterschaftsbegutachtung. Anthrop Anz. 1980;4:271–7.

[10] Gerhardt K. Zur Morphognose des Kopfes, der Ohren und der Augengegend mit grundsätzlichen Erläuterungen. Anthrop Anz. 1968;4:280–5.

[11] Burkhardt L, Burkhardt I. Die Gestaltung des äusseren Ohres als konstitutionspathologisches Merkmal. Z menschl Vererb Konstit.lehre. 1949;29:496–516.

[12] Kovacs R. L'auriculomédecine en consultation journalière. Paris: Maloine; 1983.

[13] Caspani F. Auricoloterapia. Como: red/studio redazionale; 1988.

[14] Oleson TD. Auriculotherapy manual: Chinese and Western systems of ear acupuncture. 3rd ed. Edinburgh: Churchill Livingstone; 2003.

[15] Romoli M. A contribution to the study of new areas of the ear lobe for the treatment of migraine and cephalalgia with acupuncture. Brno: 1st Czechoslovak Congress of Acupuncture; 3–6 June 1981.

[16] Durinyan RA. Anatomy and physiology of auricular reflex therapy. Scand J Acup Electroth. 1986;3–4:83–91.

[17] Romoli M, Mazzoni R. The validation of a new system of transcription of acupuncture points on the ear: the Auricular Sectogram (submitted for publication).

[18] Nogier PFM. Traité d'auriculothérapie. Maisonneuve; 1969.

[19] Iida M, Sakai M. A statistical study of fistula auris congenita in Japan. Tokai J Exp Clin Med. 1997;3:133–6.

[20] Pearson AA. Developmental anatomy of the ear. In: English GM, editor. Otolaryngology, vol. 1. Philadelphia: Harper & Row; 1985. 1–66.

[21] Deadman P, Al-Kafaji M, Baker K. A manual of acupuncture. Journal of Chinese Medicine Publications; 1998.

Chapter 4

Inspection of the outer ear

INTRODUCTION

So far, in Western countries, inspection of the outer ear has attracted little attention with the exception of the ear lobe, the diagonal crease of which has been thoroughly studied in patients with cardiovascular risk (see section entitled 'The diagonal ear lobe crease or Frank's sign' later in this chapter).

The only Western physicians to show an interest in auricular morphology have been those practicing Rudolf Steiner's (1861–1925) philosophy of anthroposophy. Steiner wrote:

> *The ear portrays our past and reveals tendencies and weaknesses that we have carried since birth. It is the only important physiognomic organ undergoing very little change after birth.*

The physician Norbert Glas[1] proposed a physiognomic classification of the outer ear into three parts (Fig. 4.1):

1. The upper third corresponds to the 'head and the mind' and is subdivided into three different parts; the descending part of the helix (a) corresponding to the 'shape and the strength of the erect body'; the upper part of the helix (b) corresponding to the 'capacity and strength of the mind'; the rising part of the helix (c) corresponding to the 'internal energy'. A large, thin and softened helix in (a) therefore suggests rickets, a lymphatic constitution and a tendency towards infections and the common cold. A flattening or folding down of the helix in (b) suggests weak powers of thought, depression and learning difficulties. A folding of the helix (c), with a vertical straightening of the posterior ridge, suggests asthma, speech disorders and mental inhibition.
2. The middle third corresponds to the 'rhythmic system', meaning the respiratory system and blood circulation. If the concha is regular in shape these systems are working perfectly; a narrow concha indicates poor circulation and a weakness of the corresponding organs. For example, an upper narrow concha on the left suggests weakness of the pancreas with a tendency to diabetes.
3. The lower third, including the ear lobe, the antitragus and the intertragal notch, corresponds to the 'metabolic system' and also to the subject's reproductive capacity and willpower. An enlarged incisura intertragica therefore implies

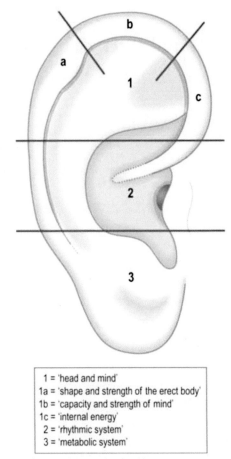

1 = 'head and mind'
1a = 'shape and strength of the erect body'
1b = 'capacity and strength of mind'
1c = 'internal energy'
2 = 'rhythmic system'
3 = 'metabolic system'

Fig. 4.1 The physiognomic classification of the ear according to anthroposophy.

hyperthyroidism and overactivity of the pancreas; a narrow incisura, on the other hand, indicates a slow metabolism and, in females, endocrine disorders, gynecological disorders and troublesome delivery.

The information given by Glas in his chapter dedicated to the specific physiognomy of the outer ear is of interest and surprising because it was gathered over a long period of time, before Nogier's discovery of auriculotherapy. The importance given by anthroposophy to the inspection of the outer ear, as to the whole face, is, however, based on considerations that differ somewhat from Nogier's representation of the body.

The French author was aware that certain skin alterations of the auricle could be found on the corresponding area of a suffering organ. He said: 'When the patient is affected by a longstanding disease, we can recognize its signature on the ear.'

He referred two clinical cases with skin alterations of the lung area.[2] The first was a patient with severe non-responding eczema of the buttocks, genitals and face. Furthermore Nogier identified a small area of eczema corresponding to the lung; this led him to suspect a tubercular origin for the eczema which afterwards responded well to the appropriate treatment. The second case was that of a patient who had been affected for several years by pneumothorax; the corresponding lung area was well recognizable on inspection because it was creased and yellowish.

The French lung area corresponds on the whole to the Chinese one (CO14 *Fei*); nevertheless, in the latter the lung has a larger representation, occupying almost the whole inferior concha. The dimensions of this area are proportional to the importance of the lung in traditional Chinese medicine (TCM); the indications for treatment are cough, chest congestion and hoarseness, but also skin disorders such as acne, itching and urticaria. Other indications are constipation and control of the abstinence syndrome as described in Chapter 1.

Even though Nogier realized the importance of skin alterations on the auricle he did not perform any systematic study nor did he invite his pupils to focus on this subject.

THE CHINESE CONTRIBUTION TO THE INSPECTION OF THE OUTER EAR

As noted in Chapter 1, the application of the principles of TCM to ear acupuncture by Chinese therapists favored an original development of this discipline. If we consider the four different diagnostic methods proposed by TCM, besides pulse and tongue diagnosis, we find examination of the patient at the top, followed by the interview, auscultation and smelling and palpation of the body. It is not by chance that palpation has been ranked last; an aphorism written by the famous physician Pien Chueh in his book *Nan Jing* (Difficult Classic) was:

the physician who knows his patient's condition through inspection examining him is a genial physician; the physician who understands his condition through auscultation and smelling is a saint; the physician who recognizes his condition through palpation is a second-rate physician.

There is no part of the body which was not the object of observation by TCM. It is plausible, therefore, that the outer ear was included in this thorough examination during past centuries.

Nevertheless, observations on the auricle were scanty compared to those on the tongue and the other parts of the face. Among signs found in Chinese classical textbooks are those related, for example, to the color of the helix[3] (Table 4.1).

Table 4.1 Some explanations of abnormal color of the helix according to traditional Chinese medicine (TCM) (after Maciocia[3])

Color of the helix	Tone	Energetic explanation according to TCM
Pale	Bright	*Yang* deficiency
Pale	Dull	Blood deficiency
Pale	Deep and 'thick'	*Qi* deficiency with Phlegm
Yellow	Bright	Damp-Heat; Heat predominates
Yellow	Dull	Damp-Heat; Dampness predominates
Greenish		Blood stasis from Heat
Greenish	Dark	Kidney-*Yin* deficiency
Bluish		Blood stasis from Cold
Red		Heat in the Lung and/or in the Heart
Red	Floating	Kidney-*Yin* deficiency with Empty-Heat

The auricular inspection proposed by Chinese acupuncturists after 1958 goes beyond a simple somatotopic diagnosis as conceived in Western countries: it reflects the concept of the human body according to the rules of TCM. The body is a united totality of contradictions. Every single part of it is closely physiologically interconnected. After the onset of disease, a local ailment reflects itself on other parts as well as on the whole, while the transformation of the whole will certainly exert an influence locally. This is the reason why Chinese acupuncturists proposed a points selection for the ear according to the *pien-cheng sih chih* method, where *pien-cheng* means grasping the essence of a disease by distinguishing the subjective and objective symptoms, and *sih chih* means treating diseases according to the principles of TCM after analyzing and synthesizing a patient's symptoms. In this way, for example, the heart and small intestine are correlated, and therefore a cardiovascular pathology will evoke a positive reaction on the ear's area for the small intestine.[4]

It is interesting to recall the different stages in the Chinese experience: the first was the confirmation of the ear's somatotopic representation of the different anatomical parts of the body through inspection, for example deformation or cartilaginous hypertrophy of the inferior crus of the anthelix in case of lumbar spondylosis or prolapsed intervertebral disk. Next came the proof that acupuncture treatment of dyschromia, telangiectasia, etc. within the somatotopic area related to a patient's disease gave good results. Then came the *pien-cheng sih chih* method with the global consideration of the ear according to TCM. The last fascinating and at the same time complex stage was to obtain elements, through auricular inspection, for eventually revealing a suspected hidden tumor.

It is possible, in my opinion, that auricular inspection as proposed by Chinese acupuncturists has not been considered essential in the West because of the almost complete lack of photographic documentation. The historical textbook of the Nanjing military headquarters was the only one in the early 1970s that contained a few color plates related to diseases of the uterus, stomach and liver. A fourth plate showed desquamation of the lung area in a case of skin disease. Nanjing's test, which has been translated into several languages, among them English[5] and Italian,[6] reports type and location of the various skin alterations observed in the different diseases. Unfortunately the description of 'positive reaction points,' as they were called by the army doctors of the Nanjing garrison, does not follow any dermatological classification and we cannot understand, for example, what 'congestive papules' or 'white small spots with reddish borders' are. The authors, however, examined about 20 000 patients by simple inspection, reaching the conclusion that when certain internal organs or local areas of the human body suffer through illness, especially organic diseases, positive reactions will appear on the corresponding regions or specific areas of the majority of the patients. These pathological changes are symbolized by changes in skin color, deformation, desquamation and papules, etc.

The general instructions recommended by the authors for correct auricular inspection are as follows:

1. Careful attention must be paid to the patient's skin which varies in summer and winter. The skin of an elderly person is not the same as that of a child. We should pay more attention to these distinctions.
2. Before observation, do not wipe, wash, lift or pull the auricle, to avoid causing discoloration of the skin or even elimination of matter which would greatly influence the accuracy of inspection. If a depressed area of the auricle is not clean, it may be wiped lightly in a given direction with a cotton swab.
3. When a positive reaction is found, the theory of *zang-fu* in TCM should be taken into consideration, and comprehensive analysis carried out by the *pien-cheng* method, to reach a diagnosis.
4. On the auricle of healthy persons there are often different manifestations such as pigmentations, white nodules, small pustules and scars from chilblains, etc. Most of these are 'false appearances'. A method for distinguishing these is: first inspect, secondly press. If pressure does not cause pain this indicates that the manifestation pertains to a 'false positive reaction'.
5. The light should be good, and natural light is preferable, though a flashlight may also be useful for appreciating the more internal parts of the auricle or its medial surface.

Points 2 and 5 are important for making a reliable inspection; as regards point 4, it is rare in our countries to find scars from chilblains. Tenderness at pressure of a skin alteration is, however, fundamental for diagnosis and may be used to treat symptoms. For example, acupuncture on a sensitive telangiectasia located within the representative area of a painful joint sometimes gives very quick and lasting relief.

Point 3 surely gives interesting indications for a general evaluation of the patient based on TCM syndromes. For example, desquamation of the lung area, as demonstrated also by Nogier, may direct the physician's attention to possible skin disorders; a telangiectasia of the liver zone may orient his diagnostic intuition also toward depression and insomnia (see p. 97). Seborrhea of the cavum conchae instead may orient the acupuncturist's diagnosis to metabolic disorders associated with food intolerance and diabetes if the pancreatic area is sensitive to pressure.

CLASSIFICATION OF SKIN ALTERATIONS OF THE OUTER EAR

Among the few Western authors who have given due importance to inspecting the outer ear and who have studied it systematically are Dr Nguyen in France and myself. Dr Nguyen has spoken about a 'lésion cutanée ponctuelle' (LCP) while I have spoken about 'skin alterations'.

One of the major difficulties in ear inspection is how to classify the auricle's skin alterations. Chinese authors limited the auricular reactions to four categories (change in color, deformation, papules and desquamation) whereas Nguyen proposed nine different categories distinguishing the following elements:[7]

- follicle (referring to sebaceous cyst)
- nevus
- angioma
- telangiectasia
- comedo
- nodule
- chondroplasia
- scar
- hair hyperplasia.

I did not feel satisfied with this classification and here propose an alternative which in my opinion includes all of the auricle's visible elementary skin lesions. In my research I was helped by a dermatologist, Antonia Pata, and together we set up a classification which includes six groups of alterations related to the vascularization, pigmentation, keratinization, cartilaginous, cutaneous and sebaceous gland structure of the auricle (Table 4.2).

Using this classification I examined 711 patients of various ages (471 females, average age 46.9 years, range 12–92, SD 17.4; 240 males, average age 45.6 years, range 12–85, SD 18.4). I photographed both ears of every patient and reported on the Sectogram those skin alterations which I could detect with my naked eye. A database was created with the following data from every patient: age, sex, symptom prompting request for help, current or past important diseases, surgical operations, traumas, location and type of skin alterations. The main aim in assembling these data was to establish if ear inspection offers any elements of specificity which could be used in the process of auricular diagnosis. The total number of skin alterations was 8828 with an average of 12.4 skin alterations per patient, range 0–35, SD 4.7; the distribution on the right and left was almost equal; 52.7% on the right and 47.3% on the left auricle. The higher rate of skin alterations was found on the anthelix followed by the helix, the ear lobe and the cymba concha. A decreasing rate was found on the cavum concha and the medial surface of the ear; on the remaining parts (tragus, triangular fossa, intertragic notch) the rate did not reach 5% of the total (Table 4.3). The total number of skin alterations varies with the age of the patient and in both sexes there is a progressive increase passing from younger subjects to patients aged 70 or over (Fig. 4.2). The outer ear therefore acts as a mirror reflecting not only diseases of single organs but also the whole ageing process of a patient's body. This process is not homogeneous on all auricular parts; indeed some of them, such as the ear lobe, anthelix, helix, tragus, antitragus and intertragic notch, show a significant correlation between age and the number of skin alterations (Table 4.4).

Another parameter which varies with age and accompanies the increasing number of skin alterations is the number of hospitalizations and, to a lesser extent, the number of surgical operations, whereas the number of traumas remains constant throughout the decades examined (Fig. 4.3). The skin alterations are not evenly distributed through the six different categories: vascular skin alterations (particularly telangiectasia and hyperemia)

Table 4.2   Classification of skin alterations (SAs) of the outer ear according to Pata and Romoli

Category	Type of SA	Pattern
SA related to vascularization	Paleness Hyperemia Telangiectasia Angioma	 – reticular telangiectasia – punctiform telangiectasia – linear telangiectasia – spider angioma – punctiform angioma
SA related to pigmentation	Dyschromia Macula Nevus	 – isolated spot – pigmented area – mixed melanin–hemosiderin area (grey, yellow, orange) – blue – melanocytic
SA related to keratinization	Dyskeratosis Dystrophy (skin is thin, lucent and fragile)	– furfuraceous scales – psoriasiform scales
SA related to cartilaginous structure	Hypertrophy (thickening) Hypotrophy (depression)	
SA related to cutaneous structure	Depressed area Crease Incisure	
SA related to sebaceous gland structure	Milium Sebaceous cyst Comedone	

correspond to 42.6% of the total followed by pigmented skin alterations (mainly nevi and maculae) corresponding to 26.2%; skin alterations of skin structure (creases and incisures) correspond to 15%. The remaining three groups follow with percentages below 5–10% (Fig. 4.4). The six categories of skin alteration have a different distribution on the 11 areas of the auricle. Telangiectasia are mostly seen on the anthelix, nevi prevalently on the helix followed by the ear lobe. Maculae have a uniform distribution on the anthelix, helix and lobe. The skin alterations of sebaceous gland structure (particularly comedones) were found mainly on the cymba conchae followed by the cavum conchae. Also depressions and dyskeratosis were found mostly on the cavum conchae. Also interesting is the comparison between the different percentage distribution throughout the six categories in the extremes of the age groups: younger people tended to have pigmented skin alterations (especially nevi) followed by vascular and sebaceous gland skin alterations (comedones), whereas in the oldest group of patients vascular skin alterations ranked first, followed by creases, incisures and pigmented skin alterations (especially maculae) (Fig. 4.5). The scantiness of skin alterations on the medial surface compared to those on the lateral surface is remarkable and only 902 (10.2% of the total) were found there. It is possible that this percentage could be higher if inspection of the medial surface were easier, if we consider that pain pressure test (PPT) tender points of this area in 325 patients were 14.4% and those with lower electrical resistance 19% of the total.

Table 4.3 Distribution of skin alterations (SAs) (summing those of the right and left ear) on the different parts of the auricle in 711 patients

Category of SA	Type of SA	Part of the auricle											
		Anthelix	Antitragus	Lower concha	Upper concha	Helix	Triangular fossa	Intertragic notch	Ear lobe	Scaphoid groove	Medial surface	Tragus	Total
Related to vascularization	Telangiectasia	964	142	300	288	294	41	4	130	154	253	3	2573
	Hyperemia	309	81	154	62	144	28	6	72	38	27	6	927
	Angioma	55	17	7	1	77	1	0	32	13	11	0	214
	Paleness	38	3	3	3	1	0	1	1	1	0	0	51
Related to pigmentation	Nevus	144	79	13	5	522	9	9	281	75	172	47	1356
	Macula	227	132	29	9	223	7	3	218	35	38	20	941
	Dyschromia	6	1	1	1	4	0	0	3	3	0	0	19
Related to keratinization	Dyskeratosis	6	4	82	35	11	24	10	13	13	11	8	217
	Dystrophy	6	2	3	3	8	0	0	2	0	2	0	26
Related to cartilaginous structure	Hypotrophy	6	2	17	18	4	2	1	7	2	302	0	361
	Hypertrophy	102	2	65	65	54	0	0	4	9	14	1	316
Related to cutaneous structure	Incisure	112	129	17	15	146	1	34	205	16	12	54	741
	Crease	2	1	1	2	9	0	0	261	0	1	18	295
	Depressed area	17	40	73	49	12	4	1	26	5	56	1	284
Related to sebaceous gland structure	Comedone	0	1	338	68	1	16	6	6	1	3	0	440
	Sebaceous cyst	3	0	40	19	2	0	1	1	0	0	1	67
	Milium	0	0	0	0	0	0	0	0	0	0	0	0
Total		1997	636	1143	643	1512	133	76	1262	365	902	159	8828

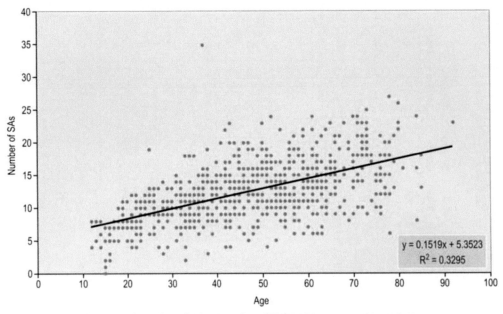

Fig. 4.2 Regression line for age and number of skin alterations (SAs) in 711 consecutive patients.

Table 4.4 Correlation in 711 patients between age and the number of skin alterations on the auricle as a whole and on its different parts

The auricle as a whole		R2	Coefficient	IC 95% for coefficient	P
		0.329	0.152	(0.136; 0.168)	<0.001
Parts of the auricle taken singularly	Ear lobe	0.251	0.050	(0.044; 0.057)	<0.001
	Anthelix	0.199	0.048	(0.041; 0.055)	<0.001
	Helix	0.088	0.026	(0.020; 0.033)	<0.001
	Tragus	0.051	0.007	(0.005; 0.009)	<0.001
	Antitragus	0.047	0.014	(0.010; 0.019)	<0.001
	Intertragic notch	0.007	0.002	(0.000; 0.003)	<0.050
	Medial surface	0.003	0.004	(−0.002; 0.011)	NS
	Lower concha	0.002	−0.003	(−0.008; 0.002)	NS
	Upper concha	0.001	0.002	(−0.002; 0.006)	NS
	Scaphoid groove	0.001	0.001	(−0,002; 0.005)	NS
	Triangular fossa	0.000	0.000	(−0,002; 0.002)	NS

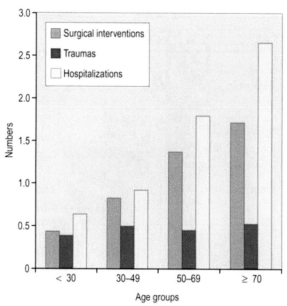

Fig. 4.3 Average number of surgical operations, traumas and hospitalizations in 711 patients according to four age groups (<30, 30–49, 50–69, ≥70 years).

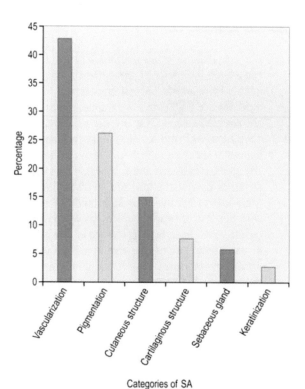

Fig. 4.4 Percentage distribution of skin alterations (SAs) in each of the six categories in 711 patients.

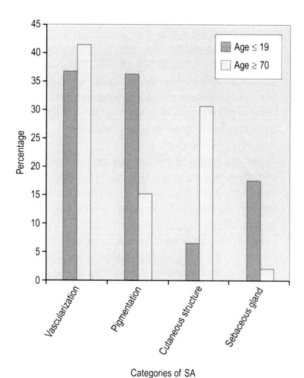

Categories of SA

Fig. 4.5 Percentage distribution of skin alterations (SAs) related to vascularization, pigmentation, cutaneous and sebaceous gland structure in the youngest age group (≤19) and in the oldest (≥70 years).

CASE STUDY

As an example of auricular inspection and correct methodology in recording skin alterations, I here report the case of an elderly woman. Considering type of skin alterations and above all their location, I could confirm the presence of some past and current health problems. In this case the difference between the richness of skin alterations on the lateral surface and their scantiness on the medial surface is clearly outlined.

The patient was a 77-year-old woman, 162 cm tall and weighing 65 kg (who in the past had weighed up to 83 kg). She had undergone the following surgical operations: appendectomy at the age of 19, uterine retroversion at age 27, crural hernia at 45, uterine–bladder prolapse at 60. She had suffered from depression when she was young and after menopause. She reported having suffered from chronic migraine for at least

50 years and even after menopause. She still suffered occasionally from attacks, mainly on the right side. She had had hypertension for at least 30 years, controlled by drugs. Some members of her family (brother, sister and nephew) had hypertriglyceridemia. Her levels of triglycerides had often been above average, reaching a maximum of 600 mg.

Her cholesterol levels had always been normal and there was no evidence of diabetes. She had had chronic lumbago in the L4–L5 herniated disk for over 20 years with recurrent sciatic and knee pain on the right side. She had also been suffering with bilateral neck pain for several years. Moreover, she suffered from gastritis and chronic dyspepsia, due also to her prolonged intake of NSAIDs. She had become increasingly deaf in recent years.

Inspection of the lateral surface of the right ear showed a series of skin alterations which can be described as follows (Fig. 4.6):

- The upper part of the ear shows a hyperemic area of the helix (sector 21 of the Sectogram); one telangiectasia and one hyperemia on the scapha and two neighboring hyperemic areas at the bifurcation of the superior and inferior crura of the anthelix. A small incisure and a few small furrows are visible respectively on the edge of the inferior crus of the anthelix and on the upper portion of the helix. The location of these skin alterations is consistent with the patient's chronic back pain and recurrent sciatic pain.
- In the central part of the ear an oval area of cartilaginous hypertrophy is visible adjoining the root of the helix and surrounded on the upper border by a linear telangiectasia. These skin alterations are consistent with the patient's gastritis and chronic dyspepsia. Below the root of the helix two sebaceous cysts are visible, one of them approaching the lung area. The sebaceous gland skin alterations of the upper and lower concha may orient the acupuncturist to suspect a hyperlipidemia (see Plate XVD) which in this case is confirmed by the increased levels of triglycerides.
- In the lower part of the ear two pigmented spots on the antitragus are visible. These can be

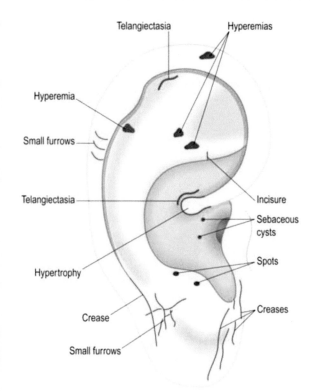

Fig. 4.6   Type and location of skin alterations in a 77-year-old female patient.

considered indicative of the patient's long history of migraine. Several creases and incisures are visible on the ear lobe: the creases are more evident on the anterior part and are consistent with the patient's hypertension, and generally speaking with her cardiovascular risk. The small crease and the furrows on the posterior part of the lobe are consistent with the patient's chronic depression and perhaps with her loss of hearing which has worsened in recent years. In spite of profuse skin alterations of the lateral surface, the medial surface shows only a few incisures on the lobe border and a deepening of the anthelix groove, relative to the patient's chronic neck and back pain.

METHODOLOGY OF INSPECTION

As recommended by the Chinese, good lighting is important and my advice is to adopt either natural light or white light, possibly employing the type of magnifying lens used by dermatologists. In photography a ring-flash easily evidences more hidden areas and gives very good images. The flash may provoke reflex vasodilatation causing a significant change in the skin alterations, especially those of vascular type. Such vasodilatation may occur particularly when touching, lifting or bending the auricle, for example during examination of the posterior part of the auricle. It is therefore advisable first of all to fully inspect the lateral part of the auricle and then the medial part, keeping the hair away. Every skin alteration must be transcribed on the Sectogram according to type and topography before taking pictures, touching the ear or applying any other subsequent diagnostic method such as the pressure pain test or electrical detection.

It is necessary to inspect both ears even if the patient reports symptoms on only one side. One must be prepared for either the right or the left ear to give information and that more often the distribution of skin alterations will be asymmetrical.

At a glance the ear can immediately offer a series of clues, especially in the elderly. Inspection in younger patients may yield fewer diagnostic elements but at the same time could lead to the discovery of tendencies as yet unknown.

Inspection generally begins at the upper part and proceeds downwards, otherwise attention can be shifted from the helix to the concha. Once the accessible parts of the ear have been inspected, the hidden parts may be lifted or bent in order to obtain further information.

As regards the possible association between particular types of skin alteration and specific disorders, caution is recommended since a particular part of the ear may carry a prevalent type of skin alteration independently of the symptom believed to be associated with it. This is the case with the concha, which is the only part of the ear with sebaceous glands. It is not surprising therefore to find a high rate of comedones in this area since, as is known, these are plugs of sebum in a dilated pilosebaceous orifice. This process which is normal in this area may have a particular meaning if it is widespread (see Plates XVIB1 and XVIB2), or if limited zones of the concha show comedones of larger dimensions (see Plate XVA).

The histological structure of this skin is possibly also associated with a higher frequency of furfuraceous scales (dandruff) in this area, which again may be a clue to a specific syndrome in the patient (see Plate XVIA).

There are, however, differences in the distribution of skin alterations which do not depend on different histological patterns of the skin or a different nervous supply. In these cases other factors may be involved such as the representation on each auricular portion of specific anatomical structures of the body. For example it is very interesting to see how variable the ratio is between the vascular and pigmentary skin alterations on the different parts of the ear which have the same innervation: the ratio is 3.6 for the anthelix; 1.4 for the medial surface; 1.1 for the antitragus; 0.7 for the helix; 0.5 for the ear lobe. These differences make sense if we look at the topography of skin alterations: the skeletal apparatus with its muscles is represented on the anthelix and the medial surface of the ear. Therefore if hyperemia or telangiectasia are found on these parts it is reasonable to suspect a chronic or recurrent disorder of the locomotor system (see Plates IIA and IVA and IVD).

If, however, macules or nevi are found on the ear lobe or the helix, they may indicate some developmental defect of the spine and the cranial bones, or a tendency to mental disorders such as depression (see Plates XA, B, C, XIC and XIID).

Moreover, if we consider skin alterations related to cutaneous structure, such as depressed areas, creases and incisures, and their relative percentage of distribution on the different parts of the ear we find 6.5% and 7.6% on the anthelix and the medial surface of the ear, 11% on the helix and 26.7% and 39% respectively on the antitragus and the ear lobe. In my opinion incisures or creases of the antitragus or the ear lobe may be associated with symptoms related to a loss of function or to aging of the central nervous system (Plates XIIB and XIIIA, B, D).

As regards the topography of skin alterations, a reliable diagnostic clue becomes available if the area in which the skin alteration is located overlaps with the accepted representation of the corresponding anatomical part. In some cases, unfortunately, the expected correspondence is not found and incomplete overlapping of these areas may be misleading. This is the case, for example, of neighboring structures such as those pertaining to the lower and upper limbs. In the case of Plate IIIA, the telangiectasia appeared to overlap with the Chinese representation of the knee, but instead the patient had had a carpal syndrome for several months. We should by no means feel disappointed, but try with our medical knowledge to verify diagnosis through clinical judgment and the help of diagnostic instruments, imaging techniques and laboratory tests available in our profession.

One of the issues in inspection is to make an appropriate analysis of the various skin alterations observed in order to find the combination closest to diagnosing the current health problems of the patient. For example, to take notice of a diagonal ear lobe crease in a patient already under treatment with antihypertensive drugs may be less important than finding signs of an unexpressed depressive disorder. Since knowledge on the areas of the ear of possible use in the treatment of mental disorders is incomplete, I will present my considerations on this topic, which I consider to be very important, in a specific section later in this chapter.

DOES INSPECTION HAVE THE SAME VALUE IN ALL SECTORS OF THE OUTER EAR?

For all the following observations and analyses I have restricted the number of patients to the 357 that I had examined over the preceding 3 years.

If we consider the mean number of skin alterations on the right and left ear we obtain respectively 7.5 and 6.7. We would therefore expect a uniform distribution among the different sectors but this is not always the case. If we make a spatial cluster analysis[8,9] of the total number of skin alterations on the right and left ears, regardless of sex, we may observe that there are some specific sectors with a significantly higher concentration. Figure 4.7 shows a distribution of skin alterations on the right ear which is quite uniform throughout from sector 3 to sector 19; on the left ear, there are two main groups of sectors on the upper and lower part of the auricle with a significantly greater cluster of skin alterations compared to the mean of the remaining sectors (Table 4.5A). It is possible that the reduced concentration of skin alterations on the remaining parts of the upper and lower conchae may be related to the more difficult visual access to these areas. Another possibility is that uneven or asymmetrical distribution of skin alterations in some sectors may be due to chance. This phenomenon in my opinion is worth particular consideration

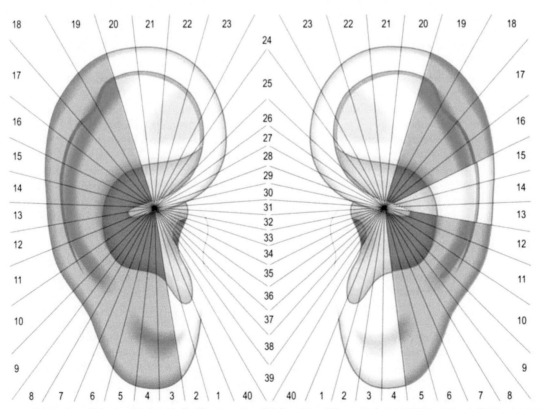

Fig. 4.7 Distribution of the total amount of skin alterations (SAs) on the right and left ear of 711 patients. The sectors with a significantly higher concentration of SAs at cluster analysis are colored.

Table 4.5A Sectors in which the number of skin alterations in 357 patients was significantly higher than the average of points per sector according to the Getis-Ord local statistic Gi[8,9]

	Sectors	Z	P
Right ear	3–19	4.35	<0.001
Left ear	5–12	3.42	<0.001
	16–19	3.01	<0.005

because it seemingly happens also if we apply the pain pressure test (PPT) (see Fig. 5.5) and electrical skin resistance test (ESRT) (see Fig. 7.1) in diagnostic procedures.

The application of Nogier's alignment principle to the inspection of the ear may furthermore add some elements to the issue of asymmetrical distribution of skin alterations. I have always been intrigued by aligned skin alterations because my clinical impression is that they can have a particular

value for diagnosis and therapy to the pertaining sector, no matter to which category they belong. It should be pointed out here that the number of skin alterations which are aligned in two or more units is not negligible as it represents 38.5% of the total.

If we go back to the issue of asymmetrical distribution of skin alterations, we can see that the concentration of alignments on both auricles is not random but favors certain sectors above others. Cluster analysis indicates that sectors 9 and 16–19 on the right ear and 8–10 and 15–19 on the left ear have a significantly higher number of alignments than the average in the other sectors (Fig. 4.8; Table 4.5B).

The majority of alignments consisted of two skin alterations (82.9%) and the minority of three (16.6%). Moreover the categories often seen in the alignment phenomenon are in decreasing order: two vascular skin alterations (see Plate IIA); one vascular and one pigmented (see Plate IXD); one vascular and one related to cartilaginous structure.

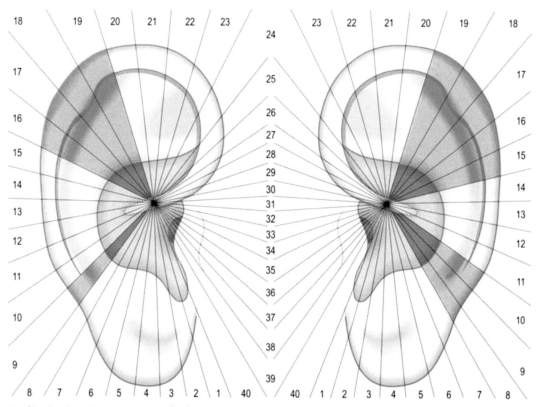

Fig. 4.8 Distribution of skin alterations (SAs) which are aligned in two or more units on the right and left ear of 357 patients. The sectors with a significantly higher concentration of aligned SAs at cluster analysis are colored.

Table 4.5B   Sectors in which the number of alignments of two or more skin alterations was significantly higher in 357 patients than the average of alignments per sector, according to the Getis-Ord local statistic $Gi^{8,9}$

	Sectors	Z	P
Right ear	9	2.25	<0.05
	16–19	3.63	<0.001
Left ear	8–10	3.56	<0.001
	15–19	2.74	<0.005

If we consider the auricular parts on which the skin alterations are more often aligned we find the same part in 23.6%, anthelix with helix or with medial surface in 21.3%, followed by lower concha with ear lobe or antitragus in 14.5%. The second group of combinations appears to be related to the frequent occurrence of musculoskeletal problems in the aging population; the latter, however, seems to be associated with the presence of psychosomatic and metabolic disorders so common in contemporary patients.

THE INSPECTION OF THE OUTER EAR IN THE LITERATURE

Before further describing some auricular signs and their possible association with patients' symptoms it is necessary to recall what has been reported on this topic.

The following signs have been the object of inspection and have been reported in the literature or presented at congresses:

1. the diagonal ear lobe crease as a sign of cardiovascular risk
2. the skin alterations of the ear lobe for identifying new areas for the diagnosis and treatment of headache
3. the skin alterations of the concha as a complementary diagnostic tool in suspecting lesions of the upper digestive system
4. the auricular nevi in suspecting skeletal abnormalities
5. the crus cymbae in suspecting renal anomalies
6. last but not least, the possibility reported by Chinese authors that inspection may be of help in indicating the presence of a hidden tumor.

1. THE DIAGONAL EAR LOBE CREASE OR FRANK'S SIGN

One of the most investigated auricular signs in the literature is undoubtedly the diagonal ear lobe crease (ELC). When Frank[10] in 1973, in a letter to the *New England Journal of Medicine*, described his 'aural sign of coronary artery disease' he cannot have imagined that he would trigger a long and unbroken series of researches all over the world. There are probably 40 or more reports and articles in the literature, written mainly by cardiologists, dealing with the following aspects of the question:

- Is ELC a reliable diagnostic sign of coronary heart disease (CHD)?
- Does it have a predictive value for cardiac events such as cardiac death, acute myocardial infarction or coronary bypass operation in high risk patients?
- Can ELC be associated with conventional risk factors such as hypertension, smoking, diabetes, cholesterol, triglycerides, obesity, etc.?
- Should ELC be considered a sign of aging of the cardiovascular system?
- Should ELC be considered an androgen-sensitive trait like baldness and ear-canal hair?

Several authors tried to answer these questions but none of them was curious enough to seek a correlation with the representation of the *homunculus* on the pinna. On the other hand only a few acupuncturists were making an effort to understand the strange topography of a sign which apparently seems totally unrelated to the representation of the cardiovascular system.

As regards the investigations carried out by cardiologists, Tables 4.6 and 4.7 report a (probably incomplete) list of articles published in the period between 1974 and 2007.[11–49] While waiting for a complete systematic review on this topic the following information can be summarized from the tables:

1. ELC manifests itself after the age of 40 but becomes more evident and frequent around the sixth and seventh decades of life, especially in males. There is a general consensus that those patients showing an ELC before 40 have a higher risk of cardiovascular disease. Also performing an age- and sex-matched comparison with non-ELC subjects, the crease seems to be significantly correlated with a higher

prevalence of CHD and a higher score of coronary stenosis in patients undergoing angiography (Table 4.6). Even in post-mortem studies there is a strong correlation between ELC with both the cardiovascular cause of death and the degree of atherosclerosis in the coronary and cerebral arteries and in the aorta (Table 4.7).

2. ELC may manifest unilaterally or bilaterally. Bilateral ELC, especially deep and clear-cut creases, seem prospectively to be associated with a lower cardiac event-free survival.[36]

3. There is often a lack of association between ELC and the conventionally accepted risk factors. This inconsistency, whenever confirmed by a systematic review, closely recalls the controversy in the literature about the real importance of these factors. Indeed, it is still suggested by different authors that 50% of patients with CHD lack any of the conventional risk factors.

This implies that other non-traditional factors could play a significant role in the development of this disease. However, the factors which seemingly show a higher association with ELC are hypertension and obesity.

4. ELC can be considered an indicator of biological age as opposed to chronological age and could be used to identify subjects who are aging more quickly than the general population. Biopsy sections from ear lobes at the site of the crease[19] report a premature destruction of elastic fibers in the skin which is similarly correlated with coronary artery disease (Fig. 4.9A, B).

5. Some articles report a possible association between CHD, ELC, ear-canal hair and male-pattern baldness. This association is supposed to be due to the long-term exposure to androgens which may facilitate the development of atherosclerosis and CHD.

Table 4.6 Study groups: association of ear lobe crease (ELC) with acute myocardial infarction (AMI) and coronary heart disease (CHD); association of ELC with the conventional risk factors. A review of the literature 1974–2007

Author	Study groups	Association of ELC with AMI/CHD	Association of ELC with conventional risk factors
Lichstein (1974)	531 patients with AMI vs. 305 patients in a control group with no clinical evidence of CHD	ELC in 47% in the first group vs. 30% in the control group ($P<0.001$)	Negative association with diabetes mellitus and hypertension. Smoking prevalent in the AMI group with ELC vs. no ELC ($P<0.005$)
Mehta (1974)	211 patients undergoing coronary angiography: 159 with CHD; 52 with normal coronary arteries	No different frequency of ELC in the two groups. The prevalence of ELC increases with age	
Christiansen (1975)	503 unselected patients admitted to a medical and a surgical department	The prevalence of ELC increases with age, but is significantly higher (46%) in patients over 50 with AMI/CHD vs. control group (31%) ($P<0.02$)	Not clearly reported prevalence ratios about hypertension, smoking and diabetes mellitus
Andresen (1976)	101 diabetic patients	ELC observed in 51.4% of patients with retinopathy compared to 7.6% with normal retinal vessels	

Continued

Table 4.6 Study groups: association of ear lobe crease (ELC) with acute myocardial infarction (AMI) and coronary heart disease (CHD); association of ELC with the conventional risk factors. A review of the literature 1974–2007—cont'd

Author	Study groups	Association of ELC with AMI/CHD	Association of ELC with conventional risk factors
Rhoads (1977)	1237 men aged 50-74 from a cross-section of the population of Hawaii	No different frequency of ELC in CHD of any type vs. asymptomatic people	Weak association of ELC with hypertension. Strong association with obesity
Kaukola (1978)	Study group A: 288 patients <65 with AMI vs. 290 normal subjects	ELC observed in 69% vs. 24% ($P<0.01$ for patients aged 30–39, $P<0.001$ for the other age groups)	Negative association between ELC and smoking, hypertension, cholesterol, triglycerides, diabetes mellitus, family history of diabetes, obesity, level of physical activity, blood group, birth place The only significant difference was for patients with ELC of study group A having a family history of premature cardiovascular disease ($P<0.01$)
	Study group B: 286 randomly selected patients undergoing coronary angiography: 200 with at least 50% stenosis in one of the main coronary arteries (CHD patients) vs. 86 without significant stenosis ($\leq$50%; non-CHD patients). Groups comparable in age	ELC observed in 72% of patients with single, double and triple vessel disease vs. 21% of patients with no significant atherosclerotic changes in coronary arteries ($P<0.001$). The prevalence of ELC increases with age and severity of the heart disease, being positive in nearly 90% of CHD patients with triple vessel disease aged 50–59 years	
Moncada (1979)	300 healthy subjects: 150 with ELC, 150 age-matched controls		Positive association of ELC with hypertension, eye ground changes and ECG ischemic findings
Kristensen (1980)	125 hypertensive patients (74 male, 51 female); 55 normotensive subjects (29 male, 26 female)		Positive association in males between ELC and hypertension ($P<0.005$)
Shoenfeld (1980)	421 consecutive patients with AMI vs. 421 controls ELC as a deep wrinkle extending for a distance greater than or equal to one-third of the ear lobe length, evaluated by an independent assessor on one or both auricles, while the subject was supine and seated ELC biopsies performed in 12 subjects	ELC observed in 77% of the AMI group vs. 40% of the control group ($P<0.05$)	Positive association between ELC and hypertension ($P<0.001$), and diabetic retinopathy ($P<0.05$) No significant association with diabetes, hypertensive retinopathy, hyperuricemia, hyperlipidemia, smoking
Chen (1982)	729 hospital staff members with bilateral ELC during a lipid profile examination		Negative correlation between abnormal serum cholesterol and ELC

Pasternac (1982)	340 selected patients undergoing coronary angiography Degree of occlusion graded from 0 to 3 (grade 1 = 30–50% reduction in the diameter of one or more of the main vessels; grade 2 = >50% reduction in one or two main vessels; grade 3 = >50% reduction in three main vessels)	Sensitivity of ELC rated 59.5%, specificity 81.9%, positive predictive value 91.1% 79 patients with ELC vs. 35 without ELC both having grade 3 of coronary occlusion ($P<0.001$)	Negative association between ELC and family history of AMI or sudden death before the age of 55, smoking, systolic and diastolic pressure, cholesterol, triglycerides, blood glucose
Gral (1983)	234 veterans (average 66 years old): 119 with ELC; 115 without	No different frequency of CHD in the two groups	No prevalence as regards body weight, diabetes, blood pressure, cholesterol, urea, creatinine, uric acid
Elliott (1983)	1000 unselected patients admitted to various hospitals: 376 with CHD vs. 624 non-CHD patients	ELC observed in 73.1% of CHD patients vs. 19.2% of non-CHD patients ($P<0.00001$)	No prevalence as regards family history, smoking, hypertension, diabetes mellitus, cholesterol
Wagner (1984)	63 unselected patients undergoing coronary angiography Association between ELC and ear-canal hair in stenosis >50% of one or more coronary arteries	ELC associated with CHD ($P<0.001$) ELC + ear-canal hair associated with CHD ($P<0.05$)	
Gibson (1986)	100 patients with aortic valve stenosis undergoing coronary angiography Degree of occlusion graded from 0 to 5 ELC scored for each side from 1 to 3 (total scoring from 0 to 6)	No correlation between ELC scoring and degree of coronary occlusion	
Toyosaki (1986)	Study group A: 1000 unselected patients 237 patients with angina pectoris and/or myocardial infarction vs. 720 patients without evidence of CHD	ELC observed in 24.5% of CHD patients vs. 4.8% of non-CHD patients ($P<0.001$)	No prevalence of obesity, hypertension, diabetes mellitus, smoking and hyperlipidemia
	Study group B: 200 patients undergoing coronary angiography 119 patients with >50% stenosis of at least one major coronary artery vs. 81 patients with normal arteries	ELC observed in 26% of patients with stenosis vs. 3.7% without ($P<0.01$)	
Brady (1987)	261 consecutive male patients with CHD undergoing coronary angiography. Unclear classification of coronary artery lesions	No different frequency of CHD in the groups with and without ELC Both CHD and ELC increase with age	

Continued

Table 4.6 Study groups: association of ear lobe crease (ELC) with acute myocardial infarction (AMI) and coronary heart disease (CHD); association of ELC with the conventional risk factors. A review of the literature 1974–2007—cont'd

Author	Study groups	Association of ELC with AMI/CHD	Association of ELC with conventional risk factors
Lesbre (1987)	172 selected patients undergoing coronary arteriography with >75% stenosis of at least one major coronary artery	ELC observed in 52.3% of patients with stenosis vs. 12.8% without ($P<0.001$)	No prevalence of obesity, hypertension, diabetes mellitus, smoking and hyperlipidemia
Kenny (1989)	125 consecutive patients undergoing coronary angiography Severity of CHD graded according to the jeopardy score: (1) normal = 0; (2) mild disease = 2–6; (3) moderate to severe disease >6	No different angiogram score between patients with and without ELC The severity of disease increases with age ($P<0.02$)	No prevalence in patients with ELC as regards gender, smoking, history of myocardial infarction, hypertension, family history of CHD, obesity
Verma (1989)	215 randomly selected patients to predict the correlation between ELC, ear-canal hair and CHD	Bilateral ELC significantly associated with documented CHD in the group 50–69 ($P<0.001$). The combination ELC + ear-canal hair is significantly associated with CHD ($P<0.005$)	
Romagnosi (1990)	290 selected subjects undergoing a blood lipid profile examination: 166 with ELC, 124 without		Negative association between ELC and blood glucose, cholesterol, cholesterol HDL-LDL, tryglicerides, apolipoprotein A1 and B
Tranchesi (1992)	Group I: 1086 consecutive patients denying myocardial ischemic symptoms and hospitalized for other reasons Group II: 338 with documented CHD ($\geq$70% stenosis at angiography)	ELC was present in 28% of group I and 65% in group II ($P<0.0001$). When adjusted for age and sex the prevalence of ELC was still higher in patients with CHD than in the control group ($P<0.001$). Observed sensitivity of ELC for the diagnosis of CHD was 65%, the specificity 72%, the positive predictive value 42% and the negative predictive value 87%	
Moraes (1992)	247 consecutive patients admitted to a general hospital Independent assessment of ELCs as running diagonally at 45° down the whole ear lobe	Significant correlation between ELC and CHD ($P<0.001$) No significant correlation between ELC and age and no prevalence in males vs. females	Negative association between ELC and hypertension, hyperlipidemia, peripheral vascular disease, stroke and smoking
Petrakis (1995)	625 white women studied for possible association of ELC with reproductive factors, use of contraceptives and menopausal estrogen, smoking, alcohol		Negative association between ELC and use of oral contraceptives, smoking and alcohol Positive association with Quetelet index (weight/height^2)

Kuon (1995)	670 patients undergoing coronary angiography studied for correlation between ELC and coronary diameter stenosis >70%	No correlation between ELC and coronary stenosis >70%	Positive association with age, overweight and hyperuricemia Negative association with diabetes, hypercholesterolemia, hyperlipidemia, family history of CHD, physical activity and smoking
Elliott (1996)	Prospective study on 264 patients of a coronary care unit followed up for 10 years Primary outcome measure: time to cardiac event (coronary artery bypass graft, AMI or cardiac death)	Significantly different cardiac event-free survival rates for patients, with or without ELC: the highest for the group without ELC; the lowest for the group with bilateral ELC; intermediate for those with unilateral ELC	
Miric (1998)	842 male patients <60 years hospitalized for the first non-fatal myocardial infarction vs. 712 patients hospitalized with non-cardiac diagnoses and with no clinical sign of CHD	Significant association between AMI and ELC in the first group	Positive association with baldness and thoracic hairiness Prevalence for males of the first group of hair graying under the age of 45
Motamed (1998)	1200 non-cardiac patients attending routine ENT clinic CHD assessed if angina or previous AMI in the patient's history	ELC observed in 48% of patients with positive history of CHD ($P<0.001$) Sensitivity of ELC 48%; specificity 88%; positive predictive value 16%	Positive correlation with family history, hyperlipidemia and smoking Negative correlation with hypertension and diabetes
Davis (2000)	1022 selected patients to determine whether ELC is a clinically useful sign of CHD or retinopathy in type 2 diabetes	Patients with ELC more likely to have CHD than those without an ELC ($P<0.02$), but the proportions with retinopathy were not significantly different in the two groups	
Dharap (2000)	Observational study on 1576 healthy male and female Malay subjects randomly selected ELC studied in upright position Three different types of ELC: I = incomplete crease, II = complete but flat, III = extensive crease		ELC present in 31.1% of males and 3.6% of females Significantly different incidence for all types of ELC ($P<0.001$)
Evrengül (2004)	415 consecutive patients undergoing coronary angiography: 296 with at least a stenosis >70% in one of three major coronary arteries vs. 119 with normal arteries	Prevalence of ELC in patients with CHD 51.4% vs. 15.1% in the control group ($P<0.001$) Sensitivity of bilateral ELC for the diagnosis of CHD 51.3%; specificity 84.8%; positive predictive value 89.4%; negative predictive value 41.2%	Positive association with hypertension and smoking Negative association with diabetes, family history of CHD, cholesterol, triglycerides, obesity

Continued

Table 4.6 Study groups: association of ear lobe crease (ELC) with acute myocardial infarction (AMI) and coronary heart disease (CHD); association of ELC with the conventional risk factors. A review of the literature 1974–2007—cont'd

Author	Study groups	Association of ELC with AMI/CHD	Association of ELC with conventional risk factors
Bahcelioglu (2005)	3722 subjects from six primary health care centers ELC grading: grade 0 = no crease at all; grade 1 = any crease <50% across the lobe; grade 2 = <100% across the lobe; grade 3 = deep and prominent crease across the whole lobe	Prevalence of ELC in males ($P<0.05$) and in patients with CHD ($P<0.05$)	Significant association between ELC grading and hypertension, diabetes and family history of CHD
Celik (2007)	130 apparently healthy subjects examined by carotid ultrasound to measure intima-media thickness (IMT) of the right common carotid artery	Higher carotid IMT in subjects with ELC compared to a group of age- and sex-matched non-ELC subjects ($P<0.0001$)	Higher prevalence in these subjects as regards hypertension and body mass index. No prevalence as regards smoking, diabetes, family history of CHD, cholesterol, triglycerides, cardiovascular medical therapy

Table 4.7 Post-mortem studies on causes of death and severity of atherosclerosis (in coronary and in cerebral arteries, and in the aorta) in patients with ear lobe crease (ELC). A review of the literature 1976–2006

Author	Cause of death and/or severity of atherosclerosis	Association between ELC and severity of atherosclerosis	Association of ELC with conventional risk factors
Lichstein (1976)	Post-mortem study on 113 consecutive patients aged 40 or older Amount of coronary sclerosis graded from 0 to 4 (1 = 25%, 4 = 100%) Degree of occlusion graded from 0 to 4 (1 = 25%, 4 = 100%)	The mean amount of coronary sclerosis was higher in patients with ELC than without ($P<0.01$) Patients with bilateral crease show a higher score than patients with unilateral crease. As regards the degree of occlusion, a trend was noted without significant difference	
Cumberland (1987)	777 consecutive autopsies performed for forensic reasons 'Significant atherosclerosis' = one or more of the three main coronary arteries with stenosis >75%	Significant correlation between ELC and 'significant atherosclerosis' ($P<0.01$) Observed sensitivity 55%; specificity 83%; positive predictive value 42%; negative predictive value 90%	
Kirkham (1989)	Post-mortem study on 303 consecutive persons The cardiovascular causes of death were classified in six groups:	Strong association between cardiovascular causes of death and ELC	Increased risk of cardiovascular cause of death in non-diabetic women with ELC

	ischaemic/hypertensive disease; abdominal aneurysm; thoracic aneurysm; calcific valvar stenosis; cor pulmonale; cardiomyopathy		
Ishii (1990)	134 autopsies on males not deceased from cardiovascular or cerebrovascular diseases Grading of atherosclerosis: mean % of intimal area with macroscopically atherosclerotic lesions in the three coronary arteries and in the thoracic and abdominal aortic segments ELC score groups: Group I = no ELC; group II = superficial ELC or not completely crossing the ear lobe; group III = deep, clear-cut crease (Fig. 4.10)	The extent of coronary and aortic atherosclerosis was higher in group III of ELC (P<0.01)	Positive association with hypercholesterolemia; negative association with systolic and diastolic blood pressure
Patel (1992)	Post-mortem study on 376 subjects over 40 Grading of coronary atherosclerosis according to maximal luminal narrowing: grade I = mild (<50%); grade II = moderate (50–75%); grade III = severe narrowing (>75%). Grading of ELC: 0 = no crease 1 = any degree <2 2a = diagonal crease >50% but less than 100% 2b = complete superficial crease 3 = complete deep crease	Significant association between severe coronary atherosclerosis and 3-grade ELC In both sexes ELC grades 2 and 3 carried a significantly increased relative risk of AMI as a cause of death Sensitivity of ELC for detecting severe coronary atheroma 62.1% for men and 69.2% for women; specificity 65.9% in men and 78.0% in women	
Edston (2006)	Post-mortem study on 520 consecutive patients Assessment was made of cause of death, of degree of atherosclerosis in the coronary and cerebral arteries and in the aorta Heart, kidney and spleen weights were assessed as well as body mass index (BMI) and thickness of abdominal fat Baldness and excessive hair in the external acoustic meatus were also noted	ELC strongly correlated with CHD in both men and women (P<0.0001), but only in men with sudden cardiac death (P<0.04) Strong correlation between ELC and degree of atherosclerosis in the coronary and cerebral arteries and in the aorta. Significantly higher heart weight in ELC patients (P<0.0001) Total sensitivity with regard to the severity of CHD 75%; specificity 64%; positive predictive value 68%; negative predictive value 72%	Positive association with thickness of abdominal fat; negative association with BMI

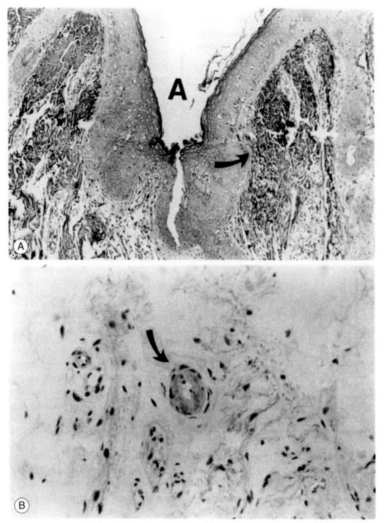

Fig. 4.9 (A) Biopsy section from ear lobe in the area of crease (A); the arrow indicates elastic-fiber tears (×100) *(with permission)*. (B) Biopsy section from area of ear lobe crease (ELC) the arrow indicates pre-arteriolar wall thickening (×240) *(with permission)*.

There are, however, some aspects which have not been considered sufficiently and which require a careful and reliable standardization of the crease. The first is that the ELC was rarely evaluated by independent observers; the second is that differences in interpretation of the crease itself may account for at least a part of the different results in comparing subjects with and without CHD. For example, it is rarely stated if the creases are observed with the patient in the upright or the supine position; the creases are more evident in the second position. What is perhaps more important is that not all the authors have reached a consensus that ELC has to be considered present if it

appears to involve the full thickness of the skin, extending entirely across the ear lobe. Only in a few articles has the crease been measured in three different degrees, as in the post-mortem study[47] shown in Figure 4.10.

However, the question that remains open for us is how to explain the topography of the crease and its relationship to the cardiovascular system. Cardiologist Yoshiaki Omura,[50] who was involved early in the observation of ear lobe creases, tried to explain the relationship between the ear lobe and myocardial abnormalities by a common neural supply. The main part of the lobe being innervated by the great auricular nerve (C2–C3), he surmised

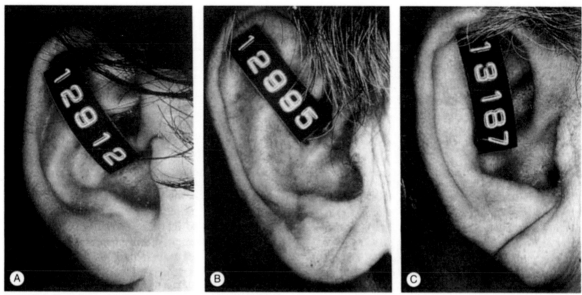

Fig. 4.10   Ear lobe crease (ELC) grading in a post-mortem study: A, B and C show representative cases that scored respectively 0, 1, 2 points *(with permission)*.

that there could be an 'unrecognized supply of small branches of nerves coming directly or indirectly from the heart'. He supported his hypothesis with the possible observation in cardiac patients of a radiating pain involving also the neck, chin and occipital area, covered indeed by the same supply, C2 and C3.

Johan Nguyen[51] instead supposed that the correlation between a sign corresponding to the representation of the face and the heart could be explained only with the theory of TCM. He quoted as an example a sentence from the classical textbook *Su Wen*, Chapter 9, 'The Heart is the source of life and the place of transformation of mental energy. Its energy manifests itself on the face.'

As regards my own opinion on this subject, I am far from being convinced that there is an easy approach to the question. I think two different topographical aspects have to be considered; the first is that the starting point of ELC, just below the intertragic notch, is constant for all types of creases. The second is the variable angle of the diagonal crease crossing the ear lobe and therefore encompassing a different surface of the anterior part of the lobe. The end point of a clear-cut crease can in certain cases reach the lowest point of the lobe or even trespass this limit backwards (see Plate XIIC); in other less frequent cases a double ELC can be observed (see Plate XIIB).

Concerning the starting point of the crease, Nogier's map does not report any point related to the cardiovascular system in this area but shows the representation of the pituitary gland on the anterior ridge of the intertragic notch; the Chinese standardization, on the other hand, reports a puzzling tooth area (LO1 *ya*) with the indication for hypotension, besides toothache and periodontitis. The indication for raising blood pressure was maintained from the ancient map of the China Academy of TCM and is actually coincident with this starting point of the crease (Fig. 4.11). The possibility that this auricular area is related to dysfunctions of the cardiovascular system may be supported by the fact that just nearby on the tragus there are further points related to the heart such as *xinzangdian* of the ancient map, located within the current area TG1, with the indications of atrial fibrillation and tachycardia. Further points for treating hypertension are currently located in the area TG2 and adrenal gland *shenshang-xian* located at the free border of the tragus between TG1 and TG2. The association of the tragus and the intertragic notch to diastolic pressure in hypertensive patients can be found in Chapter 5 (Figs 5.42, 5.43). As regards the possible association between CHD, ELC and ear-canal hair, which is supposed to be due to the long-term exposure to androgens, it is interesting from the topographic point of view that hair does not cover just the canal but also

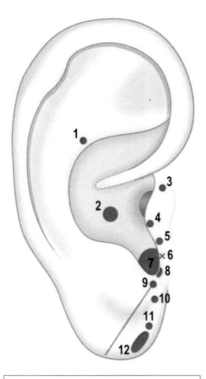

1 = heart point (French)

2 = heart area (CO15 *xin*)

3 = cardiac point (*xinzangdian*)

4 = adrenal gland point (*shenshangxian*)

5 = hypertension point (*gaoxueyadian*)

6 = ACTH point (French) (on the internal side)

7 = endocrine area (CO18 *neifenmi*)

8 = hypophysis area (French)

9 = point for raising blood pressure (*shengyadian*)

10 = aggressiveness point (French)

11 = neurasthenia point, in the anterior part of the ear lobe (LO4 *chuiqian*)

12 = fear area (French)

Fig. 4.11 Possible interpretation of ear lobe crease (ELC) by means of topographic overlapping of some auricular points according to Chinese and French arrangement of the auricle. ACTH = adrenocorticotropic hormone.

neighboring areas such as the tragus, the antitragus and the intertragic notch. All these areas appear to be involved in the regulation of neuroendocrine functions (Fig. 4.12).

In my opinion, therefore, the first hypothesis for ELC could be related to a complex disorder of the central mechanisms regulating blood pressure, with a progressively increasing resistance of the peripheral arterioles. A second hypothesis, possibly linked to the former, regards the areas of the anterior part of the ear bounded by the crease.

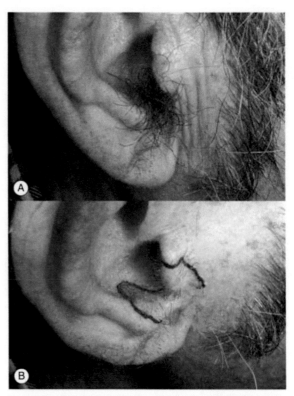

Fig. 4.12 Ear-canal hair and ear lobe crease (ELC) in a 71-year-old patient suffering with coronary heart disease (A); area of implantation of hair marked with ink (B). The patient had noticed a particularly intense growth of the hair throughout the previous 5 years.

These areas are clearly associated with the emotional state of the patient: Nogier identified a point for aggressiveness and an area for 'fear' on this part of the lobe; the Chinese called it anterior ear lobe (LO4 *chuiqian*). Besides toothache, as for LO1, the major indication for this area is 'neurosis', which was changed from 'neurasthenia', the former term used by the Chinese Academy of TCM.

The reader will allow me to make a short digression on this condition which belongs to the culture-bound syndromes of DSM IV but still survives in the Chinese Classification of Mental Disorders (CCMD-2-R).[52–54] The Chinese translation for it is *shenjing shuairuo* where *shen* is emblematic of vitality and capacity of the mind to form ideas, *jing* originally refers to the meridians and channels carrying *qi* (vital energy) and *xue* (blood) through the body. Conceptually *shen* and and *jing* are treated by Chinese people and doctors as one term, *shen-jing*, that means 'nerve' or 'nervous system'. *Shuai* means decline, degeneration, and *ruo* weakness.[54]

At the end of this digression it has to be specified that the CCMD-2-R diagnostic criteria for *shenjing shuairuo* are any of three out of five groups of symptoms such as fatigue, dysphoria (restlessness, malaise), excitement, nervous pain and sleep disturbances. This syndrome, very popular at the end of the 1980s, is nowadays less and less diagnosed by Chinese psychiatrists who now favor a diagnosis of depression.

Returning to the second hypothesis, it is possible that ELC could be associated with the particular emotional status or personality trait of patients which seem to be recurrent in those developing some form of CHD. In the past I have been impressed by the representation of the rhinencephalon drawn by René Bourdiol,[55] a neurologist who was also Paul Nogier's closest collaborator. He dedicated his doctoral thesis to the interpretation of the different neural anatomical structures of the part of the CNS involved in 'reaction behavior' in humans. He described at least four neurophysiological systems:

- the 'olfactory' brain, or rhinencephalon proper
- the 'sexual' brain, regulating aggression and certain compulsive behavioral traits
- the 'anamnesic' brain, enabling the retention of past experiences

- the 'reactional' brain, orientating the individual (Fig. 4.13).

Bourdiol's observations, even if not supported by any experimental data, urged me to measure at least one parameter, the anxiety level, in subjects bearing a mono- or bilateral diagonal crease completely crossing the ear lobe. With colleagues, I therefore carried out a survey on 258 consecutive subjects in my practice: 143 with unilateral or bilateral ELC (86 males, 57 females); a control group of 115 without ELC (57 males, 58 females).[56] We measured the anxiety level with the IPAT anxiety scale questionnaire (ASQ) which proposes 40 items with the total score ranging from 0 to 80.[57] The exclusion criteria for this study were the intake, even if temporary, of psychotropic drugs and the presence, in the clinical history of the patient, of previous myocardial infarction, angina pectoris or evidence at ECG of abnormal Q waves, or ST segment and T wave abnormalities. The anxiety scores in the group with ELC and in the control group showed a parallel tendency: higher in the females and decreasing from the fifth to seventh decade (Fig. 4.14). The mean anxiety scores of the two groups were compared by sex and decade using the *t*-test. The differences were all highly significant ($P<0.001$). The conclusions of the article were:

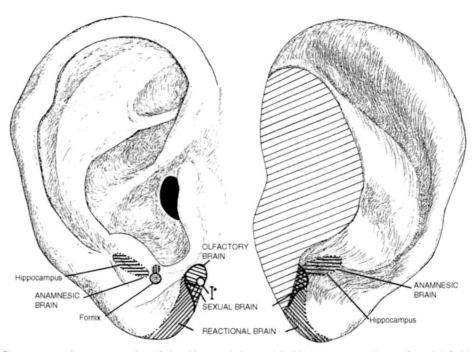

Fig. 4.13   The somatotopic representation of the rhinencephalon and limbic system according to Bourdiol *(with permission).*

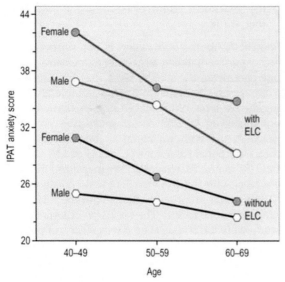

Fig. 4.14 IPAT anxiety scores per decade and sex in asymptomatic subjects with ear lobe crease (ELC) (dots) compared to controls without ELC (hexagons).

Anxiety and coronary risk seem to have a common biological mechanism which is possibly responsible for the appearance of the crease in the course of years. The crease indeed is not present at birth, manifesting itself only in the fifth decade or so and shows its highest prevalence in the years following. We are not able to explain how and why the crease appears. Ear acupuncture may give us a key to interpreting this phenomenon, presuming the existence of somatotopic areas of the CNS on the ear lobe.[56]

When our article was published 20 years ago the relation between type A behavior, anxiety and CHD had long been recognized in the Western world. The type A personality (formulated by Friedman and Rosenman as the 'coronary-prone behavior pattern') was very popular as it included several characteristics of the 'modern' man such as aggressiveness, time urgency, excessive competition, striving for achievement, restlessness, hostility, etc.[58] A little more than 20 years after our article the relationship between CHD and depression and anxiety was clearly underlined in a survey carried out in 38 US states on 129 499 adults aged 45 years and over, performed by a behavior risk factor surveillance system. Patients with a history of cardiovascular disease (including CHD and stroke) were more likely than those without to experience current depression and to have a lifetime diagnosis of depressive disorders or anxiety disorders.[59]

There are, however, several aspects of current research which are of interest for this subject such as the relationship of trait negative emotions to high-frequency heart rate variability (HF-HRV) which is considered a specific indicator of parasympathetic cardiac autonomic function related to premature cardiovascular morbidity and mortality.[60]

Current research indicates that trait anxiety, abnormalities of sympathetic activity, endothelial dysfunctions and insulin resistance may increase the risk of atherosclerosis and cardiovascular disease.[61–63]

2. THE INSPECTION OF THE OUTER EAR IN THE CASE OF HEADACHE

One of my first systematic studies on auricular diagnosis was presented at the 1st Czechoslovak Congress of Acupuncture held in Brno in June 1981. This was also the first opportunity for me to introduce a preliminary version of the Sectogram. An article was then published with the title 'A contribution to the study of new areas of the ear lobe for the diagnosis and treatment of essential headache'.[64] I drew my inspiration from Oleson's original work on auricular somatotopic mapping of musculoskeletal pain[65] and I examined the outer ears of 102 consecutive patients suffering with headache. All observable skin alterations in the areas corresponding to Oleson's representation of the head and neck were reported on the Sectogram (sectors 7–9) (Fig. 4.15). At the time of my study I was still far from applying the first International Classification of Headache Disorders issued later in 1988. I classified headaches according to the 'chronopathological' classification of Francesco Sicuteri, a leading authority in those years. The classification subdivided headaches into accessional, chronic accessional, continuous and cluster headaches. In my group of 102 patients 70.5% were affected by accessional headache which nowadays could be considered as migraine with the recent classification (HIS 2004); 17.6% by chronic accessional headache and 0.8% by continuous headache; both the latter nowadays could be considered as chronic migraine. Only three patients out of 102 had a clear pain pattern of cluster headache.

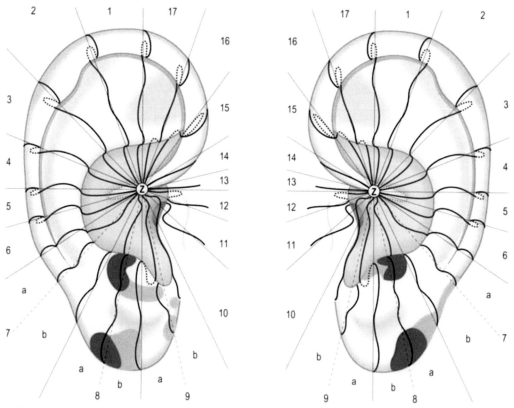

Fig. 4.15 Distribution of skin alterations on the right and left ear in 102 consecutive patients suffering with headache (areas with higher concentration of skin alterations in red; areas with lower concentration of skin alterations in pink) *(courtesy of Marco Banti).*

Altogether 491 skin alterations were found, on average 4.8 per patient; the results of our study were as follows:

1. Skin alterations were distributed on the whole of the ear lobe and were not limited to the antitragus as was commonly believed when treating headache disorders. Actually the total number of skin alterations located on the peripheral zones of the ear lobe and on the antitragus were in a ratio of 2:1; sector 8 (a and b) held the highest concentration of skin alterations, 47.6% of the total on the right ear, and 55.3% of the total on the left ear.
2. Pigmented skin alterations were present in a higher concentration than vascular skin alterations (on average 47.8% to 38.7%). These findings were quite different from the general trend which indicates the prevalence of vascular over pigmentary skin alterations (see Fig. 4.4).

A sex- and age-matched group of patients without migraine indeed showed a lower prevalence of pigmentary skin alterations.

3. Distribution of skin alterations in the sectors (7–9) was significantly associated with the lateralization of pain during migraine attacks. Fifty-six patients with bilateral or alternating headache without prevalence of pain showed no differences in distribution of skin alterations on the right and left ear; instead 46 patients with recurrent or prevalent pain on one side showed a higher concentration of skin alterations on the same side ($P<0.01$).

The conclusions of this first study were that the areas to be included when diagnosing headache were more numerous than presumed and that the pigmentations of the antitragus and ear lobe could represent a sign of headache disorders (see Plate IXA).

The skin alterations were mainly distributed on the same side of the pain or bilaterally if headache did not show any prevalence of pain. I interpreted this finding as an indication for therapy since ear acupuncture could be presumed to be more effective if carried out on the same side as the pain.[64]

3. THE INSPECTION OF THE OUTER EAR IN DIGESTIVE DISORDERS

The second diagnostic study with the inspection was carried out at the department of endoscopy at the hospital of my city. I examined 175 consecutive patients with digestive complaints of different kinds before they underwent gastroscopy. Again drawing inspiration from Oleson's work on auricular somatotopic mapping of musculoskeletal pain, I tried to identify the areas on the concha related to disorders of the upper digestive tract. I was the blind observer and had to answer the following two questions: (i) could auricular inspection of the concha suggest the existence of whatever lesion? (ii) could the topography of the visible skin alterations suggest the lesion of a specific part of the upper digestive tract?

In 144 (82.3%) of the group of 175 patients I was able through inspection to confirm the positive diagnosis of the gastroscopy; for 17.7%, however, results were non-concordant: in 21 patients (12%) inspection was positive and gastroscopy negative; in 10 patients (5.7%) inspection was negative and gastroscopy positive. The first group was composed of 10 patients affected by anxiety and depression, regularly taking variable doses of benzodiazepines and antidepressant drugs; two had liver disease; one had gallstones; eight were apparently healthy. The second group was composed of considerably younger patients affected by recent digestive disorders. The first information I acquired from this study was that also dysfunctions or somatoform disorders could induce a change in auricular skin and that sufficient duration of symptoms was necessary for diagnosis through auricular inspection to be made possible.[66]

Regarding the second question on how to correlate the location of skin alterations on the ear with the site of lesions found at gastroscopy, we first excluded patients with multiple lesions, then selected 86 patients with only one type of lesion located on the following parts of the upper digestive tract:

1. lower third of the esophagus and cardia
2. lesser curvature of the stomach and antrum pyloricum
3. greater curvature of the stomach and gastric fundus
4. pyloric canal
5. anterior wall of duodenal bulb
6. posterior wall of duodenal bulb
7. duodenal bulb at the whole.

We noted at first a prevalent distribution of skin alterations on the right concha (65.6%); this prevalence was significantly associated with the first and second anatomical site ($P<0.001$) whereas the third showed a higher concentration of skin alterations on the left auricle ($P<0.05$).

As regards the duodenum we found some interesting differences concerning the site of lesions of the bulb (pars superior duodeni). Eleven patients affected by an ulcer of the anterior–superior wall of the bulb had a significantly higher number of skin alterations on the right ear whereas 10 patients with an ulcer of the posterior–inferior wall of the bulb had a higher number of skin alterations on the left ear. A control group of 11 patients with duodenitis affecting the whole duodenal bulb showed no differences of distribution. With t-test the difference was significant ($P<0.005$).

The second information I acquired from this study was that the outer ear reflects chronic ailments prevalently of the corresponding side of the body. In the case of a system such as the upper digestive tract, which we imagine to be located along the midline of the body, the representation of the different parts on the right and left ear can be very variable.

This diagnostic approach can be helpful with patients presenting puzzling symptoms, as in the following case.

CASE STUDY

A 65-year-old lady had been suffering for 4 months with intermittent pain of the left posterior thoracic area. The usual routine examinations, ECG and chest X-ray as well as ultrasound of the upper abdomen were negative. An X-ray of the thoraco-lumbar spine showed degenerative changes of the lower thoracic tract which could explain the patient's recurrent pain. The patient had no digestive complaints nor had she noticed a variation of symptoms related to the intake of food. Nevertheless the analgesic medication with NSAID prescribed by her GP had been ineffective up to the time she contacted me for trying acupuncture. I examined her ears and was surprised to find two telangiectasia of the left concha where the Chinese locate the stomach area (CO4 *wei*) and the French locate the duodenum (Fig. 4.16A). I examined her back which was stiff but frankly not painful on flexion, extension and lateral bending. Trying the skin-rolling test of Maigne, gently taking a fold of the skin between my thumb and forefinger, I found a thickened and hypersensitive area on the left side of her chest, corresponding to the seventh to eighth thoracic dermatomes (Fig. 4.16B). I also found a tender point very close to the observed telangiectasia on which I carried out the needle-contact test (NCT) (see Ch. 8) for a few seconds: the hypersensitive areas disappeared in the following minute. I did not treat this patient with acupuncture as I was uncertain about the diagnosis; nevertheless I prescribed ranitidine which indeed was effective in the following days. Gastroscopy evidenced a non-perforating ulcer of the posterior wall of the bulb. Therapy with ranitidine was therefore continued and the thoracic pain did not recur.

4. THE INSPECTION OF THE OUTER EAR IN THE CASE OF SKELETAL ABNORMALITIES

For several years I have been fascinated by melanocytic nevi of the outer ear. Two observations stimulated my interest: the first was that nevi were among the few skin alterations noticeable in children and young people. The second was that nevi were not randomly distributed on the auricle but concentrated on specific areas innervated prevalently by trigeminal and cervical nerves. For example if we consider the distribution of nevi on the different parts of the auricle in 711 patients we can see that the helix is in first place with 38.5%, and the upper and lower concha in last place with only 1.3% (Table 4.8). One possible reason for this striking difference is that this part of the ear, innervated mainly by the tenth cranial nerve, is not concerned with the 'emigration' of melanocytes. According to what is still accepted as a hypothesis, these cells emigrate to the epidermis and derma from the lateral ridges of the neural plate as the ridges join to form the neural tube. Congenital nevi are present within the first 6 months of life; acquired nevi appear later and peak in number during the second and third decades of life, but involute spontaneously by the seventh to ninth decades.[67]

I too observed this phenomenon on the auricle and have presented it in Figure 4.5.

The richness of the distribution of these nevi on the helix led me to consider the possible

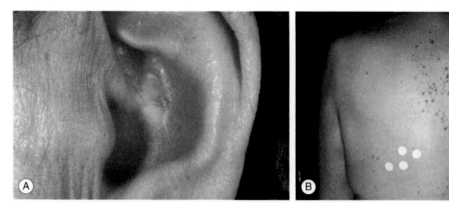

Fig. 4.16 (A) Double telangiectasia of the left concha in a 65-year-old female affected by intermittent posterior thoracic pain on the left side in duodenal ulcer of the posterior wall of the bulbus. (B) Hypersensitive areas at skin-rolling test of the left thoracic area in the same patient.

Table 4.8 Distribution (%) of melanocytic nevi on the different parts of the auricle in 711 subjects

Part of the auricle	Nevi distribution
Helix	38.5%
Ear lobe	20.8%
Medial surface	12.7%
Anthelix	10.6%
Antitragus	5.8%
Scaphoid groove	5.5%
Tragus	3.5%
Upper and lower concha	1.3%
Other parts	1.3%
Total	100%

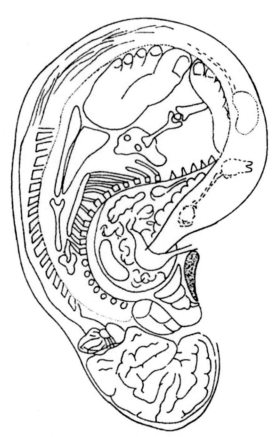

Fig. 4.17   Representation of the spinal cord on the helix according to Nogier *(with permission)*.

associations between this still puzzling part of the ear and some skeletal abnormalities such as scoliosis which must be considered, as is well known, a three-dimensional deformity of the spine in which lateral deviation combines with vertebral torsion.

The Chinese auricular map does not give too much importance to the helix areas HX9 *lunyi* to HX12 *lunsi* which start from the lower border of the helix tubercle and end overlapping with the tail of the helix. The indications of these areas are coincident and concern fever, tonsillitis and infections of the upper respiratory tract. The verity of these correlations is highlighted in Figure 9.15.

Nogier's opinion about the significance of the helix had been postponed until 1977 when, after much consideration and clinical application, he thought of its possible representation of the spinal cord[68] (Fig. 4.17). His hypothesis is very interesting as the helix appears to be involved in several neurological conditions such as, for example, neuropathic pain of herpes zoster (see Fig. 3.20).

Seeking an association between melanocytic nevi and scoliosis I was helped by the article of Bañuls[69] who found a significantly higher number of nevi on the body in a group of patients with scoliosis compared to a control group ($P<0.001$). The same author also assumed that a genetic factor could influence the segmental arrangement of multiple nevi, both of congenital and acquired origin.[70]

The possibility that a segmental arrangement of nevi could also exist on the auricle urged me to study two groups of boys and girls; the first from the Centre for Prevention of Scoliosis of the Pro Juventute Foundation in Florence; the control group from the pupils of a state secondary school of the same city. Clinical scoliosis was ruled out applying Adam's forward bending test which is proved to be the best non-invasive clinical test for evaluating scoliosis.[71]

A preliminary report on the association between melanocytic nevi and skeletal malformations was presented at the 5th International Symposium of Auriculotherapy and Auriculomedicine in October 2006.[72]

The final unpublished data concerned 311 subjects: 190 girls (average age 12.8 years, SD 1.6, range 6–16) and 121 boys (average age 12.9 years, SD 1.7, range 8–18). All subjects were examined by an orthopedist who specialized in scoliosis:

203 of them showed skeletal abnormalities, 108 were considered normal. The skeletal disorders were classified into the following four categories:

- idiopathic scoliosis (when a structural, lateral, rotated curvature of the spine was demonstrated) in 133 subjects
- compensatory scoliosis (when the lateral curvature was associated with a pelvic obliquity on the frontal plane related to a leg length discrepancy) in 37 subjects
- combined idiopathic and compensatory scoliosis in 11 subjects
- combined scoliosis and kyphosis in 22 subjects.

All observable nevi were transcribed on the Sectogram and a first evaluation was made on the total number of nevi in the four categories and in the control group (respectively 2.04 and 1.56 nevi). With t-test for independent samples we found a significant difference ($P<0.05$). If in the first two categories we weigh the sectors with a significantly higher concentration of nevi compared to the control group, we may find sectors 4, 6, 10, 18, 19 and 24 in the group with compensatory scoliosis (on the left of Fig. 4.18A) and sectors 15, 17 and 18 in the scoliosis group (on the right of Fig. 4.18A). If we assume that the sectors in the scoliosis group correspond to the representation of the thoracic spine, for the first group we should assume that the outspread distribution of nevi may correspond to other structures, thereby confirming the different pathogenesis of these conditions. Comparing the two groups, in the first group we found a significantly higher concentration of nevi on the ear lobe in sectors 3–6 ($P<0.005$) and on the helix in sector 20 ($P<0.001$) (on the left of Fig. 4.18B).

The first information we obtained from this evaluation was that a reduced number of nevi (<2), in boys and girls aged 10–14, may indicate a low risk

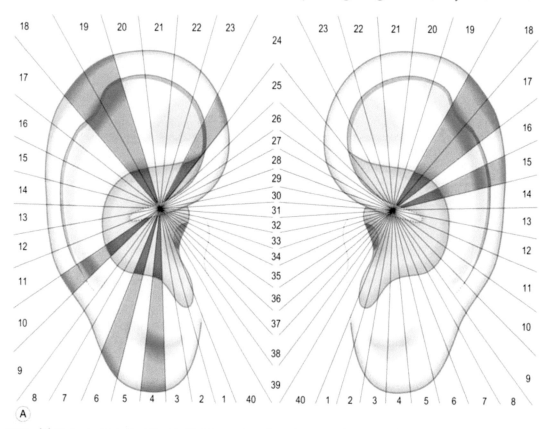

Fig. 4.18 (A) Sectors with a significantly higher concentration of nevi compared to control group in 170 girls and boys (average age 12.8 years): 37 subjects with compensatory scoliosis (on the left); 133 subjects with idiopathic scoliosis (on the right).

Continued

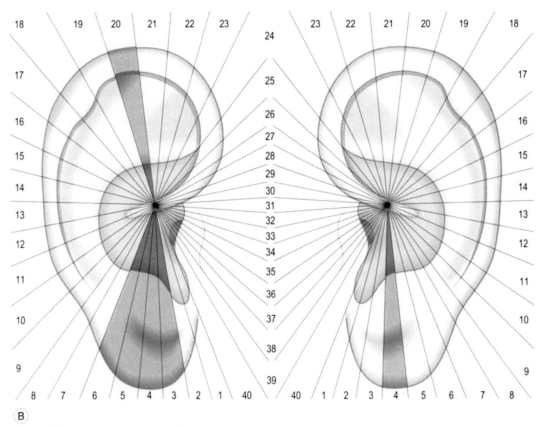

Fig. 4.18, cont'd (B) Sectors with a significantly higher concentration of nevi in the same subjects with compensatory scoliosis compared to idiopathic scoliosis (on the left); sector 4 has a significantly higher number of nevi in boys and girls who have worn fixed or mobile bite-plates compared to control (on the right).

of skeletal abnormalities; a higher average number of nevi (≥ 2), however, may be associated more frequently with a skeletal abnormality of the spine.

The second information we obtained was that a deformity of the spine is not only associated with a distribution of nevi on the helix and the anthelix, parts which we commonly presume to be related to the spinal cord and the vertebral column, but it also reflects an evident extension on portions of the ear lobe which are presumed to be the representation of the cranial bones and the central nervous system.

We formed a hypothesis about the particularly striking differences between the groups with idiopathic and compensatory scoliosis, and carried out a further analysis on the whole group of 311 boys and girls, at first as regards the wearing of fixed or mobile bite-plates for orthodontic–esthetic purposes. A large percentage of these

young subjects (54.5%) had worn these plates for a longer or shorter time and we compared the total number of nevi in this group with a group of boys and girls who had never worn this kind of appliance. We did not find a significant difference (the average number of nevi was respectively 1.98 and 2.03), but we found that sector 4 had a significantly higher concentration of nevi in the first group ($P < 0.001$) (on the right of Fig. 4.18B).

Our hypothesis was that the nevi located on the ear lobe (sectors 3–6) may be the representation of asymmetries of the central nervous system and the cranial bones, often related to craniomandibular disorders (see Plates XC and XD). As the compensatory scoliosis group was characterized by a short-leg syndrome we made an analysis regarding also this issue.

We had the opportunity, for a second study involving the same group of subjects, to measure both lower limbs with various techniques (visual and instrumental) with the aim of ascertaining the intra- and inter-rater reliability of each method. The visual inspection of pelvic obliquity and the correction of it using lift blocks under the short leg in the standing position and the visual appreciation of tibial and femoral shortening following the classical orthopedic examination[73] proved to be the best diagnostic tools. The examination was performed by two independent observers and gave some unexpected results as 181 of 311 girls and boys showed various short-leg patterns. A right or left short tibia or femur was found in 51.9% in this group, followed by the combination of short tibia and short femur on the same side in 32.6%. In a minority of cases a further combination was found of short tibia and femur on the opposite side: 21 subjects showed a right short tibia and a left short femur; 7 showed a left short tibia and a right short femur (in total 15.5%). These cases were excluded from the analysis and in the remaining group of 153 girls and boys we compared first the total number of nevi with the rest of the subjects showing a symmetrical length of the lower limbs. The difference was significant since the average number of nevi was respectively 2.1 and 1.6 ($P<0.05$).

Applying paired samples t-test to the distribution of nevi on the right and left ear, we obtained a significantly higher number of nevi on the right ear in case of right short tibia ($P<0.05$) and in all categories comprehending a short tibia or femur of the right lower limb ($P<0.02$). The left short tibia

and the short femur, however, did not show any difference (Table 4.9A).

The hypothesis that an incomplete growth of the bones of the lower limb could be associated with an asymmetrical distribution of nevi on the auricle was subsequently verified in a group of adults in my practice, in whom skeletal growth was complete.

I examined 127 consecutive adults (average age 35.8 years, range 18–69, SD 12.8) bearing at least one nevus on their ears, in both standing and lying positions. In the latter position I measured the distance twice between the anterior inferior iliac spine (AIIS) and the medial malleolus with a tape-measure. I calculated the average of two measurements, which appears to have acceptable validity and reliability when used as a screening tool.[74]

I found 79 subjects with a shorter leg (42 on the right and 37 on the left) with an average number of 4.6 nevi, and 48 subjects with equal length of the lower limbs with an average of 3.1 nevi; the difference was significant ($P<0.001$). Considering the distribution of nevi on the auricle according to the various short-leg patterns, we obtained a significantly higher number of nevi on the right ear for the right short leg and in a similar way a higher number of nevi on the left ear for the left short leg ($P<0.001$). Only 10 subjects with short right femur did not show any difference (Table 4.9B). If we report the location of all nevi corresponding to the short side (left side of Fig. 4.19), whether right or left, we may visually better appreciate their greater number compared to the contralateral side

Table 4.9A   Short-leg patterns and distribution of nevi on the right and left ear in 153 girls and boys with an average age of 12.9 years

	Number of subjects	Average number of nevi on the right ear	Average number of nevi on the left ear	P
Right short tibia	28	1.18	0.64	<0.05
Left short tibia	31	1.45	1.13	NS
Right short femur	20	0.55	0.55	NS
Left short femur	15	0.73	0.67	NS
Right short tibia and right short femur	44	1.32	1.00	NS
Left short tibia and left short femur	15	0.93	0.87	NS
All categories (right short tibia or right short femur)	92	1.14	0.79	<0.02
All categories (left short tibia or left short femur)	61	1.15	0.95	NS

Table 4.9B   Short-leg patterns and distribution of nevi on the right and left ear in 79 adults with an average age of 34.7 years

	Number of subjects	Average number of nevi on the right ear	Average number of nevi on the left ear	P
Right short tibia	15	3.80	2.07	<0.02
Left short tibia	17	1.47	2.82	<0.05
Right short femur	10	1.90	1.40	NS
Left short femur	13	1.38	3.08	<0.002
Right short tibia and right short femur	17	3.06	1.59	<0.05
Left short tibia and left short femur	7	1.14	3.00	<0.05
All categories (right short tibia or right short femur)	42	3.05	1.71	<0.001
All categories (left short tibia or left short femur)	37	1.38	2.95	<0.001

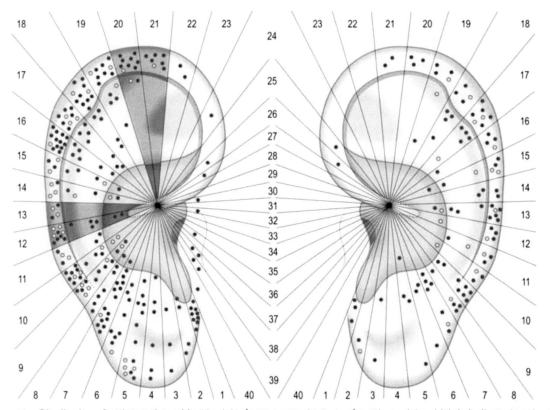

Fig. 4.19   Distribution of melanocytic nevi in 79 adults (average age 34.7 years) on the auricle which is ipsilateral to the side of the short leg (on the left); distribution of nevi on the contralateral auricle on the right. The sectors with a significantly higher number of nevi in case of short femur or short tibia are colored. Dots = lateral surface; circles = medial surface.

(right side of Fig. 4.19). What is interesting is the distribution of the nevi on the auricle: in the first rank is the helix with 31.6%, followed by the ear lobe with 24.9% and the medial surface with 18.6%. If, however, we sum all nevi belonging to the helix, whether located on its lateral or its medial side, we obtain 43.6% of the total. The full importance of the helix has yet to be revealed and meanwhile we must be satisfied with collecting further fragments of the mosaic. I could not understand, for example, why sectors 12 and 13, which consistently belong to the topographic representation of the neck, should carry a significantly higher number of nevi in case of short tibia and femur. On the other side it is perhaps easier to interpret the higher number of nevi on sector 20 for the short tibia ($P<0.05$) and on sector 21 for the short femur ($P<0.005$). Both sectors may indeed be related to the representation of the lower limb according to Nogier's map and the Chinese standardization (left side of Fig. 4.19).

In the case of Plate XB, the 43-year-old lady pictured showed at least four nevi on the left ear and only one on the right. The pelvic obliquity in a standing position, the visual appreciation of a short left tibia and the measurement of the distance between the AIIS and the medial malleolus were consistent with the finding of a ~13 mm shorter left leg.

From this second series of analyses some further elements emerged relating to the possible role of auricular nevi indicating, on the same side of the body, developmental or growth defects of the skeletal system as in the case of short-leg syndrome. However, follow-up observation should be carried out on the same subjects over time, starting from infancy, to distinguish the congenital nevi from those acquired and to understand if their appearance can be associated with musculoskeletal disorders manifesting themselves at puberty or in adulthood.

5. THE CRUS CYMBAE IN SUSPECTING RENAL ANOMALIES

The crus cymbae has been described in Chapter 3 as a possibly dominant morphological trait consisting of a more or less raised and extended ridge in the upper concha.

Nogier wrote on this subject in 1956 describing the case of a young lady whom he had been treating since she was 16 years old because she was suffering from hypertension of unknown origin. He said:

one day on inspection of the ears I saw an anomaly of the kidney area (in the upper part of the concha) shaped like a vertical cartilaginous ridge. As the patient was a young girl suffering with hypertension and slight albuminuria I concluded that she probably had a congenital anomaly of the kidney manifesting itself on the corresponding auricular area.[75]

Nguyen[76] tried to verify this possibility examining 45 consecutive subjects bearing crus cymbae and 80 (40 male and 40 female) patients of a control group without this sign.

For each patient he recorded the following data: previous surgery of the urinary tract; previous syndromes/symptoms of the urinary tract such as kidney diseases, calculi, prostate diseases and hematuria; previous recurrent urinary infections needing further diagnosis with imaging techniques. He found 13 patients (28.9%) in the first group compared to 6 (7.5%) in the control group who had undergone surgery for prostate adenoma (8 cases), renal cystic disease (2 cases), bladder papilloma (2 cases) and cystocele (1 case). The other patients bearing crus cymbae had various symptoms such as recurrent bladder infection, hematuria, suspected renal colic with or without calculi, etc. What is perhaps interesting in Nguyen's observational study is the surprisingly high number of anomalies of the genitourinary tract. Indeed two females aged 35 and 63 years, had, respectively, a ureteropelvic duplication and a non better defined congenital anomaly of the uterus. Furthermore a male subject aged 54 suffering with recurrent urinary infection had a son with a ureteral duplication.

Unfortunately I did not come across as many cases as Nguyen, therefore my experience on this subject is not of much value. In a couple of cases, however, I could demonstrate a nephroptosis with a downward displacement of the kidney and in some other cases recurrent urinary infection with calculi, without any demonstration of congenital anomalies, as in the case in Figure 4.20.

What is interesting in Nogier's case report is the further confirmation that the first representation of the kidney area was indeed on the upper concha where the Chinese still locate the kidney (CO10 *shen*). It is still not clear why, in the contemporary French map, the kidney and the ureter (but not the bladder) have been shifted to the ascending part of the helix.

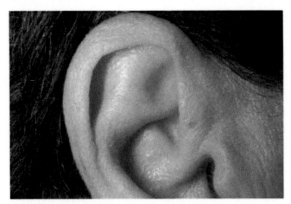

Fig. 4.20 Crus cymbae in a 43-year-old female affected by recurrent urinary infections and calculi.

6. IS THERE ANY FOUNDATION FOR SUSPECTING THE PRESENCE OF A TUMOR BY MEANS OF AURICULAR INSPECTION?

There are some articles in the literature about this odd and apparently out of place aspect of diagnosis. Given the enormous diagnostic possibilities offered today by the various imaging techniques it would appear to be completely unnecessary to rely also on the inspection of the outer ear in cases of tumor. Nevertheless it is still feasible that a tumor could be hidden and diagnosis made too late. This may, and in fact does, occur often in the following cases: the subject is asymptomatic and does not consider it necessary to consult a physician; the subject has no time or is not willing to participate in prevention campaigns, for example for breast, colon or prostate cancer; the subject presents unclear symptoms for which he has not yet completed all the tests focused on excluding such a possibility. In any case the chance of an acupuncturist being approached by a patient with a hidden tumor, asking to be treated for example for pain presenting due to a primary neuromuscular disorder, is not so remote. As the information needed for preventing cancer is vast and involves several aspects of a person's life, it is perhaps possible to obtain some clues also from an auricular inspection.

In Western countries only Nguyen and I have published case reports of patients with tumors: Nguyen found, in the case of adenoma of the prostate gland, a nodule of the French area of representation of the ureter, and a sebaceous cyst in the fossa ovalis corresponding to the Chinese representation of the uterus.[77]

In my first article dedicated to the topic of inspection (with Vettori) I published two case reports of lung cancer. A circumscribed atrophic area with desquamation in the first case and an atrophic depressed area in the second case were visible in the middle of the lower concha on the same side as the lesion.[78]

The China Academy of TCM and several authors such as Zhu Dan[79] have published numerous articles on this topic and identified two main specific tumor areas, n. I and II, on the ear lobe and the helix. These areas, according to different authors, have a variable extension: the former corresponds to sectors 4–9, the latter to sectors 15–19 of my Sectogram.

Li-Chun Huang[80] wrote about area n. II, describing 'a dark grey color, dark brown color or a color of fly droppings which will fade if pressed; and small nodule(s) in specific area II indicate a tumor in the body'. The China Academy of TCM named the areas *zhongliuteyiqu* I and II respectively, but a further area (III) was also proposed on the back of the helix precisely overlapping n. II (Fig. 4.21). Another three points shortly named tumor (*zhongliu* 1, 2 and 3)

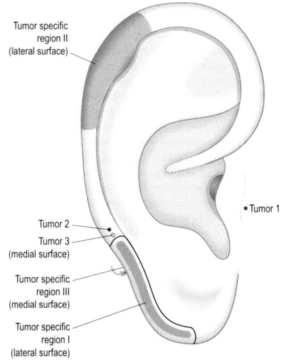

Tumor specific region II (lateral surface)

Tumor 2

Tumor 3 (medial surface)

Tumor specific region III (medial surface)

Tumor specific region I (lateral surface)

• Tumor 1

Fig. 4.21 Representation of tumor-specific areas I–III and tumor points 1–3 according to the China Academy of TCM.

were located by the China Academy, the first on the tragus, the remaining two on sector 10: number 2 on the lateral surface of the helix, number 3 on the medial surface, about 2 mm below the former. Other areas have been proposed by Zhu Dan for an early diagnosis of tumor, such as the representation of the internal ear, subcortex, endocrine, adrenal cortex and gluteus muscles. The standardization process has almost completely abandoned these representations and retained only one zone, Lower Tragus (TG2 *xiaping*).

We designed a project to verify if the assertions of the Chinese authors made before standardization had been of some significance or not. Two pupils, Miriam Manetti and Gianfranco Matera, independently examined a series of consecutive patients in the departments of oncology at their hospitals. For each patient, age, sex, histology and stage of the tumor were recorded and each visible skin alteration was then photographed and recorded on the Sectogram. A preliminary communication on this research was presented as a poster at the European Traditional Medicine (ETM) International Congress held on 4–6 October 2007 in Vinci.[81]

The number and the type of skin alterations of 165 patients with various types of cancer were compared with those of a sex- and age-matched group of patients of mine without any current or past history of tumor. As regards the distribution of skin alterations in the two groups we found no significant differences for tumor area I (sectors 15–19) and tumor areas II and III (sectors 4–9). We therefore could not confirm the specificity of these areas in the diagnosis of tumor. Nevertheless our research was not useless as we found some striking differences for some particular skin alterations such as angioma.

It has to be remembered that angioma is itself an extremely common benign tumor, made up of newly formed blood vessels, and resulting from the malformation of angioblastic tissue during fetal life. The angioma usually seen on the auricle are tiny and have a diameter of 1–5 mm; when pressed with the fingertip they characteristically disappear and reappear. My impression, in singular cases, that this sign could be associated with some kind of tumor was confirmed by this larger observational study. The number of these vascular skin alterations was 1.54 in the cancer group vs. 0.44 in the control patients ($P<0.001$). Not all types of tumor showed the same tendency to manifest

angioma on the auricle; especially tumors of the breast, lung, colon, stomach and the genitourinary system seemed to show a higher concentration on the helix, anthelix and ear lobe. The confounding aspect of these observations is that frequently angioma tend to develop on parts of the ear which apparently are not the representation of the corresponding site of the tumor. Only in some cases of breast, lung and stomach tumor did we find this kind of correspondence.

Despite the small numbers of patients ranked according to different types of cancer, which are a limiting factor for any further analysis, we can nevertheless notice that the sectors where angioma are located may still have a relation to the corresponding somatotopic areas according to Nogier's alignment principle. If we consider, for example, the distribution of angioma in two groups of 11 patients with cancer of the lung and colon we can see that, despite their apparent similarity, in the first group (on the left of Fig. 4.22) there is a higher number of angioma on the lower concha and the antitragus whereas in the second group they tend to spread toward the superior part of the helix (on the right of Fig. 4.22). An advisable strategy, in case the reader were to dedicate himself to this type of observation, could be not to rely too much on single sectors but to take account of larger parts of the ear. For example, in the case of breast cancer, 20 patients out of a total of 32 (62.5%) showed particularly tiny angioma especially on the lower half of the anthelix and helix (on the left of Fig. 4.23), some of them coinciding with Nogier's and the Chinese representation of the chest (see Plate VIIID). Moreover, if we consider patients with benign adenomas of the thyroid gland we can see that there is a basic overlapping in the distribution of angioma (on the right of Fig. 4.23).

This study is continuing with the aim of identifying a possible specificity of angioma for particular types of cancer. Some provisional conclusions can be reported:

1. The specific tumor areas proposed by the Chinese do not show a different concentration of skin alterations in cancer and control patients. The sectors thought to be specific when presuming the presence of a hidden tumor probably have per se a higher concentration of skin alterations as shown in Figure 4.7.

2. Cancer patients have a higher number of angioma compared to the control group, but

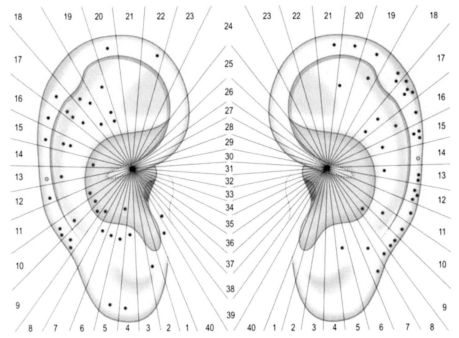

Fig. 4.22 Location of angioma in 11 patients with lung cancer (on the left) and in 11 patients with cancer of the colon (on the right). Dots = lateral surface; circles = medial surface.

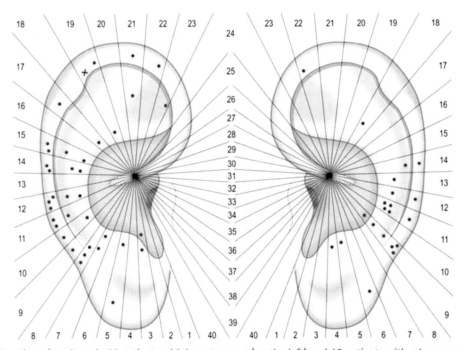

Fig. 4.23 Location of angioma in 20 patients with breast cancer (on the left) and 10 patients with adenomas of the thyroid gland (on the right). The cross on the upper helix (on the left) indicates an angioma of the internal (hidden) border.

probably only specific types of tumor show a higher rate of this skin alteration.

3. Also patients declaring benign tumors such as adenomas of the thyroid and prostate (see Plate VIIIA), adenomas and papillomas of the breast (see Plate VIIIB, C) and uterine myomas in their case history may show a larger number of angioma compared to control patients.

4. Angioma tend, however, to be concentrated on areas which do not coincide with the presumed representation of the affected organ. Sometimes there is a segmental representation on the helix which roughly follows a subdivision of the abdominal and thoracic organs. Therefore cancer of abdominal organs such as the colon, kidney or prostate perhaps could be represented more in the upper part of the ear, while cancer of the thoracic organs such as the lung instead could be represented more on the lower part of the ear.

5. However, no information can be given as regards the issue of laterality in the distribution of angioma. Seemingly, in the case of lesion of one of two coupled organs and/or in the case of metastases of one side of the body, a higher distribution of angioma can be foreseen on the auricle located on the same side. Nevertheless a much larger sample of patients is needed to clarify this issue.

The reader will allow me to add a last consideration on this subject about the interesting association of stasis of Blood and tumors in TCM. According to Maciocia:[82]

> abdominal masses are always characterized by either stagnation of qi or stasis of Blood, the former being non-substantial and the latter substantial masses. In addition to stagnation, there may also be Phlegm. However, in all cases of abdominal masses there is always an underlying deficiency of qi. Deficient qi fails to transport and transform and, leading to stagnation of qi and Blood, it allows masses to form.

FURTHER OBSERVATIONS NOT YET REPORTED IN THE LITERATURE

As reported in the validation of auricular diagnosis in Chapter 9, the inspection of the outer ear seems to give better results than the other two methods commonly used, namely the pain

pressure test (PPT) and the electrical skin resistance test (ESRT). This section reports unpublished data on the possibilities offered by inspection for diagnosing different syndromes, with the aim of giving practitioners a simple tool for integrating diagnostic procedures with their patients. The following paragraphs are based on the observation of 325 patients, evaluated between 2004 and 2007, examined blindly with the three methods mentioned above. For the methodology applied the reader is invited to consult Chapter 9.

I have always felt the urge to find one or more clues to cast light on the issue of whether acupuncture is of value in treating mental disorders. In my opinion this is a promising field for research but different reasons have hampered its growth. One of the reasons may be the reduced and incomplete terminology adopted by textbooks of acupuncture. In an article published in 2005 with the title 'Why is clinical research on acupuncture in psychiatric disorders so lacking?'[83] I reported, with colleagues, the results of a survey among 67 GPs and 42 psychiatrists; 50.7% of the first group and 26.2% of the second had regularly practiced acupuncture for at least 3 years. The colleagues were invited to rate all symptoms, listed in two Chinese textbooks published approximately 20 years apart (1975[84] and 1997[85]), among the therapeutic indications for every acupuncture point, as primarily psychological/psychiatric, psychosomatic or somatic. The symptoms were considered prevalently somatic by the majority of colleagues. A consistent interpretation of a psychological/psychiatric term was reached in the first textbook for the following 11 conditions: hysteria, schizophrenia, mental disorder, mania, anorexia, anxiety, neurasthenia, neurosis, insomnia, dream-disturbed sleep, poor memory; only six terms reached an agreement in the second text: mania, depression, anorexia, irritability, insomnia, globus hystericus.

The conclusions of my survey were that:

> even in recent years Chinese acupuncture books report a reduced and incomplete list of psychological/psychiatric terms compared to medical literature. This may be one of the reasons for the apparent lack of interest in the West for controlled clinical trials evaluating acupuncture's effect on psychiatric disorders. Potential researchers in this field should include patients according to the internationally accepted classifications of

mental disorders and choose an adequate acupuncture treatment according to the syndromes of TCM.

As regards ear acupuncture the situation was no better than that of acupuncture until a few years ago. Recently, however, in the West, several trials have been published applying different types of auricular stimulation such as acupuncture, acupressure, press needles and *Vaccaria* seeds, mainly for anxiety and insomnia, and to a lesser extent for phobias and depression.[86–97]

POSSIBLE SIGNS ASSOCIATED WITH MENTAL DISORDERS

As a general practitioner and an acupuncturist, in my observation of the outer ears of hundreds of people a year I took the following signs into consideration because I felt they were of special clinical value:

1. depressed areas and incisures of the upper part of the ear lobe
2. incisures and drills of the antitragus and the scapha
3. nevi of the anterior part of the ear lobe
4. comedones of the lower concha
5. telangiectasia of the upper and lower concha.

These signs were compared in two groups of patients: the first group bore the specific sign; the other did not and was considered a control group. The groups were always compared, when possible, for *t*-test for independent samples.

1. Depressed areas and incisures of the upper part of the ear lobe

These are quite similar to those reported in Chapter 3 (Fig. 3.10) as descriptive non-hereditary characters referred to in the literature by anatomists and anthropologists. Depressions and incisures in this area may be more or less evidenced; in two out of three cases they are tender to PPT (Fig. 4.24, numbers 1 and 2) (see Plates XIIC and XIID). My clinical intuition has always been that this area could be associated with mood disorders. In effect 75.8% of patients bearing one of these signs, compared to the control group (43.5%), declared or confirmed depression or symptoms consistent with this diagnosis. The difference was highly significant

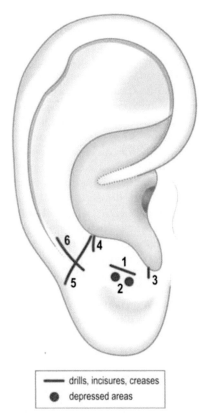

— drills, incisures, creases

● depressed areas

Fig. 4.24 Depressed areas, grooves and incisures of the upper and posterior parts of the ear lobe. For their possible clinical significance see the text.

using Student's *t*-test (*P*<0.001). Insomnia, which is one of the important symptoms accompanying mood disorders, was also represented more in the first group (51.5%) compared to the control group (34.9%) but did not reach a significant level. It has to be noticed that this area coincides with Nogier's representation of the hypothalamus and partially with the Chinese temple area (AT2 *nie*), both of which also report partially consistent indications such as headache, insomnia and dizziness. Anxiety and related disorders such as panic attacks and phobias on the other hand showed no significant differences. In conclusion, this area appears to be important for the diagnosis of mood disorders. In all probability it should be included in any treatment for regulating mood (see also Chapters 5 and 7).

2. Deepening of the anthelix–antitragus notch and/or deepening of the final part of the scaphoid groove

These have been considered together because they are both aligned on sectors 8 and 9 and are supposed to have similar significance (Fig. 4.24, numbers 4 and 6). Out of 78 patients, 49 showed the first pattern and 11 the second, and 18 showed both patterns. My intuition that they were associated with sleep disorders proved to be exact: in effect 61.5% of subjects bearing one or both of these signs were bad sleepers compared to 28.7% of the control group ($P<0.001$). Depression was also represented more in the first group (64.1%) than in the control group (41.3%); but the difference did not reach a significant level. In this area, at the transition line from the groove of the scapha to the ear lobe, we find the historical point that Nogier named 'Jérôme' or point of joy, which he considered effective in sleep disorders and depression. Nogier named this point after Hieronymus Bosch (d.1516) who in his famous painting 'The Garden of Earthly Delights' depicted a devil indicating this point with the tip of a lance. It has to be remembered that the subject of this painting is problematic, but most scholars interpret it as a hostile view of a life devoted to the pleasure of the senses. This area is important also for the Chinese because both the above mentioned incisures end in the Chinese occiput area (AT3 *zhen*) which has several indications such as headache, neurasthenia, dizziness, asthma, etc. In a minority of cases there is a third deepening/incisure, on the anterior part of the antitragus, which seems associated with sleep disorders; this area overlaps with the Chinese forehead (AT1 *e*) whose indications are indeed headache, sinusitis and insomnia (Fig. 4.24, number 3). In conclusion the sites observed seem to be further important areas in the diagnosis and treatment of either depression or sleep disorders. What may be of interest for the practitioner is the fact that especially the first two deepenings may be related to spinal disorders not only of the cervical tract, but also of the lumbosacral tract. Indeed, 40 patients (51.3%) with sciatic pain showed this sign compared to 36% of the control group. Two main hypotheses can be put forward to explain the association between these signs and spinal pain: in the first, cervical and lumbar pain may be the expression of postural dysfunctions which could be related to craniomandibular disorders; in the second, pain and muscular stiffness may be considered as physical complaints in somatization disorder accompanying depressed mood.

3. Nevi of the anterior part of the ear lobe

On this part of the ear the French and Chinese schools reached the greatest degree of consensus as regards the diagnosis and treatment of psychological/psychiatric conditions. Nogier located his points for aggressiveness and fear in this area; the Chinese located their anterior ear lobe (LO4 *chuiqian*) to treat neurasthenia, *shenjing shuairuo* (see section above on the diagonal ear lobe crease). Further points, however, received particular attention, such as the hypertension point *gaoxueyadian* on the inferior part of the tragus, coinciding with the 'tranquilizer point' according to Oleson and the 'Lexotan area' of the inferior part of the ear lobe according to Bahr.[98]

My hypothesis was that as well as the diagonal ear lobe crease the presence of nevi in this area could also be associated with higher levels of anxiety (see Plate XIA). In this hypothesis I was of course influenced by Bourdiol's representation of the limbic system[55] and by the results of my study on higher levels of anxiety in patients bearing a diagonal ear lobe crease (see Figs 4.13, 4.14). I first made a comparison with Student's *t*-test between 104 patients bearing at least one nevus of the ear lobe and 221 patients without. I found no difference in the number of nevi in asthenia and in mental disorders such as anxiety, depression, insomnia, phobia and panic attacks. However, performing a second comparison in 31 patients bearing at least one nevus on the anterior part of the lobe (sectors 1–2) I found a significant prevalence of depression and phobia ($P<0.005$). Therefore my hypothesis that nevi of the anterior part of the lobe could be associated prevalently with a particular trait for anxiety could not be confirmed. In conclusion, a tendency to depression seems prevalent in subjects bearing nevi of this part, together with abnormal fear and migraine. It should be remembered that Nogier's master point for headaches is located on the anterior border of the lobe, which is especially indicated for migraine (see Fig. A1.17).

4. Comedones of the lower concha

Comedones of the lower concha have always been a favorite topic of research for me for various reasons. The coincidence of their area of distribution, especially with the Chinese lung area, oriented me at first to skin problems. The large lung area (CO14 *fei*) has several indications regarding dermatological conditions such as acne, itching, urticaria, condylomata but also symptoms of the coupled large intestine according to TCM, such as constipation. Later I decided to see if I could verify whether a particular concentration of comedones in the upper part of the lower concha could be correlated with anxiety disorders such as panic attack and phobic behavior leading to the avoidance of feared objects or situations (see Plate XVA). The area concerned is related to the Chinese mouth (CO1 *kou*) and esophagus (CO2 *shidao*). It is enlightening that the indications given by Chinese authors to the latter go beyond esophagitis to 'globus hystericus'. This term has long been left out of any internationally recognized classification of mental disorders but it has to be remembered that 'hysteria of anxiety' was a psychoanalytical concept introduced by Sigmund Freud for describing a type of hysteria in which anxiety manifested itself as a phobic reaction. As regards the corresponding representations on Nogier's map, we find the esophagus and part of the stomach which do not seem to be related to any specific psychiatric problem. Table 4.10 shows the broad range of symptoms which are variously related to the presence of comedones of the lower concha. In this group we find especially anxiety disorders such as panic attack (25%) and phobic reaction (70%), compared to, respectively, 9.8% and 31.3% of the control group; this area of the ear does not, however, correlate with depression and insomnia.

In conclusion, the finding of comedones in the lower concha may hold different meanings, but the most important in my opinion is the diagnosis in these subjects of phobic behavior and a tendency to panic attacks. The diagnosis is further strengthened if the area concerned is detectable also by PPT and electrical detection; indeed treatment with acupuncture may have not only a symptomatic effect on anxiety, but also help in preventing further panic attacks. Furthermore, interesting are the correlations with irritable bowel syndrome, allergy, food intolerance and dermatitis. The following case has been enlightening for me thanks to a follow-up of 20 years (see Plates XVIB, C, D).

Table 4.10 Disorders significantly associated with the presence of comedones of the lower concha in 325 patients

Disorder	Comedones of the lower concha (60 patients)	No comedones (265 patients)	P
Phobia	42	83	<0.001
Panic attack	15	26	<0.001
Depression	31	121	NS
Insomnia	18	101	NS
Irritable bowel syndrome	48	121	<0.001
Allergy	29	80	<0.001
Food intolerance	24	60	<0.001
Dermatitis	19	33	<0.001

CASE STUDY

A 48-year-old female affected by migraine, gastroesophageal reflux disease associated with a sliding hiatus hernia, irritable bowel syndrome (IBS), asthenia and depression had for 3–4 weeks demonstrated dystrophy of the triangular fossa and the anthelix of the left auricle. Comedonic plaques were noticeable on the inferior concha (Plate XVIB).

Relevant findings from the patient's history are allergy to dust and familial hypercholesterolemia with recently diagnosed gallstones.

Two years later, after a careful and prolonged elimination from the diet of wheat, yeast, dairy products, beef and coffee, the dystrophy had disappeared and the comedones were decreased in number even if they appeared of greater size (Plate XVIC). At this time migraine, asthenia and depression had responded well to this elimination, and constipation and symptoms of gastroesophageal reflux had improved.

Twenty years later the patient had been stable as regards her medical conditions only when managing her food intolerances well. The skin disorders of the auricle did not reappear and only some residual telangiectasia were visible on the cardia area (Plate XVID).

5. Telangiectasia of the concha

These are very frequent and 161 (49.5%) out of 325 patients had at least one telangiectasia (average 1.7) on this area. It should be remembered that the concha is the only part of the body where the vagus nerve emerges at the surface. Therefore every bit of information gathered at this level regarding diseases and dysfunctions of the internal organs is important. Chinese authors give much more importance to the representation of the bowels and organs than Westerners. They often start the examination of the ear from the concha. Thus when we find telangiectasia on this area, in agreement with the principles of TCM, we should pay attention also to symptoms which do not directly express organic disease. Telangiectasia, however, do not appear regularly over the whole surface of the concha: for example the area facing the external acoustic meatus (sectors 1–2) rarely shows telangiectasia; the same applies to sectors 23–25, but here the scarcity could result from the difficulty of accessing this area for inspection. If we make a cluster analysis we find an asymmetrical distribution of sectors with a significantly higher number of telangiectasia on sectors 13–15 on the right and 12–13 on the left ear. On the right there is a good correspondence with the Chinese liver (CO12 *gan*) (see Plates VA and VIB), as with the Chinese spleen (CO13 *pi*) on the left. We may be surprised, however, to notice the reverse situation on the French map: on the right, sectors 13–15 correspond better to the pancreas and spleen; on the left, sectors 12–13 correspond better to the liver. This difference should never confuse the reader because in the topographical anatomy of the body, the liver keeps its predominant location on the right and the pancreas and spleen have an evident location on the left. What is nevertheless important in my opinion is to remember that on Nogier's original maps the spleen was located below the liver, in the same position where Chinese maps still represent it (see Figs 1.9 and A1.12). The faithful acceptance of Nogier's historical map explains why Chinese authors continue to interpose the liver between the pancreas and

spleen, even if the corresponding meridian does not separate these organs. As regards telangiectasia covering sectors 9 and 10 on the left and 9 on the right as well, it could be supposed that they are associated with some symptoms/dysfunctions of the chest area. If we were to outline the disorders which in 52 patients bearing bilateral telangiectasia of the concha are significantly more represented than in the control group, we would be surprised by their heterogeneity. A higher concentration of telangiectasia is in fact found not only for visceral disorders or symptoms such as IBS, gastritis or dyspepsia (see Plates VB and XIVA), but also for asthenia and anxiety disorders (see Plate VD). Therefore telangiectasia of the concha may express also a tendency toward somatization disorders which have occurred over a period of several years. If we consider patients with telangiectasia only on the right or left ear, we may obtain further information. For example, in 56 patients presenting one or more telangiectasia on the right concha I found, besides the disorders listed above, a significant prevalence of liver disorders and depression ($P<0.001$). Therefore in this case too a link to TCM could be sought, because syndromes such as *Qi* stagnation of Liver or *Yin* deficiency of Liver, according to TCM, can be responsible for both depression and insomnia.

FURTHER SIGNS TO BE OBSERVED ON THE OUTER EAR

Signs were:

1. scales of the concha
2. sebaceous cysts of the concha
3. hypertrophy of the root of the helix
4. groove of the anthelix
5. groove of sector 8
6. drills of the helix.

For this second series of signs two groups of patients were again compared; one bore the specific sign; the other did not and was considered a control group.

1. Scales of the concha

Scales of the concha are often encountered at the inspection of the concha. Sometimes we may come across scales of psoriasis which are flakes of stratum corneum, typically silvery white and lamellated. A further type of scale, called furfuraceous (Latin *furfura*, branlike, scaly), is, however, more often visible in the concha; this type is fine and loose and sometimes detaches during use of the algometer for the pressure pain test (PPT) (see Plate XVIA). It is interesting to note that scales and comedones, even if covering the same areas of the concha, are rarely concomitant. Indeed only in 8 out of 47 patients with more or less extended scales did I also find areas of comedones nearby or interposed. Comedones and scales, as distinct basic dermatological lesions, could therefore represent a clue to different symptoms or tendencies to specific diseases. In the case of scales, dermatitis as well as allergy are still important but the most significant differences found were those regarding dyslipidemia, diabetes and hypothyroidism. Unlike comedones, scales do not have a significant association with symptoms of the psychological/psychiatric area. Scales therefore point to metabolic disorders and it is noteworthy that a diet which improves levels of blood sugar and cholesterol in a metabolic syndrome may clear up or markedly reduce this sign.

2. Sebaceous cysts of the concha

These are rarely seen; however, they may stimulate the attention of the therapist as they may be associated with hyperlipidemia and cholesterol gallstones (see Plate XVD).

3. Hypertrophy of the root of the helix

This has undoubtedly been one of my favorite topics of research. Twenty years ago it was quite common to meet elderly people with a marked cartilaginous hypertrophy causing a rise in the root of the helix. They had usually been suffering from a peptic ulcer over a long period of their life and quite often had undergone Billroth II surgery. After the appearance on the scene of ranitidine there were fewer and fewer people showing a marked hypertrophy (see Plate XIVA); nevertheless I was able to observe a less marked sign in 52 (16%) patients out of 325. This area belongs both to the Chinese ear center (HX1 *erzhong*) and stomach (CO4 *wei*); in Nogier's map it includes the representation of the duodenum, gallbladder and part of the stomach. My impression that this sign could be associated with disorders of the upper digestive system was substantially exact: 53.8% of patients bearing this sign suffered with dyspepsia compared

to 30.4% of the control group; 38.5% compared to 17.9% of the control group had had recurrent gastroduodenitis treated with drugs such as ranitidine and omeprazole.

4. Grooves of the medial surface of the auricle

Grooves of the medial surface of the auricle are often visible, as 137 (42.1%) out of 325 patients showed at least one groove or cartilaginous hypotrophy. This is the most frequent sign to be detected when bending the auricle forwards during inspection. The groove of the anthelix is normally present on the back of the auricle but may appear in some patients as enlarged and deepened. Given the hypothesis that the medial surface of the ear is the representation of anatomical structures of the back of the body, we may assume that the groove of the anthelix is the representation of spinal muscles. Chronic disorders of the lumbosacral tract causing recurrent pain and increasing muscular stiffness could therefore act in a reflex manner on this normally present groove, causing significant enlargement and deepening. I put forward the hypothesis that patients with a deep unilateral or bilateral groove were more affected by back problems as well as hip and knee pain. My hypothesis was partially correct as 47.4% of patients with sciatic pain showed this sign compared to 34% of the control group ($P < 0.005$). Back pain without irradiation to the legs, however, showed no differences. Hip pain could not be considered because the number of patients was too small; patients with knee pain, however, showed a deep groove in 27% compared to 17.6% of the control group ($P < 0.005$). The other symptoms taken into consideration, such as neck pain, cervical–brachial and shoulder pain, showed no significant difference.

There are different patterns of groove: the most frequent is a bowl-shaped depression 8–10 mm in diameter corresponding exactly, on the lateral surface, to the Chinese gluteus (AH7 *tun*) which carries the indications of sciatica, gluteal myofascial pain and pain in the lower extremities (Fig. 4.25, number 1; and see also Plate XIVD). This bowl-shaped depression is often not alone and is combined in 67.1% with other skin alterations such as telangiectasia, maculae and cartilaginous hypertrophy on the same side or bilaterally. It is interesting to note that this bowl-shaped depression corresponds perpendicularly to the representation of

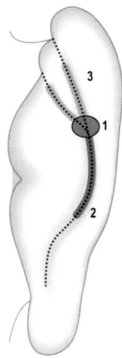

Fig. 4.25 Different aspects of the groove of the anthelix. For their possible clinical significance see the text.

the thoracolumbar tract of the spine. Another frequent pattern of this sign is grooves extending caudally and involving the thoracic and cervical tract of the spine (Fig. 4.25, number 2; and see Plate XIVC). Patients with this sign often have multiple disk lesions caused by lifting heavy loads or by non-ergonomic posture at work. Another less frequent pattern is grooves of the superior and inferior crura of the anthelix which continue upwards from the above-mentioned bowl-shaped area (on the right of Fig. 4.25, number 3). Both are the expression of myofascial pain of the posterior thigh and knee arising from muscles such as gluteus minimus, biceps femoris, gastrocnemius and popliteus.[99] It is understandable therefore that a knee pain, without any documented lesion of traumatic origin, could be localized especially on the superior crus in an area which corresponds, on the lateral surface, more consistently to the Chinese knee (AH4 *xi*) (see Fig. A1.2). However, if we were to consider the standardized areas crossed by the groove of the anthelix, we would notice that neither for heart (P1 *erbeixin*), spleen (P3 *erbeipi*) nor liver (P4 *erbeigan*) do the Chinese report indications for back and sciatic pain. Knee pain could perhaps

be related to the Spleen and Liver meridian covering the internal side of the articulation and having several points to treat relative disorders. However, we must agree that Chinese maps do not remotely consider the possibility of the existence of a somatotopic representation of the body on the medial surface of the auricle corresponding to that on the lateral surface.

In conclusion, the groove of the anthelix in its various patterns may point to several spinal disorders, especially those involving the muscles of the lumbosacral spine and the muscles of both the pelvic and the scapular–humeral girdle.

5. Diagonal groove of sector 8

The diagonal groove of sector 8 (Fig. 4.24, number 5), corresponding to the line of demarcation between the ear lobe and the remaining part of the auricle lying behind, has already been described by the anatomists as a morphological variation (see Fig. 3.10 and Ch. 3). The groove is placed very close to the above-mentioned incisures and drills of the antitragus and scapha, but seems to have a different origin and also consistently different associated symptoms. Nogier's map reports the representation of the cerebellum on the upper part of this groove, and some German authors report several points for treating dizziness and Ménière's disease on this line.[100,101] My hypothesis was that patients carrying this sign could suffer from vertigo and other otologic–vestibular disorders. Indeed, 59.1% of the patients bearing this sign had suffered from vertigo in the past compared to 17.8% of the control group ($P<0.001$). The same significant difference occurred in patients with tinnitus (45.5% vs. 5% of the control group) ($P<0.001$). A diagonal groove of sector 8, as expected with the above described deepening of the anthelix–antitragus notch, was more frequently associated with depression in comparison to the control group, but the difference was not significant.

6. Incisures/drills of the helix

These are rather rare, but are nevertheless very interesting signs because they are involved in the aging process (see Fig. 4.5). It is difficult to know whether this sign can be attributed more to the aging of the vascular, neural and musculoskeletal systems separately or as a whole. With common musculoskeletal symptoms such as lumbago and cervical pain, this is probably the reason why

I could not find any significant difference in 48 patients bearing this sign on one or both auricles when compared to the control group. The helix, as the representation of the spinal cord, according to Nogier, seems often to be involved in neuropathic pain syndromes such as herpes zoster (see Fig. 3.20) or chronic pain as in the case of herniation of the intervertebral disk or as the outcome of vertebral fractures. The two following clinical cases are examples of incisures or marked drills of the helix associated with different musculoskeletal disorders.

CASE STUDY 1

A 70-year-old male patient had fractured the joint of his right ankle falling from a tree 5 years previously. When the photographs shown in Figure 4.26A1 and A2 were taken the patient had been suffering for 3 months with increasing lumbar pain on the right side. Inspection showed a marked incisure of the right helix (see arrows)

corresponding to sectors 15–18 which was very tender at pain pressure test (PPT). The application of ASP semi-permanent needles on these points was very effective against the pain. The imaging diagnosis carried out afterwards with tomography showed the outcome of a presumed fracture of the L1 vertebra (Fig. 4.26B, C). This case is interesting in my opinion as it represents a dissociation between the early manifestation of auricular skin alterations before an evident pain syndrome was experienced by the patient.

CASE STUDY 2

A 73-year-old male patient had been affected for at least 20 years by persistent neck pain and stiffness with frequent dizziness. The patient did not suffer from hypertension or hyperlipidemia which could be considered as a frequent co-factor

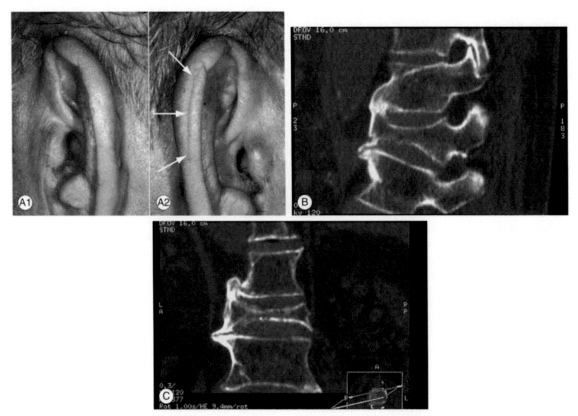

Fig. 4.26 (A2) Long incisure of the upper part of the right helix in a 70-year-old male patient with a compression fracture of L1 in his past history. (B, C) CT multiplanar reconstruction of L1 in the same patient: moderate impingement on spinal cord and reactive osteophytosis of the vertebral body, in sagittal view (B); in coronal view (C) (courtesy of Dr Gianna Zanfranceschi).

in the elderly. Auricular inspection showed a series of incisures mainly on the left helix, on the inferior part (Fig. 4.27A), some of which were sensitive to PPT (Fig. 4.27B). An X-ray and a CT multiplanar reconstruction of the cervical spine showed marked degenerative changes of all cervical vertebrae with a narrowing of the intervertebral foramina, especially on the left-hand side (Fig. 4.27B, C).

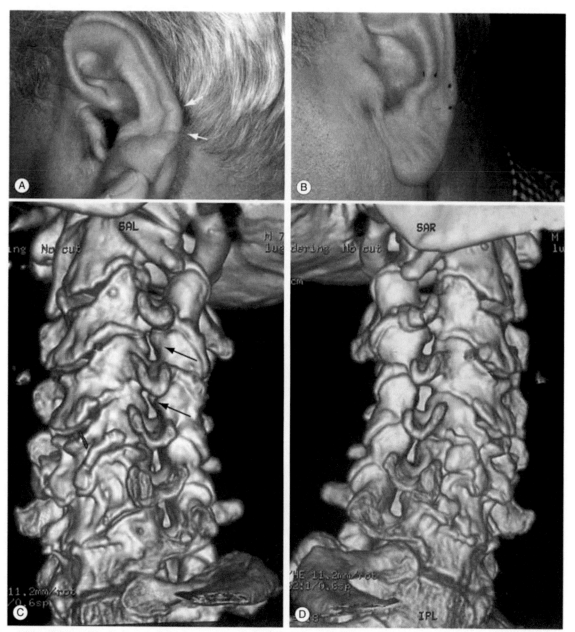

Fig. 4.27 (A) Multiple incisures of the lower part of the helix (see arrows) in a 73-year-old male patient with chronic neck pain and dizziness. (B) Multiple tender points marked with ink identified in the same patient with PPT. (C, D) CT multiplanar reconstruction of cervical spine in the same patient: degenerative disease with narrowing of all intervertebral foramina especially on the left side (see arrows); left oblique sagittal view (C); right oblique sagittal view (D) *(courtesy of Dr Gianna Zanfranceschi).*

WHAT INFORMATION CAN INSPECTION OF THE CHINESE SHEN MEN AND WIND STREAM AREAS YIELD?

In some cases the acupuncturist can identify zones which do not have anatomical descriptions but functional or metaphorical names. This is the case for Shen men (TF4 *shenmen*) and Wind stream *fengxi* at the juncture of areas SF1 and SF2.

1. **Shen men** was probably described for the first time by Dr Xu Zuo-Lin of Beijing and located on the upper part of the posterior third of the triangular fossa (see Fig. 1.11).

Shen means mind, spirit, consciousness; *men* means door, gate. This name is familiar to acupuncturists because meridian point HT7 bears the same name. As known, this point is located on the transverse wrist crease, in the small depression between the pisiform and ulnar bones. HT7 calms the spirit, regulates and invigorates the heart. Auricular Shen men has a similar activity to HT7, but shows a broader range of therapeutic effects which Dr Huang[80] classified in the following order:

- relieving pain (it was one of the most commonly used points for auricular acupuncture anesthesia or hypalgesia)
- relieving convulsion
- relieving cough
- relieving asthma
- relieving itching
- relieving vomiting
- tranquilizing the mind
- lowering blood pressure
- reducing heart rate
- relieving sore throat.

Even if TCM concepts and the indications of HT7 can help us to appreciate the value of auricular Shen men, there is in my opinion an issue regarding the physiological explanations for this area. Neither Nogier nor his pupil René Bourdiol ever accepted this point because apparently it had no anatomical or embryological consistency. Nevertheless, Shen men was progressively accepted and introduced in several Western maps. Even so, the puzzle still remains and only hypotheses can be put forward. My observations on this topic went essentially in two directions: first I took into consideration the segmental topography of Shen men

by means of Nogier's alignment principle; then I clinically examined patients who bore a particular sign in this area.

As regards the hypothesis about the correspondence of Shen men to a specific part of the body, we can assert that this area is covered by Nogier's radii of TH12–L2 (see Fig. 3.19). A second segmental clue comes from the overlapping of other anatomical structures, as, for example, in the case of Figure 4.28, a young man with a painful inguinal hernia who had a cluster of very sensitive points overlapping with the Shen men area. Immediately after intervention the tenderness began to reduce and a day later it had completely disappeared. If we consider the segmental innervation of the inguinal zone of the abdominal wall, we see again the twelfth thoracic and first lumbar segment.

A third segmental clue, which in my opinion may explain the complex influence of Shen men, is the anatomy and functions of the sympathetic system in the abdomen. This system is located at the level of the first and the second lumbar

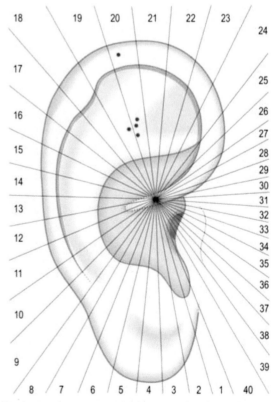

Fig. 4.28 Tender points in 24-year-old patient before surgery for acute inguinal hernia.

vertebrae and was called the 'intestinal brain' by the ancient anatomists. Several ganglia and plexuses, variable with respect both to their number and to their exact location, lie on the ventral surface of the aorta and surround the origins of the celiac and superior mesenteric arteries, extending caudally as far as the level of origin of the renal arteries. All these plexuses are continuous cranially and caudally with other subsidiary plexuses creating a large neural supply to organs and anatomical parts such as the aorta, diaphragm, stomach, liver, small and large intestine, adrenal gland, kidney, ovary, etc.

From the clinical point of view, I tried to obtain further information from observing a particular telangiectasia of the Shen men area which corresponds to a penetrating branch of the posterior auricular vein accompanying the homonymous artery (see Plates IVC and VIA). I found a one-sided or bilateral telangiectasia in 84 (16.6%) out of a group of 506 patients examined blindly. As this telangiectasia is often a longstanding skin alteration and does not bleed on puncture, I thought it could be a sign of chronic dysfunctions and diseases. Therefore I noted from the patients' case histories recurrent symptoms and the relative duration. I was not surprised to find lumbar–sciatic pain ($P<0.001$) most often, and knee pain very near to significance, since Shen men is very close to representations of both the lumbar spine and the knee joint. Other symptoms which do not have a topographic correlation with the neighboring zones seem more related to pain syndromes and functional disorders such as dysmenorrhea, tension type headache and dyspepsia (Table 4.11). Out of 84 patients, 41.8% had at least one tender point close to the telangiectasia and 39.5% at least one point of reduced electrical resistance (Agiscop with modality −).

In conclusion, it can be said that if we assume that the Shen men area does not correspond to a macroscopic anatomical structure, we need to imagine for it the representation of a system regulating several functions of the body. In my opinion we could presume this area to be connected with an essential part of the autonomic nervous system. If we accept this hypothesis, the abundance of indications described by Chinese authors for this area becomes more intelligible. Moreover, treatment of the Shen men area seems promising in patients with vegetative disorders of psychosomatic origin.

2. **'Wind stream'** is one of the few metaphorical names retained by the Chinese standardized nomenclature for a point called *fengxi* which is located at the juncture of scapha areas SF1 and SF2. In 1989 the China Academy of TCM considered this point rather as an area overlapping SF2; its function was to eliminate Wind-dampness and reduce itching. Several hypotheses can be put forward regarding the possible correlations with meridian points LI4 *hegu* and LI11 *quchi* which are often sensitive at palpation in cases of allergy. The common indications for *fengxi* are urticaria, eczema, allergic rhinitis and bronchial asthma. This is the area in which Marc Yu has located his 'hypersensitive point' which he indicated for all forms of hypersensitive condition.[102]

In my opinion the larger size of the urticaria area proposed by the China Academy of TCM seems to fit its diagnostic importance better (see Fig. 5.29). This area, extending itself caudally to the elbow zone and including the aligned portion of the helix, is in my experience one of the most important for confirming an allergic condition or for offering

Table 4.11 Disorders significantly associated with the presence of telangiectasia of the *shen men* area in 506 patients

Disorder	Telangiectasia of *shen men* area (79 patients)	No telangiectasia (427 patients)	P
Lumbar-sciatic pain	42	158	<0.001
Dysmenorrhea	12	24	<0.001
Tension type headache	24	83	<0.05
Allergy	33	127	<0.05
Dyspepsia	37	140	<0.05

Table 4.12   Disorders significantly associated with the presence of telangiectasia and/or hyperemia of the *fengxi* area in 325 patients

Disorder	Telangiectasia and/or hyperemia of *fengxi* area (84 patients)	No telangiectasia or hyperemia (241 patients)	P
Allergy	46	64	<0.001
Food intolerance	38	46	<0.001
Constipation	37	64	<0.001
Dermatitis	21	31	<0.001
Phobias	40	85	<0.05

indications, in an apparently symptom-free subject, of a predisposition to the future development of allergies. Moreover, despite the uncertain boundaries that prevail between food allergy and food intolerance, I consider this area to be associated also with a tendency towards hypersensitivity to food. The inspection of the outer ear, but also the PPT or the electrical examination of the outer ear, may be useful in this type of preventive diagnosis.

With regard to the inspection of the outer ear, care must be taken in identifying a vascular skin alteration such as hyperemia and telangiectasia in the area of the wrist and the elbow (see Plate IIIA). The corresponding part on the opposite surface of the ear seems to carry this sign more frequently (see Plate IVB) and I found it in 54.7% of patients with documented allergy and 45.2% of subjects with suspected food intolerance. The relative percentages of the control population without this sign were respectively 26.5% and 19.1% and the difference was highly significant ($P<0.001$). A further significant prevalence was also found in patients with constipation and dermatitis ($P<0.001$) (Table 4.12). It is surely not necessary to remind the reader that most perceived adverse reactions to food are not immune mediated and are not reproducible. This issue is made worse by the fact that the non-conventional methods used for diagnosing food intolerance are often unproven. Common symptoms such as headache, fatigue, difficulty in concentrating, myalgia, arthralgia, bloating, stomach ache and loose stool thus risk being insufficiently considered or being classified as a psychosomatic disorder. When examining the patient we should take into consideration the possibility that at least some of the symptoms may be associated with hypersensitivity or intolerance to one or more types of food. In this first phase questionnaires and scales may help the general practitioner as well as the patient who is invited to 'remember' some of these associations.

In conclusion, the practitioner, detecting a hyperemia or telangiectasia on the Chinese *fengxi* area or on the corresponding area on the medial surface, may be able to confirm the patient's allergy or suspect a tendency to it. The same findings may be of help in identifying patients with food intolerance, especially if the areas mentioned are sensitive to PPT or show a reduced electrical resistance.

References

[1] Glas N. Das Antlitz offenbart den Menschen. Vol 1. Stuttgart: Mellinger Verlag; 1992.

[2] Nogier P. Die Akupunktur der Ohrmuschel. DZA. 1957;7–8:87–93.

[3] Maciocia G. Diagnosis in Chinese medicine. Edinburgh: Churchill Livingstone; 2004.

[4] Compiling Group of Nanking Military Headquarters. Ear acupuncture. Shanghai: People's Publishing House; 1973.

[5] Practical ear-needling therapy. Hong Kong: Medicine and Health Publishing; 1982.

[6] Roccia L. Agopuntura auricolare cinese. Saluzzo: Minerva Medica; 1978.

[7] Nguyen J. Sémiologie des LCP auriculaires. Mens Med Acup. 1982;92:853–60.

[8] Getis A, Ord JK. The analysis of spatial association by distance statistics. Geographical Analysis 1992;24:189–206.

 [9] Ord JK, Getis A. Local spatial autocorrelation statistics: distributional issues and an application. Geographical Analysis 1995;27:286–306.

[10] Frank ST. Aural sign of coronary artery disease. New Engl J Med. 1973;289:327–8.

[11] Lichstein E, Chadda KD, Dayanand N et al. Diagonal ear lobe crease: prevalence and implications as a coronary risk factor. New Engl J Med. 1974;290:615–6.

[12] Mehta J, Hamby RI. Diagonal ear lobe crease as a coronary risk factor. N Engl J Med. 1974;291:260.

[13] Christiansen JS, Mathiesen B, Andersen AR et al. Diagonal ear lobe crease in coronary heart disease. N Engl J Med. 1975;293:308–9.

[14] Andresen AR. Diagonal ear lobe crease and diabetic retinal angiopathy. N Engl J Med. 1976;21:1182–3.

[15] Rhoads GG, Klein K, Yano K et al. The earlobe crease sign of obesity in middle-aged Japanese men. Hawaii Med J. 1977;36:74–7.

[16] Kaukola S. The diagonal ear-lobe crease, a physical sign associated with coronary heart disease. Acta Med Scand. 1978;619(Suppl.):1–49.

[17] Moncada B, Ruíz JM, Rodríguez E et al. Ear-lobe crease. Lancet 1979;1(8109):220–1.

[18] Kristensen BO. Ear-lobe crease and vascular complications in essential hypertension. Lancet 1980;1(8162):265.

[19] Shoenfeld Y, Mor R, Weiberger A et al. Diagonal earlobe crease and coronary risk factors. J Am Geriatr Soc. 1980;27:184–7.

[20] Chen WC, Zhao TM, Xue W et al. Ear-lobe crease, high serum cholesterol and human leukocyte antigen, risk factors in coronary artery disease. Chin Med J. 1982;95:839–42.

[21] Pasternac A, Sami M. Predictive value of the ear-crease sign in coronary artery disease. CMA Journal 1982;126:645–9.

[22] Gral T, Thornburg M. Earlobe crease in a cohort of elderly veterans. J Am Geriatr Soc. 1983;31:134–6.

[23] Elliott WJ. Earlobe crease and coronary artery disease: 1,000 patients and review of the literature. Am J Med. 1983;75:1024–32.

[24] Wagner RF, Reinfeld HB, Wagner KD et al. Ear-canal hair and the ear-lobe crease as predictors for coronary-artery disease. N Engl J Med. 1984;311:1317–8.

[25] Gibson TC, Ashikaga T. The ear-lobe crease sign and coronary artery disease in aortic stenosis. Clin Cardiol. 1986;9:388–90.

[26] Toyosaki N, Tsuchiya M, Hashimoto T et al. Earlobe crease and coronary heart disease in Japanese. Heart Vess. 1986;2:161–5.

[27] Brady PM, Zive MA, Goldberg RJ et al. A new wrinkle to the ear-lobe crease. Arch Intern Med. 1987;147:65–6.

[28] Lesbre JP, Castier B, Tribouilloy C et al. Signe de Frank et maladie coronarienne. Ann Cardiol Angéiol. 1987;1:37–41.

[29] Kenny DJ, Gilligan D. Ear-lobe crease and coronary artery disease in patients undergoing coronary arteriography. Cardiology 1989;76:293–8.

[30] Verma SK, Khamesra R, Mehta LK et al. Ear-lobe crease and ear-canal hair as predictors of coronary artery disease in Indian population. Ind Heart J. 1989;2:86–91.

[31] Romagnosi G. Piega diagonale del lobo auricolare e rischio coronarico: studio dei parametri biochimici in una popolazione non selezionata. Padova: Tesi A. I.R.A.S.; 1989–1990.

[32] Tranchesi B, Barbosa V, Albuquerque CP et al. Diagonal earlobe crease as a marker of the presence and extent of coronary atherosclerosis. Am J Cardiol. 1992;70:1417–20.

[33] Moraes D, McCormack P, Tyrrell J et al. Ear-lobe crease and coronary heart disease. Ir Med J. 1992;4:131–2.

[34] Petrakis NL. Earlobe crease in women: evaluation of reproductive factors, alcohol use, and Quetelet index and relation to atherosclerotic disease. Am J Med. 1995;4:356–61.

[35] Kuon E, Pfahlbusch K, Lang E. The diagonal earlobe crease for evaluating coronary risk. Z Kardiol. 1995;84:512–9.

[36] Elliott WJ, Powell LH. Diagonal earlobe crease and prognosis in patients with suspected coronary artery disease. Am J Med. 1996;100:205–11.

[37] Miric D, Fabijanic D, Giunio L et al. Dermatological indicators of coronary risk: a case-control study. Int J Cardiol. 1998;67:251–5.

[38] Motamed M, Pelekoudas N. The predictive value of diagonal ear-lobe crease sign. Int J Clin Pract. 1998;5:305–6.

[39] Davis TM, Balme M, Jackson D et al. The diagonal ear-lobe crease (Frank's sign) is not associated with coronary artery disease or retinopathy in type 2 diabetes: the Fremantle Diabetes Study. Aust N Z J Med. 2000;30:573–7.

[40] Dharap AS, Sharma HS, Than M. Ear-lobe crease: incidence in a healthy Malay population. Anthrop Anz. 2000;3:309–15.

[41] Evrengül H, Dursunoülu D, Kaftan A et al. Bilateral diagonal earlobe crease and coronary artery disease: a significant association. Dermatology 2004;209:271–5.

[42] Bahcelioglu M, Isik AF, Demirel B et al. The diagonal ear-lobe crease as sign of some diseases. Saudi Med J. 2005;6:947–51.

[43] Celik Ş, Erdoğan T, Gedikli Ö et al. Diagonal ear-lobe crease is associated with carotid intima-media

thickness in subjects free of clinical cardiovascular disease. Atherosclerosis 2007;192:428–31.

[44] Lichstein E, Chapman I, Gupta PR et al. Diagonal ear-lobe crease and coronary artery sclerosis. Ann Intern Med. 1976;85:337–8.

[45] Cumberland GD, Riddick L, Vinson R. Earlobe creases and coronary atherosclerosis – the view from forensic pathology. Am J Forensic Med Pathol. 1987;1:9–11.

[46] Kirkham N, Murrels T, Melcher DH et al. Diagonal ear-lobe crease and fatal cardiovascular disease: a necropsy study. Br Heart J. 1989;61:361–4.

[47] Ishii T, Asuwa N, Masuda S et al. Earlobe crease and atherosclerosis: an autopsy study. J Am Geriatr Soc. 1990;38:871–6.

[48] Patel V, Champ C, Andrews PS et al. Diagonal ear-lobe crease and atheromatous disease: a post-mortem study. J R Coll Phys. 1992;26:274–7.

[49] Edston E. The earlobe crease, coronary artery disease, and sudden cardiac death. Am J Forensic Med Pathol. 2006;2:129–33.

[50] Omura Y. The effects of electrical and non-electrical acupuncture on cardio-vascular and nervous systems, and pre- and post-acupuncture evaluation of patients, including valuable visible diagnostic signs, such as the 'abnormal cardio-vascular sign of the ear lobules'. Acup Electrother Res. 1978;3:223–50.

[51] Nguyen J, Lambert G, Diem Chi T. Valeur sémiologique du sillon du lobe de l'oreille: revue générale et discussion. Rev Fr Méd Trad Chin. 1984;103:467–70.

[52] Chinese Medical Association and Nanjing Medical University. Chinese Classification of Mental Disorders. 2nd ed., revised (CCMD-2R). Nanjing: Dong Nan University Press; 1995.

[53] Lee S. Cultures in psychiatric nosology: the CCMD-2-R and international classification of mental disorders. Cult Med Psych. 1996;20:421–72.

[54] Lee S. Diagnosis postponed: Shenjing Shuairuo and the transformation of psychiatry in post-Mao China. Cult Med Psych. 1999;23:349–80.

[55] Bourdiol RJ. Elements of auriculotherapy. Moulins-les-Metz: Maisonneuve; 1982.

[56] Romoli M, Tordini G, Giommi A. Diagonal ear-lobe crease: possible significance as cardio-vascular risk factor and its relationship to ear-acupuncture. Acup Electrother Res. 1989;14:149–54.

[57] Krug SE, Scheier IH, Cattel RB. IPAT anxiety scale ASQ. Champaign (Illinois): Institute for Personality and Ability Testing; 1976.

[58] Rosenman RH, Friedman M, Straus R et al. A predictive study of coronary heart disease: the Western Collaborative Group Study. JAMA. 1964;189:15–26.

[59] Fan AZ, Strine TW, Jiles R et al. Depression and anxiety associated with cardiovascular disease among persons aged 45 years and older in 38 states of the United States, 2006. Prev Med. 2008;5:445–50.

[60] Bleil ME, Gianaros PJ, Jennings JR et al. Trait negative affect: toward an integrated model of understanding psychological risk for impairment in cardiac autonomic function. Psychosom Med. 2008;3:328–37.

[61] Narita K, Murata T, Hamada T et al. Associations between trait anxiety, insulin resistance, and atherosclerosis in the elderly: a pilot cross-sectional study. Psychoneuroendocrinology 2008;3:305–12.

[62] Narita K, Murata T, Takahashi T et al. The association between anger-related personality trait and cardiac autonomic response abnormalities in elderly subjects. Eur Arch Psychiatry Clin Neurosci. 2007;6:325–9.

[63] Narita K, Murata T, Hamada T et al. Interactions among higher trait anxiety, sympathetic activity, and endothelial function in the elderly. J Psychiatr Res. 2007;5:418–27.

[64] Romoli M, Poggiali C, Vettori F. A contribution to the study of new areas of the ear lobe for the diagnosis and treatment of essential headache. Min Riflessoter Laserter 1984;2:61–82.

[65] Oleson TD, Kroening RJ, Bresler DE. An experimental evaluation of auricular diagnosis: the somatotopic mapping of musculoskeletal pain at ear acupuncture points. Pain 1980;8:217–29.

[66] Romoli M, Poggiali C, Candidi Tommasi A et al. Inspection of the outer ear and diagnosis of diseases of the esophagus, stomach and duodenum. Min Riflessoter Laserter 1987;1:7–14.

[67] Kincannon J, Boutzale C. The physiology of pigmented nevi. Pediatrics 1999;4(Suppl. 2):1042–5.

[68] Nogier PFM. Handbook to auriculotherapy. 2nd ed. Brussels: SATAS; 1998.

[69] Bañuls J, Climent JM, Sanchez-Paya J et al. The association between idiopathic scoliosis and the number of acquired melanocytic nevi. J Am Acad Dermatol. 2001;1:35–43.

[70] Bañuls J, Ramon R, Guijarro J et al. Segmental arrangement of multiple, partly congenital, and partly acquired melanocytic nevi. Eur J Dermatol. 1998;8:80–2.

[71] Cote P, Kreitz BG, Cassidy JD et al. A study of the diagnostic accuracy and reliability of the Scoliometer and Adam's forward bend test. Spine 1998;7:796–802.

[72] Romoli M, Matucci C. L'inspection de l'oreille en acupuncture auriculaire: corrélations entre les pigmentations mélaniques et les dysmorphies squelettiques. Fifth International Symposium of

Auriculotherapy and Auriculomedicine. Lyons: 4–8 October 2006.

[73] McRae R. Clinical orthopaedic examination. Edinburgh: Churchill Livingstone; 1976.

[74] Gurney B. Leg length discrepancy. Gait Posture 2002;15:195–206.

[75] Nogier P. Le pavillon de l'oreille. Zones et points réflexes. Bull Soc Acup. 1956;20:51–7.

[76] Nguyen J, Lambert G, Trong Khanh N. Valeur sémiologique de la segmentation de la conque cymba: étude clinique et hypothèses sur la LCP génèse. Rev Fr Méd Trad Chin. 1984;105:594–7.

[77] Nguyen J. La nature de la lesion cutanée ponctuelle (LCP) a-t-elle sa valeur sémiologique propre? Rev Fr Méd Trad Chin. 1983;96:85–98.

[78] Romoli M, Vettori F. Alterations in the skin of the auricle and correlation with chronic diseases. Min Riflessoter 1982;73:725–30.

[79] Zhu Dan, Tian Ming. Changes of visual findings, electric features and staining of auricles in malignant tumor patients. J Trad Chin Med. 1996;16(4):247–51.

[80] Huang Li-Chun. Auriculotherapy – diagnosis and treatment. Bellaire: Longevity Press; 1996.

[81] Manetti M, Romoli M, Fiorentini GM. The skin alterations at the inspection of the outer ear in oncologic patients. Vinci: European Traditional Medicine (ETM) International Congress; 4–6 October 2007.

[82] Maciocia G. The practice of Chinese medicine. Ch. 28, 'Abdominal masses'. Edinburgh: Elsevier; 2008.

[83] Romoli M, Fiorio R, Rogora GA et al. Why is clinical research on acupuncture in psychiatric disorders so lacking? Considerations and suggestions based on a survey among Italian GPs and psychiatrists. Min Med. 2005;3(Suppl. 2):7–13.

[84] Academy of Traditional Chinese Medicine. An outline of Chinese acupuncture. Beijing: Foreign Languages Press; 1975.

[85] Advanced textbook on traditional Chinese medicine and pharmacology. Vol. IV. Beijing: New World Press; 1997.

[86] Chen HY, Shi Y, Ng CS et al. Auricular acupuncture treatment for insomnia: a systematic review. J Altern Complement Med. 2007;6:669–76.

[87] Suen LK, Wong EM. Auriculotherapy with magnetic pellets produces longitudinal changes in sleep patterns of elderly patients with insomnia. J Altern Complement Med. 2007;3:306–7.

[88] Cabioglu MT, Ergene N, Tan U. Electroacupuncture treatment of obesity with psychological symptoms. Int J Neurosci. 2007;5:579–90.

[89] Mora B, Iannuzzi M, Lang T et al. Auricular acupressure as a treatment for anxiety before extracorporeal shock wave lithotripsy in the elderly. J Urol. 2007;1:160–4.

[90] Karst M, Winterhalter M, Münte S et al. Auricular acupuncture for dental anxiety: a randomized controlled trial. Anesth Analg. 2007;2:295–300.

[91] Wang SM, Punjala M, Weiss D et al. Acupuncture as an adjunct for sedation during lithotripsy. J Altern Complement Med. 2007;2:241–6.

[92] Barker R, Kober A, Hoerauf K et al. Out-of-hospital auricular acupressure in elder patients with hip fracture: a randomized double-blinded trial. Acad Emerg Med. 2006;1:19–23.

[93] Wang SM, Gaal D, Maranets I et al. Acupressure and preoperative parental anxiety: a pilot study. Anesth Analg. 2005;3:666–9.

[94] Wang SM, Maranets I, Weinberg ME et al. Parental auricular acupuncture as an adjunct for parental presence during induction of anesthesia. Anesthesiology 2004;6:1399–404.

[95] Kober A, Scheck T, Schubert B et al. Auricular acupressure as a treatment for anxiety in prehospital transport settings. Anesthesiology 2003;6:1328–32.

[96] Suen LK, Wong TK, Leung AW et al. The long-term effects of auricular therapy using magnetic pearls on elderly with insomnia. Complement Ther Med. 2003;2:85–92.

[97] Wang SM, Kain ZN. Auricular acupuncture: a potential treatment for anxiety. Anesth Analg. 2001;2:548–53.

[98] Bahr FR. Primitivrezepte und medikamenten-vergleichbare Punkte in der Ohrakupunktur. DZA. 1978;4:109–12.

[99] Travell JG, Simons DG. Myofascial pain and dysfunction – the trigger point manual. Vol. 2. Baltimore: Williams and Wilkins; 1992.

[100] Lange G. Akupunktur der Ohrmuschel. Schorndorf: WBV; 1987.

[101] Pildner von Steinburg R, Pildner von Steinburg D. Die Behandlung der zentralen vestibulären Dysfunktion mittels Akupunktur (Reflextherapie). HNO Praxis Heute 1983;3:161–7.

[102] Yu M. Auricular acupuncture. Academy of Chinese Acupuncture; 1987.

Chapter 5

The pressure pain test

INTRODUCTION

In his tireless work on the nature of the auricular representation of the body Paul Nogier used a variety of methods to obtain what he called the 'reactional information' of every subject. Both evoked pain in the pinna at palpation and the application of cold and heat were repeatedly used for diagnostic purposes. For example he used the cold test, applying a rod of cold copper on the anthelix to localize any vertebral blockage. In this case he often found a reduced cold sensation on the representation of the vertebrae concerned which disappeared as soon as the blockage had been corrected with manipulation.

Nogier nevertheless realized that the most readily available technique for determining the reactivity of auricular reflex points was palpation and pressure pain test (PPT) applied to specific areas of the auricle. He wished, however, to approach this topic scientifically, so with his collaborator Bourdiol set up an experiment which is easy to realize and reproduce and which is now part of the history of ear acupuncture[1] (Fig. 5.1). The procedure was as follows:

1. The auricular area representing the thumb was first repeatedly tested with the pressure-probe to ensure it was not sensitive.
2. A clamp was placed on the tip of the thumb so that the subject experienced a local sensation of pinching. During the next few minutes the somatotopic area of the thumb became sensitized and one point was hyperalgesic at palpation, while the other areas remained neutral.
3. In the minutes following removal of the clamp, the auricular point lost its tenderness and repeated application of the pressure-probe no longer evoked any pain.

This experiment by Nogier and Bourdiol was repeated by Alimi[2] applying functional magnetic resonance imaging (fMRI). The aim of the study was to examine the hypothesis that there are specific neurophysiological connections between ear acupoints and the central nervous system (CNS). A dynamometric clamp was calibrated at 2 kg/cm² to induce a nociceptive stimulation of the thumb. To identify the auricular reflex points, instead of the pressure-probe an electronic microvoltmeter (Pointoselect DT+, manufactured by Schwa-medico) was used, selecting the points

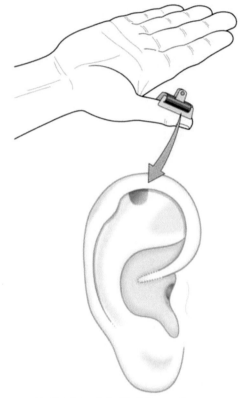

Fig. 5.1 Nogier-Bourdiol's historic experiment on evoked pain on the pinna *(with permission)*.

which had a variation of more than 3 SDs from the basic value of the auricular potential for every subject. Five paradigm stimulations were performed and real time fMRI brain signals were recorded in 10 healthy volunteers:

1. at rest
2. during tactile stimulation of the right thumb at a frequency of 2 Hz
3. during tactile stimulation of the right auricular thumb representation identified previously by electrical detection
4. after the insertion of three gold needles to a depth of 3 mm into the right thumb auricular site, without stimulation
5. during mechanical stimulation of the needles at 2 Hz frequency.

The recordings lasted 5 minutes, with alternating periods of stimulation and rest, for 30 seconds each. To avoid any interference between the different signals, there was a 10-minute rest period between every sequence.

The results of Alimi's experiment were that for 9 out of 10 subjects the stimulation of the needles produced a significant MRI signal, superimposed on that obtained by tactile stimulation of the thumb, on the presumed somatotopic projection of the thumb in the S1 somesthesic area. In three subjects recordings were obtained bilaterally; two of them showed the same phenomenon during tactile stimulation of the thumb.

We tried to repeat Alimi's work reintroducing Bourdiol's procedure: the auricular area representing the thumb was tested repeatedly 2 hours before fMRI with the pressure-probe to ensure its insensitivity.[3] By immediately afterwards applying a dynamometric clamp calibrated at 2 kg/cm^2, we identified the most tender point in the thumb area and marked it with ink. The subjects were right-handed healthy volunteers and we chose the left non-dominant thumb for the experiment. The following six recording sequences were carried out:

1. at rest
2. during active movement of the left thumb (Fig. 5.2A)
3. during tactile stimulation of the left thumb at a frequency of 2 Hz (Fig. 5.2B)
4. during the pressure stimulation of the left auricular thumb point with a blunt probe of 1 mm^2 (Fig. 5.2C)
5. after the insertion of a titanium semi-permanent ASP needle, without stimulation
6. during the mechanical stimulation of the needle at a frequency of 2 Hz (Fig. 5.2D).

Figure 5.2A shows the activation of motor region M1 on the contralateral (right) side during sequence 2; Figure 5.2B shows the activation of the primary

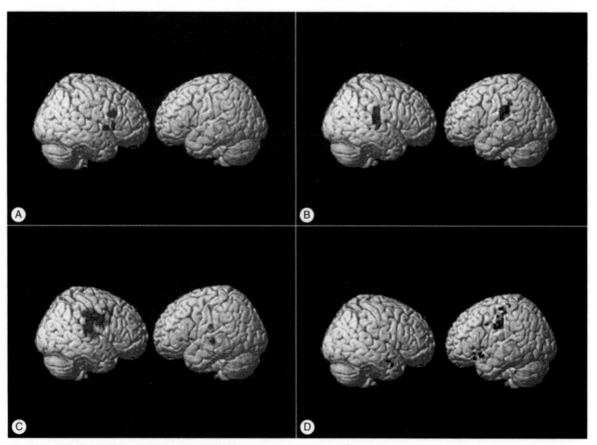

Fig. 5.2 Cerebral activity recorded with fMRI in a 30-year-old female: (A) during active movement of the left thumb; (B) during tactile stimulation of the left thumb; (C) during the pressure stimulation of the left auricular thumb point; (D) during the mechanical stimulation of the needle placed on it. *(Courtesy of William Liboni, Gradenigo Hospital, Turin, Italy.)*

somatosensory cortex S1, during sequence 3, on the contralateral but also on the ipsilateral (left) side. The acupressure stimulation of the left auricular thumb point in sequence 4 as well as the mechanical stimulation of the inserted needle in sequence 6 demonstrate that the information is processed in several areas: the right somatosensory S1–S2 and frontal–prefrontal supplementary motor area cortices are activated during acupressure, whereas the ipsilateral primary somatosensory and motor areas are more focally activated during sequence 6.

In our first cases we found that the stimulation of the auricular thumb point produces a more diffused activation than the tactile stimulus or the motion of the thumb. At the present time we find that the insertion of the needle in our cases demonstrates that the information is processed overall on somatosensory areas ipsilaterally or in both hemispheres. Our research is still ongoing and we do not know yet how far our findings will overlap with those of Alimi. Functional MRI does indeed appear to be an interesting method for deeper acquaintance with the reflex activity on the CNS induced by auricular stimulation, but of course the observation of a higher number of cases is necessary.

THE PALPATION OF THE AURICLE

Palpation of the outer ear can be carried out by anyone. Even the patient can learn to find the sensitive points of his auricle easily and massage them for relieving, for example, musculoskeletal pain.

Palpation can be carried out with the patient lying down, which is the ideal position for inducing maximum relaxation; it can also be done with the patient in the sitting or standing position. For all these positions it is best if the therapist places himself behind the patient and presses both ears simultaneously and symmetrically between the thumb and the index finger. The therapist should regulate the pressure according to the patient's sensitivity: certain people react only to strong pinching, whereas others react to the slightest compression. The whole pinna should be explored, taking care to follow all of the cartilaginous irregularities. When such investigation is rendered impossible through the anatomy, for example at the level of the concha, one may press bilaterally with the index fingers, being careful to do this in an identical fashion.

Identifying a painful point at palpation is a good start in the examination of a patient but there are several aspects to be considered before proposing a diagnostic hypothesis. The first issue to clarify is the exact meaning of the identified area: for example we do not know if the area is the expression of an acute problem or of a chronic, recurrent disorder. Another possibility is that the painful point could represent a symptom hitherto not manifested.

Sometimes a persistent sensitivity of the auricle may indicate a functional disorder: in this case it is important to verify possible tenderness of the auricular zones such as the concha, the incisura intertragica, the ear lobe, etc. which are more often related to visceral, endocrinal and psychosomatic disorders. It is obvious that Chinese acupuncturists give a lot of importance to these areas since traditional Chinese medicine (TCM) is able to reveal dysfunctions before they manifest.

Another important aspect is the variability in the number of detected areas and their relation to the tender points of the auricle to which to apply therapy. The number of painful points identified by thumb and index finger palpation is very variable and depends on several factors such as the general sensitivity of the subject, the number of symptoms and districts involved, the intake of drugs, etc. I examined 92 consecutive patients from my general practice and randomly alternated palpation and the PPT with a commercially available pressure-probe of 250 g maximal pressure (Sedatelec). The reason for the random application was to exclude any possible mutual interference between the two methods. The number of painful areas, however, ranged from 0 to 21 (average 5.1) but was not significantly different from the average of tender points (average 5.7). Each area could contain from 1 to 4 sensitive points, but what is interesting in my research is that only in 55.7% of the identified areas could I isolate at least 1 tender point.

The meaning of this observation is that for every case the therapist should try to localize the points hidden in each tender area at palpation; however, in about half of the cases he will not detect any point at all. It is possible, however, that a repeated examination of the area with the pressure-probe or the application of an instrument with higher maximal pressure (for example 400 g) may finally detect one or more tender points.

CASE STUDY

A 37-year-old female patient came for examination because she had been suffering with persistent headache of the frontal and nuchal region for a week. She was in her 20th week of pregnancy and did not wish to take any painkillers. She had never suffered from migraine before nor had any member of her family. The palpation of her auricles evidenced in total nine tender areas, three on the right (A) and six on the left (B) (Fig. 5.3). Four of these areas hid a tender point: three of them were directly related to her pain syndrome; the fourth, on the left stomach area, was included into treatment because she had suffered frequently with dyspepsia, both before and during pregnancy. Her pain score was 7 on the verbal numeric scale (VNS) at the beginning, and dropped to 4 after treatment, but a further point was needed (see arrow) for the pain to disappear.

As regards the areas which did not hide any tender point, I interpreted these as important, but less important with respect to the current pain syndrome. The two left areas of the right ear were correlated with the period of anxiety and worry experienced by the patient in relation to problems at work and especially with her husband's health problems: he had undergone a heart operation some months before. The spleen area (or alternatively the area of Nogier's sympathetic cervical ganglia) was also correlated with the patient's emotional problems: indeed her pulse frequency was 95–100/m. The last areas to interpret were those of the large intestine and hemorrhoids on the left helix which I correlated with her current constipation and a tendency to piles which was undemonstrated but possibly associated with pregnancy.

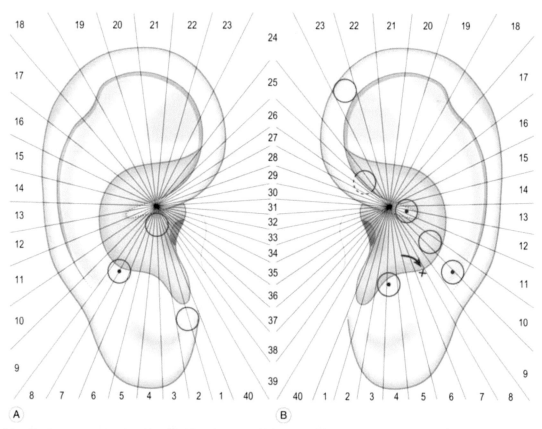

Fig. 5.3 Tender areas and points identified in a 37-year-old female, with, respectively, the thumb-index finger technique (circles) and pressure-probe of 250 g maximal pressure (dots). The arrow indicates a tender point on the internal (hidden) border of the antitragus.

WHAT IS THE SIGNIFICANCE OF A PAINFUL POINT ON THE EAR?

This question is not easy to answer since there are several confounding factors which may influence the tenderness of the auricle. Nevertheless we can assume that a healthy person, well balanced from the psychophysical point of view, shows a reduced number of tender points at PPT. We cannot, on the other hand, accept the reverse statement, since there are people who in certain circumstances, or for particular diseases, demonstrate a negative auricle.

Another confounding factor may be related to the normal functions of the body. Portnov, for example, observed that in 90% of healthy subjects the bladder point was sensitive. It was, however, sufficient to invite these people to empty their bladders to see an evident reduction of this tenderness.[4]

A further example is Bourdiol's[1] observation of a variation in auricular reactivity during digestion; in the hours following ingestion of food he was able to describe the auricular areas sensitized subsequently by the digestive process such as stomach, duodenum, gallbladder, liver, etc.

To verify the hypothesis that a healthy subject has a lower number of points compared to other subjects with any type of disorder, I examined a consecutive group of patients attending my general practice. My aim was to find a possible association between the presence of sensitive points and the scoring of the General Health Questionnaire (GHQ), developed by Goldberg for the screening of minor mental disorders in the field of general and community medicine. It is an easily understandable questionnaire, validated in several languages, which proposes a series of questions on general health during the preceding weeks. A significant correlation was found between the intensity of the health disorder and the GHQ scores.[5,6]

I examined 121 consecutive subjects of my practice with the reduced form of GHQ (30 items) and I obtained a significant regression line between the number of tender points and the GHQ score (Fig. 5.4). We may therefore assume that a tender point does not indicate only the suffering of the corresponding structure of the body, but more generally a psychophysical indisposition which may be only slightly expressed.

WHAT IS THE AVERAGE PAIN THRESHOLD FOR PRESSURE ON THE AURICULAR POINTS?

So far, a systematic study of the pain threshold of the different parts of the ear has never been carried out. One reason is perhaps that a consensus has

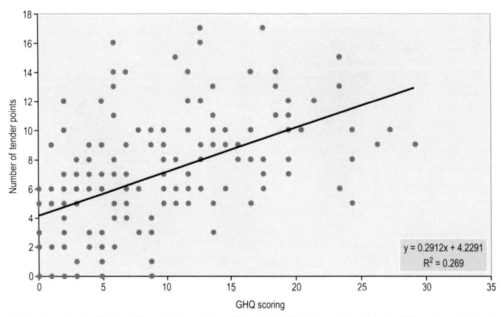

$y = 0.2912x + 4.2291$
$R^2 = 0.269$

Fig. 5.4 Regression line between GHQ scoring and the number of auricular tender points in 121 consecutive subjects.

never been reached on the methods to measure the degree of sensitivity felt when pressure is applied. Probably the simplest way is to ask the patient to indicate the point which is especially tender with either 'Now' or 'There'. Alternatively, we could use the same range of numerical or verbal responses used by Oleson in his historical article on auricular diagnosis (see Fig. 9.1). He proposed a score of 1–4: 1 for low-level tenderness; 2 for medium-level tenderness; 3 for high-level tenderness; and 4 for extremely high-level tenderness. It is also worth noting the behavior of the patient reacting to the application of the pressure-probe by knitting his brows or demonstrating the well-known 'grimace sign' described by Nogier.

As regards the pressure-probe invented by Nogier, this was composed of a small piston with a cross-section of 1 mm^2 attached to a standardized spring. Practitioners consistently use pressure-probes which exert an intermediate pressure such as 250 g and try to apply them on the majority of the ears they examine. That means that in the case of a particularly sensitive person they will apply half or less than half of the pressure allowed by the instrument, whereas in patients with a high threshold they will probably unconsciously add more than 250 g of pressure.

I have always been concerned about the issue of how to determine the real sensitivity of auricular points. With this in mind I made a preliminary identification of tender points on 41 unselected consecutive patients with Sedatelec's pressure-probe of 250 g maximal pressure. The points were marked with ink and tested again with a Lutron digital dynamometer (model FG 5000 A) which is able to record a pressure from 0 to 5 kg with a precision of 1%. The tip of the probe was blunt and had the same diameter as the above mentioned probe (about 1 mm).

The points tested were 173 (on average 4.2 per patient). Each of them was retested three times consecutively and the average pressure was retained for comparison. I was rather surprised to find that the average threshold of the points was 468 g, almost double that supplied by the blue '*palpeur*' (pressure-probe) which I use regularly in my daily work. The pain threshold was, however, not the same for the different parts of the auricle: the cartilaginous parts in fact showed a higher threshold compared to the non-cartilaginous parts (for example 590 g in the anthelix vs. 385 g in the ear lobe).

The therapist should therefore be aware of this issue and possibly adopt more than one probe, as advised by Nogier himself. For example the complete Sedatelec set is composed of pressure-probes with 130, 400 and 600 g of pressure. It is essential when conducting clinical research to rely on adjusted commercially available instruments rather on self-made pressure-probes.

Another characteristic of the pain threshold of an auricular point is that it may vary when using the probe repeatedly: the threshold usually increases and this reset is probably due to the stimulation provoked by the PPT itself. This phenomenon, which is observable in almost every patient, has also been called 'relativity of tenderness'. In my opinion it is not given sufficient consideration by those conducting clinical research, but may represent an interesting method for selecting points for treatment in a hierarchical order (see section 'Which strategy should be used in selecting points?' in Chapter 10).

ARE THERE OTHER TECHNIQUES FOR EXPLORING THE PINNA WITH THE PRESSURE-PROBE?

Another interesting technique consists of sliding the probe across the skin surface of larger areas of the outer ear. When the tip of the instrument encounters local swellings and cellulite there is a slowdown and sometimes a halt in the sliding movement. Sometimes the area concerned is sufficiently consistent to allow the tip of the probe to jump it. Exactly in these areas one or more sensitive points are hidden which have to be discovered point by point, smoothly and without abruptness, holding the probe perpendicularly to the skin. The combination of sliding–pressure allows the practitioner to save time when he is examining the patient blindly or when the symptoms described by the patient are not clear.

WHAT IS THE GENERAL DISTRIBUTION OF TENDER POINTS ON THE OUTER EAR?

The regular use of the sectogram allows the practitioner to record each patient's location of points from one session to the next.

Since 325 patients examined blindly presented an equivalent number of tender points on the right ear and on the left ear (average 4.2 and 4.4), it would be natural to expect too a fairly equal distribution of points on both ears. This was not the case in my group of patients. Cluster analysis showed an asymmetrical distribution with a larger number of sectors of high value on the left ear (Fig. 5.5).

These asymmetries, which also emerge when applying electrical detection methods, seem to have different origins: the higher concentration of points on the craniocervical area of the body (sectors 5 and 8–11) and on the thoracolumbar area (17–19) may be explained by the relevant number of people who say they have suffered backache and neck pain at least once in their life.

Another hypothesis is that these sectors could correspond to dysfunctions of the autonomic nervous system (ANS) which constantly accompany several health disorders. Even if the ANS seems homogeneously spread out on the whole body we can suppose that some parts of it have a major representation on the auricle, such as the cranial parasympathetic and the cervical sympathetic systems

on sectors 5–11 and the abdominal sympathetic system, also called 'abdominal brain', on sectors 17–19.

The larger number of sectors of high value on the left ear may indicate lateralization phenomena possibly associated with the laterality of cerebral functions of the human brain such as language, handedness, etc. (see Ch. 9).

THE ROLE OF PPT IN IDENTIFYING AREAS RELATED TO SYMPTOMS COMMONLY MET IN PRACTICE: THE MUSCULOSKELETAL SYSTEM

My diagnostic work throughout this chapter is not aiming to replace the existing maps but rather to help the practitioner to detect in every patient the most sensitive points related to his ailments. Musculoskeletal pain disorders are ranked first because they account for 32.7% of the total symptoms identified in my group of 506 patients.

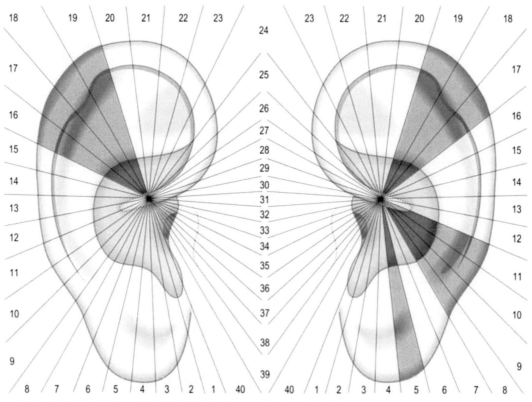

Fig. 5.5 Distribution of tender points and sectors of high value in 325 patients.

There are some important issues which have not yet been fully resolved, for example the different representations of the lower limb and the 'shorter' representation of the lumbar and cervical tract of the spine.

THE REPRESENTATION OF THE LOWER LIMB

The experienced acupuncturist knows very well that the representation of the lower limb is quite different in the French and the Chinese schools of thought. The Russian school, represented by Ruben Durynian, agreed with the Chinese and located the lower limb on the upper branch of the anthelix. The French map shows clearly that the lower and upper limb are separated by a neutral area, whereas on the Chinese map they are represented as being close together. The latter somatotopic arrangement is very similar indeed to that drawn by Bachmann in the first historical map of the ear (see Fig. 1.9). Some other drawn parts coincide with the later Chinese map, as for example the toe (AH2 *zhi*), whereas others coincide with the later French map, such as the heel; the knee was, however, reproduced on the boundary line between the fossa triangularis and the anthelix.

I would also like to direct the reader's attention to some other somatic areas of Bachmann's drawing which were faithfully reproduced on the standardized Chinese map, such as shoulder (SF4 and SF5 *jian*), clavicle (SF6 *suogu*), abdomen (AH8 *fu*) and chest (AH10 *xiong*) (see Fig. A1.2).

I made my contribution to the question of the representations of the lower limb by identifying the tender points using a pressure-probe of 250 g on selected patients affected by pain disorders on the different parts of the lower limb. Figure 5.6 shows the tender areas related to heavy coxarthrosis (nine cases), knee sprain (10 cases), ankle sprain (10 cases) and toe pain of traumatic origin (12 cases). As can be seen, the distribution of tender points, even in such small groups of patients, allows the identification of some partially overlapping areas which extend themselves from the fork of the upper and lower branch of the anthelix to the internal border of the helix. The axis of orientation of these areas lies in the middle, between the Chinese and French representations of the lower limb: it is possible therefore that both representations are valid, but also that the point to treat for a specific disorder needs to be identified case by

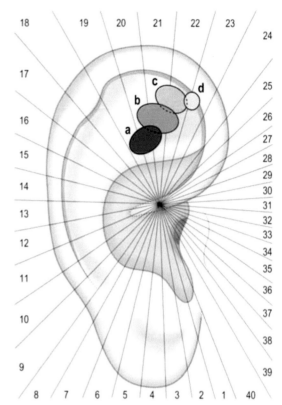

Fig. 5.6 Representation of some parts of the lower limb affected by painful disorders: a = osteoarthritis of the hip joint; b = knee sprain; c = ankle sprain; d = toe pain of traumatic origin.

case. Another possibility, however, is that different parts of the anatomical structure represented on the ear may have a different topography coinciding more with one map than with the other. This hypothesis was forwarded by Caterina Fresi using the needle contact test (NCT) for identifying the origin of knee and ankle pain. From her study it is possible that a knee pain caused by the injury of the medial capsule–ligament complex may sensitize sectors 21 and 22, whereas a disorder of the lateral complex may sensitize sectors 20 and 21. In a similar way a lesion of the medial malleolus of the ankle may correspond to sector 22, whereas the lateral malleolus appears to be represented more on sector 21 (see Fig. 8.5).

THE REPRESENTATION OF THE THORACOLUMBAR SPINE

As regards the 'shorter' representation of the thoracolumbar spine on the Chinese maps, the divergence with Bachmann's reproduction of the spine is still mysterious. The puzzle is that both schools agreed with the representation of sciatic nerve but never reached a consensus on the representation of these parts of the spine. Nogier carried out what is probably the most accurate study, identifying single vertebrae of the thoracolumbar tract, one by one, through his system of radii centered on point 0 (see Fig. 3.19). Chinese acupuncturists, on the other hand, on the maps published before standardization, placed the lumbosacral vertebrae where Nogier located the thoracic tract of the spine. The neurophysiologist Durynian reproduced the thoracolumbar spine in his work in a similar way to the Chinese maps. On the standardized map the lumbosacral vertebrae (AH9 *yaodizhui*) occupy a large area of the anthelix which is separated from the sciatic area by the gluteus area (AH7 *tun*). This area seems to be a key area for the treatment of every kind of backache, even if Bachmann drew the gluteus point very close to that which was historically cauterized for sciatic pain.

I have always been intrigued by this issue, asking myself why the Chinese spine was 'shorter' than the French one. Racial differences were absolutely not to be considered, whereas a different interpretation of back pain could be presumed. It should be remembered that lumbago arising from the facet joints of the thoracolumbar region is indeed common and erroneously attributed to pathological changes in the lower back.

One of the authors who has faced this issue systematically for many years is Robert Maigne.[7,8,9] He demonstrated that this pain commonly stems from the irritation of the lateral branch of the posterior ramus of the lower thoracic and/or the first lumbar spinal nerves, carrying motor and sensory fibers. Classically the cutaneous innervation of the lower lumbar and gluteal regions has been attributed to the cutaneous branches of L1–L2–L3. Anatomical dissections have shown, however, that the cutaneous innervation of the gluteal region originates more often from the lateral branches of the posterior rami of the nerves of T11–T12–L1[7] (Fig. 5.7).

From the clinical point of view Maigne indicated that the palpation of the iliac crest, where the lateral branches emerge on the surface, evokes a sharp pain which is similar to the patient's complaint. In these areas he also noted a thickening and hypersensitivity of the skin and the subcutaneous tissues, folding them gently between the thumb and forefinger (skin-rolling test).

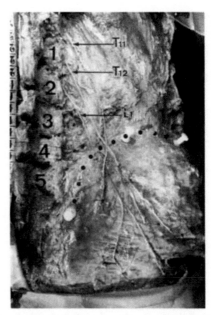

Fig. 5.7 Anatomical dissection showing the lateral branches of the posterior ramus of T11, T12 and L1 spinal nerves crossing the iliac crest and innervating the upper part of the gluteal area. The iliac crest is marked with black dots and white pins *(with permission of Robert Maigne).*

Maigne confirmed the relation between the thoracolumbar tract of the spine and the iliac–gluteal region by a diagnostic block, injecting a solution of procaine 1 cm lateral to the spinal process directly into the joint region. After the injection, when the diagnosis of 'thoracolumbar junction syndrome' (TLJS) was correct, the backache disappeared and the skin-rolling test was subsequently negative. Maigne[8,9] examined 320 patients with lumbago and found 138 patients with TLJS, 120 with low back pain (L4–L5 or L5–S1) and 62 of mixed origin.

Before the diagnostic block, however, he systematically examined the spine segments from T9 to L5 with the patient prone. One of the most reliable methods for determining the source of pain was pressure applied by the thumb on the spinal processes both vertically and laterally, either from right to left or vice versa. Once a clear tenderness was elicited on one side, the contralateral side was challenged with the so-called 'opposed thumbs technique' on the upper and lower level (Fig. 5.8). As one of these movements provoked

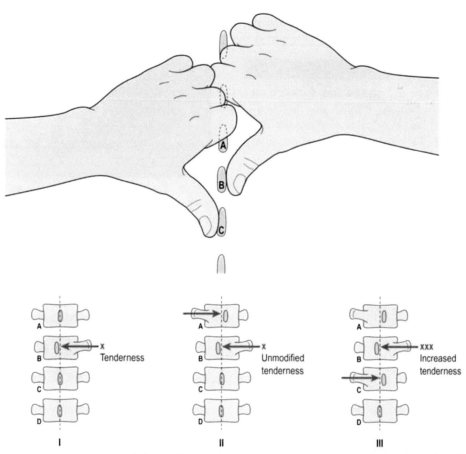

Fig. 5.8 'Opposed thumbs technique' of Maigne for the diagnosis of 'minor intervertebral derangement' (MID). The application of thumbs on spinal processes B and C is represented in the upper part; tenderness is elicited in (I); tenderness in (II) is unmodified with opposed thumbs on A and B; tenderness in (III) is increased with opposed thumbs on B and C *(with permission of Robert Maigne).*

an increase in pain, the involvement of the two vertebrae was diagnosed by Maigne as a 'minor intervertebral derangement' (MID). In the group of 138 patients with TLJS mentioned above, 59.4% presented one MID, 26.1% two MID and 14.5% three MID. The first group showed MID at various levels, but in 75.6% the vertebrae involved were T11–T12 and T12–L1 (Table 5.1).

It has to be remembered that an MID with a chronic irritation of the anterior branch of the 12th thoracic and 1st lumbar spinal nerves may also provoke referred pain in the abdomen which may be erroneously attributed to ovary, appendix or kidney.

When considering how to contribute to the issue of the 'short' lumbar spine I realized that the only possible way was to check the tenderness of the auricle before and after manipulation. Therefore I

Table 5.1   Location of the 'minor intervertebral derangement' (MID) according to Maigne in 82 patients with thoracolumbar junction syndrome (TLJS)

MID	Level	%
MID (1 level)	T9–T10	4.9%
	T10–T11	12.2%
	T11–T12	41.5%
	T12–L1	34.1%
	L1–L2	7.3%
	Total	100%

identified the MID with the opposed thumbs technique proposed by Maigne in a series of consecutive patients with possible TLJS. To ascertain the exact level of MID I placed in some patients a small metal disc 5 mm in diameter on the most painful spinal process before performing X-ray, as in the following case:

CASE STUDY

A 34-year-old male patient had been suffering for a few days from lumbago without pain radiating to his legs; the pain manifested abruptly after he lifted a weight. The most tender spot at pressure was on the right side corresponding to the spinal process of T11 (see the metallic disc in Figure 5.9). On the auricle of the same side I found one tender point on the anthelix and a second aligned on the helix (Fig. 5.10). After manipulations of the spine, as recommended by Maigne in rotation and extension for the relief of thoracolumbar disorders, the point on the anthelix lost its tenderness whereas the point on the helix remained partially sensitive.

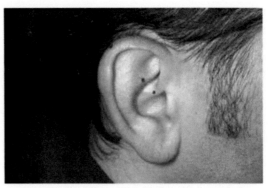

Fig. 5.10   Tender points of the helix and the anthelix, aligned with Nogier's point zero, in the same patient before manipulation.

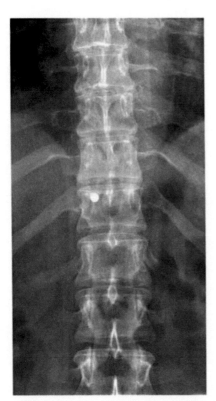

Fig. 5.9   A metal reference marker indicates the identified MID, before spinal manipulation of the thoracolumbar junction, in a 34-year-old male with lumbago without sciatic pain.

This experience permitted me to study a consecutive series of 10 male patients (average age 36.2 years) with lumbago and MID at the level of T11–T12, detecting the tender points before and after the manipulations described in the case study. Before manipulation two-thirds of the points were concentrated on sectors 18 and 19, especially on the anthelix (on the left of Fig. 5.11). After manipulation the total number of points decreased to 44.5% and only sector 19 maintained a higher concentration of points with respect to the other sectors (on the right of Fig. 5.11).

As a control group for my observations I examined 10 male patients (average age 47.6 years) with sciatic pain due to a disk lesion in L5–S1. The tender points were concentrated before the manipulation on sectors 21 and 22 (on the left of Fig. 5.12); after manipulation only sector 22 maintained a higher concentration of points (on the right of Fig. 5.12).

My results appear therefore to support Nogier's hypothesis regarding the representation of the thoracic and lumbar tract, but support also the importance of the Chinese gluteus area on which several tender points overlap, related to either TLJS or sciatic syndrome.

THE REPRESENTATION OF THE CERVICAL SPINE

A minor issue concerns the cervical tract of the spine which seems, like the lumbar tract, to be 'shorter' both on Nogier's and the Chinese map.

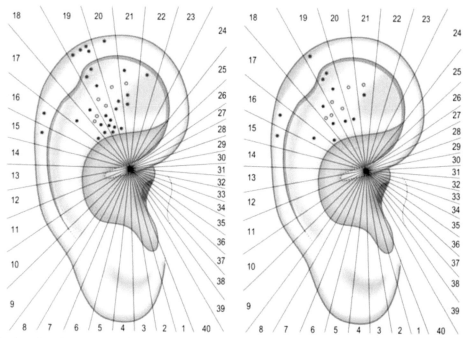

Fig. 5.11 Tender points in 10 male patients, average age 36.2 years, with lumbago associated with an MID in T11–T12, before manipulation (left) and after manipulation (right). Dots = lateral surface; circles = medial surface.

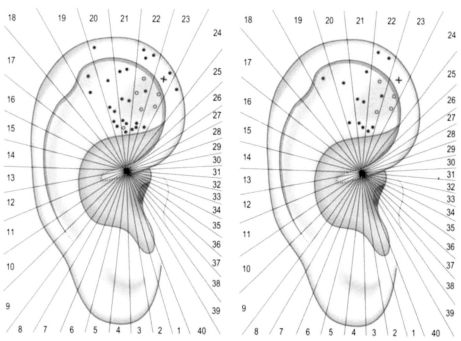

Fig. 5.12 Tender points in 10 male patients, average age 47.6 years, with sciatic pain associated with a L5–S1 disk lesion, before manipulation (left) and after manipulation (right). Dots = lateral surface; circles = medial surface; crosses = internal (hidden) border.

It is possible that the cervicothoracic junction could be represented higher up on the anthelix and the scapha.

My deductions regarding this subject derive from both inspection and pain pressure testing. The former helps us to be aware of the presence of a greater level of telangiectasia, incisures and cartilaginous hypertrophic areas, as expected. For example, in Plate XIVB we have the case of a 60-year-old female who had been suffering from chronic neck pain for many years: a large part of the anthelix showed a thickening of the cartilage and a swelling of the subcutaneous tissues. The affected part of the anthelix was very sensitive to palpation and several points were identified on its surface with the pressure-probe.

The more cranial representation of the lower cervical vertebrae may be appreciated in Figure 5.13 which relates to five female patients with a mean age of 58.2 years suffering from cervical syndrome and radiation of pain consistent with a disk lesion at C6–C7. The distribution of tender points was mainly on sectors 12 and 13 (on the left of Fig. 5.13). In the case of a disk lesion at C7–T1 related points would probably be found above the horizontal line on sectors 14 and 15.

Regarding the cervical spine, for diagnostic and therapeutic purposes we must not forget the points on the internal border of the anthelix related to whiplash syndrome (on the right of Fig. 5.13). Depending on the modalities and strength of impact we may find one or more tender points in this area (representing the cervical sympathetic plexus according to Nogier and Bourdiol) which are very effective on accompanying symptoms such as headache and dizziness (Fig. 5.14).

THE ETIOLOGICAL PUZZLE OF FIBROMYALGIA

The diagnostic criteria of the American College of Rheumatology (ACR) for fibromyalgia syndrome include widespread musculoskeletal pain, morning stiffness and muscle fatigue for at least 3 months,

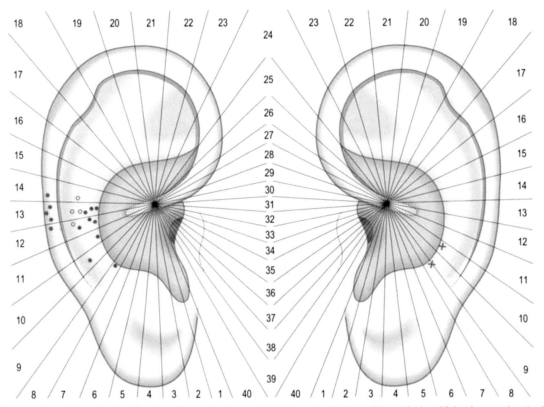

Fig. 5.13 Tender points in five female patients, average age 58.2 years, suffering with cervicobrachial pain associated with a disk lesion in C6–C7 (left); and tender points in a patient with whiplash syndrome (right). Dots = lateral surface; circles = medial surface; crosses = internal (hidden) border.

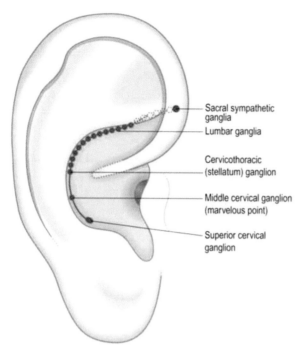

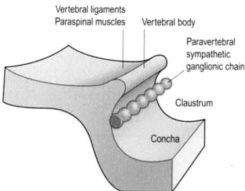

Fig. 5.14   Representation of the sympathetic ganglionic chain according to Bourdiol *(with permission).*

accompanied by pain on palpation in at least 11 of 18 anatomically defined painful tender points.[10] Other well known symptoms commonly observed are non-restorative sleep, depressive/anxious mood, fatigue and headache. The National Arthritis Data Workgroup[11] reviewed published analyses from available national surveys and provided a prevalence estimate for the US of 5.0 million adults suffering with fibromyalgia. The etiology of fibromyalgia is as yet unclear and a co-morbidity has been described with irritable bowel syndrome

(IBS), depression, chronic fatigue syndrome and tension-type headache.

Current hypotheses center on atypical sensory and pain processing in the CNS and dysfunction both of skeletal muscle nociception and autonomic nervous system.[12] Seemingly therapies targeting central pain mechanism should give the best results; this is the reason why the US Food and Drug Administration recently approved pregabalin as the first specific medication for fibromyalgia syndrome.

As regards acupuncture, the systematic review of Mayhew and Ernst[13] concluded cautiously that 'the notion that acupuncture is an effective systematic treatment for fibromyalgia is not supported by the results from rigorous clinical trials. On the basis of this evidence, acupuncture cannot be recommended for fibromyalgia'.

As regards ear acupuncture and fibromyalgia, however, an interesting experiment is currently being carried out by my assistant Dr Riccardo Mazzoni on a group of patients who are members of Scudo Amico (Association for Fibromyalgia) in our city. In a still ongoing pilot study he included 16 selected patients for observation, according to the diagnostic criteria of the ACR (15 females and 1 male with an average age of 49.1 years), and treated them with ear acupuncture. Three patients dropped out of the study: one became pregnant during the therapeutic course and two others had an increase of the severity of pain during the first sessions. The remaining 13 patients received 10 weekly sessions of ear acupuncture. Figure 5.15 shows the distribution of tender points at the first treatment (on the left) and at the last treatment (on the right).

As is visually appreciable, 70% of the points lost their tenderness during the course of the therapy and this variation was accompanied by an evident improvement of scoring in the two scales adopted: the Psychological General Well-Being index (PGWB), a specific function and symptom questionnaire, and the Regional Pain Score (RPS).[14]

Two aspects are interesting in Mazzoni's preliminary observations and are worthy of further exploration: the first is that most points are located on the scapha and particularly on the internal border of the helix. Nogier made the hypothesis that this part of the auricle could be the representation of the intermediolateral nuclei of the lateral horn, the cells of which give rise to the preganglionic sympathetic outflow.

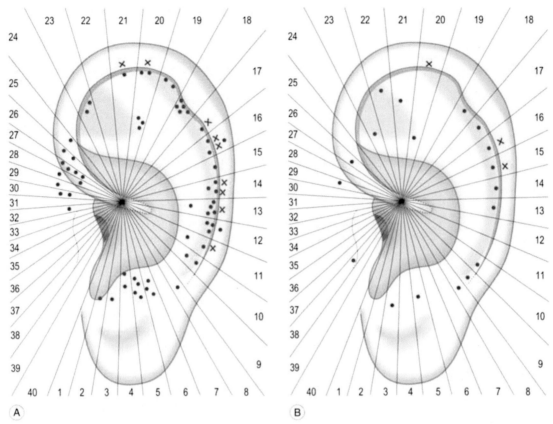

Fig. 5.15 Representation of the tender points in 13 patients with fibromyalgia, at the beginning (A) and at end (B) of a therapeutic course. *(Unpublished data, with permission of Mazzoni).* Dots = lateral surface; crosses = internal (hidden) border.

This line of points, very close to the helix, has been defined by Lange[15] as the 'vegetative groove' and was supposed by the author to be essential for regulating the functions of a disturbed segment of the body according to Nogier's principle of alignment.

The second interesting aspect is that while routinely examining some immunological parameters, high titers (between fifteen- and a hundredfold normal levels) of IgG of cytomegalovirus were found in 14 of the 16 patients. In addition, in two patients a high IgG level of the Epstein–Barr virus was documented. These findings may be fortuitous or may represent a further factor in the etiological puzzle of fibromyalgia. Some authors[16] have indeed reported the possibility that viral infection or vaccination may be associated with this syndrome: the symptoms of fibromyalgia, such as myalgia and fatigue, would therefore appear to overlap considerably with those of a viral or atypical infection.

PSYCHOLOGICAL/PSYCHIATRIC AREAS DETECTED BY PPT

INTRODUCTION

The treatment of mental disorders would seem to be a promising field for acupuncture but there are some important issues which have slowed down research and hindered clinical application. One of these concerns the terminology and international classification of mental disorders (DSM IV) which is being accepted only gradually by Chinese physicians (see also section entitled 'The diagonal ear lobe crease or Frank's sign' in Ch. 4). For example, several textbooks on ear acupuncture still use outdated or obsolete terms such as neurasthenia, neurosis, hysteria and only a few authors use recent terms such as anxiety and/or depression.[17-19]

The reader may consult Figure A1.16 and check for the terms adopted in the standardization process. He will agree that the list of psychological/psychiatric terms is reduced and still incomplete. For example, the indication for depression has been adopted only for the liver area. The situation does not look any better if we examine Nogier's psychological points which appear to be more the result of a process of anecdotal evidence built up over time rather than systematic research on auricular areas and their association with specific mental disorders. The classical points identified by Nogier are those for fear and aggressiveness on the anterior part of the ear lobe; the Jérôme point for depressive disorders on the transition zone between the scapha and ear lobe; the anxiety point on the stomach area; and the internal border of the anthelix for treating dysfunctions of the vegetative system. Something else to remember is the historical line connecting the point of aggression with the so-called omega points which were presumed to regulate psychological stress (ω), visceral stress (ω1) and somatic stress (ω2). A further point for regulating mood was presumably the representation of the hypothalamus on the posterior part of the antitragus[20,21] (see Fig. A1.15).

The neurophysiologist Durinyan,[22,23] presenting an original somatotopic arrangement of the CNS, offered me some interesting clues for the development of my research in the psychosomatic area. He circumscribed the antitragus and the intertragic incisure in the same functional area, considering them as related to the hypophysis, the hypothalamus and the reticular formation (Fig. 5.16). Durinyan's intention was probably to attribute a greater extension to this area, according to the principle of the *homunculus* on the auricle. Interesting, moreover, on his map, are the representation of the frontal lobe on the anterior part of the ear lobe and the representation, in a totally different position to Bourdiol's, of the limbic system on the posterior part of the ear lobe and on the junction with the scaphoid groove (see Fig. 4.13).

STRESS RESPONSE AREAS

Even 20 years ago, when my interest in psychosomatic disorders began to develop, I was disappointed by the lack of rationale and consensus on

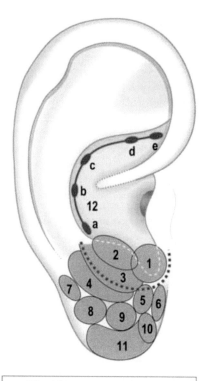

1 = hypophysis
2 = hypothalamus
3 = reticular formation
4 = limbic system
5 = thalamus
6 = frontal lobe
7 = vestibular projections of the cortex
8 = auditory projections of the cortex
9 = visual projections of the cortex
10 = motor projections of the cortex
11 = somatovisceral projections of the cortex
12 = the main sympathetic ganglia: from superior cervical ganglion (a) to lumbar ganglia (e)

Fig. 5.16 Representation of the CNS according to Durinyan. The thick dotted line circumscribes a very large functional area related to the pituitary-hypothalamic system and the reticular formation.

many of the above-reported points/areas. In particular, with a few exceptions, I could not find points which could be clearly defined as having an anxiolytic or antidepressant effect. I became aware, however, when systematically using a pressure-probe to examine patients with symptoms of possible psychosomatic origin, that the auricle presented a more or less constant sensitivity in some specific areas. I started therefore to study the auricular 'stress response' of those patients who associated the onset of symptoms such as tachycardia, dyspepsia and IBS with some particular stressful life events that had occurred in the previous months. Applying tools such as the Paykel scale[24] for life events I was able to measure the number of stressful events that had occurred in the previous 6 months and their objective impact using a five-point scale. I added a distress scale, Kellner's Symptom Rating Test (SRT),[25] which is a combination of subscales scoring anxiety, depression, somatization and inadequacy.

A group of 50 patients with one or more of the functional symptoms mentioned above, for which all possible investigation had been negative, were compared to 20 volunteers without any of those symptoms.[26]

The first group, which I called the 'stress group', showed an average of 2.2 life events compared to 0.9 in members of the control group ($P<0.001$); measuring the number of events scoring a higher objective impact (3–5), as proposed by several studies, I obtained an average of 1.8 events compared to 0.8 in the control group ($P<0.001$). All 70 subjects were submitted to 4 weekly sessions of ear acupuncture and to a control after 6 weeks. The stress group had on average 5.3 tender points compared to 2.4 of the control group; the higher sensitization of the first group was significantly different ($P<0.001$). At the baseline the total score of the SRT was, as expected, higher in the stress group; but the treatment reduced the SRT score significantly at each session from the first to the third. In the control group, however, it was reduced significantly only after the first session.

The first information I obtained from this study, published several years before those of Wang,[27,28] was that ear acupuncture may have a rapidly balancing effect on parameters such as anxiety, depression and somatization. This positive effect is more pronounced in patients with stress-related symptoms, but also measurable in apparently symptom-free subjects.

As one of the characteristic aspects of ear acupuncture during a therapeutic course is the progressive, sometimes very fast drop in the number of tender points, I expected the same effect to occur in the subjects in my stress group. I was surprised to find that the reduction of points was slow and became significant only after the third session. In my opinion this slow fall of sensitization could be related to the time necessary for the body to come out of the stress response and regulate its negative effects on the endocrinal and immune systems.

This hypothesis may be supported by the fact that stress response seems to sensitize the auricles on recurrent areas and some of them have a significantly higher number of points. I identified in 50 subjects with stress response at least nine areas with a variable concentration of points (Fig. 5.17): the first ranked area (number 5, summing 44.9% of the total in the stress group) may be associated with both Triple Energy (CO17 sanjao) and the neighboring endocrinal area (CO18 neifenmi) of the standardized map. This area corresponds to the representation of the hypophysis for Durinyan and the representation of the hypothalamus for Bourdiol (Fig. 5.18). In second place I identified area number 4 (16.3% of the total) on the tragus, which may be associated with the adrenal gland shenshangxian or Nogier's adrenocorticotropic hormone (ACTH) point on the internal wall of the tragus. Next came area number 6 (8.8% of the total), which is rather a broad one overlapping with both the heart (CO15 xin) and spleen (CO13 pi) zones, corresponding on Bourdiol's map to the upper cervical sympathetic ganglia (see Fig. 5.14). In decreasing order came the other zones on the

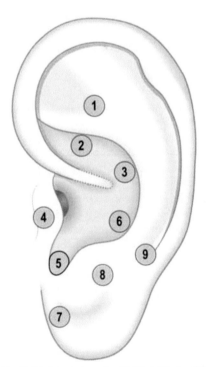

Fig. 5.17   Stress response areas in 50 patients with at least one symptom of possible psychosomatic origin according to Romoli.

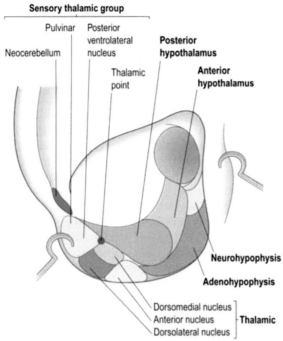

Sensory thalamic group

Pulvinar   Posterior ventrolateral nucleus   **Posterior hypothalamus**

Neocerebellum

Thalamic point   **Anterior hypothalamus**

Neurohypophysis

Adenohypophysis

Dorsomedial nucleus
Anterior nucleus   **Thalamic**
Dorsolateral nucleus

Fig. 5.18 Representation of the pituitary-hypothalamic system on the intertragal incisure according to Bourdiol (with permission).

anterior part of the ear lobe, on the Shen men area, etc. (Table 5.2).

The conclusions of my study were as follows:

The stress response seems to activate certain areas of the outer ear most of which are innervated by the vagus nerve. According to some anatomists, this nerve's field does not limit itself to the cavum and cymba conchae but includes also the tragus and triangular fossa. This sensitization of a parasympathetic territory seems to be in contradiction to the supposed liberation of catecholamines on tissue receptors under stress. But if we consider acupuncture a 'regulation therapy' there is no real sympathetic–parasympathetic contradiction here. The areas of higher density of points are located on the cavum conchae and particularly on the Sanjiao area. We do not know why this area has the name of a meridian whose points are indicated for treatment of dysfunctions of the digestive and the genitourinary systems. It is interesting to note that Sanjiao area borders on other important points such as the 'adrenal gland' and 'endocrine'. Its role, despite its name, seems therefore related to neuroendocrine structures of the brain. Its sensitization during a stress reaction could therefore be consonant with the commonly accepted theoretical and experimental model of stress in which the hypothalamus–hypophysis–adrenal cortex axis is activated.

Table 5.2 Distribution of the total tender points identified in the stress group during 4 consecutive weekly sessions of ear acupuncture and in the follow-up 6 weeks later

Location	No. points right ear	No. points left ear	Total points	%
	Stress group (50 subjects)			
Area 1	36	53	89	6.6%
Area 2	10	14	24	1.8%
Area 3	17	47	64	4.8%
Area 4	77	142	219	16.3%
Area 5	189	415	604	44.9%
Area 6	53	65	118	8.8%
Area 7	69	24	93	6.9%
Area 8	32	21	53	3.9%
Area 9	9	5	14	1.0%
Other	30	38	68	5.0%
Total	522	824	1346	100

For information on the asymmetrical distribution of points with a higher significant concentration on the left, especially for areas 5 and 6, the reader should look at the section entitled 'The symmetrical/asymmetrical distribution of the points on the auricles' in Chapter 9.

SLEEP DISORDER AREAS

A recent survey on sleep disorders in the general population indicated rates of 56% in the US, 31% in Western Europe and 23% in Japan. About 50% of subjects with sleep disorders had never taken any steps to resolve them and the majority of respondents had not spoken to a physician about the problem.[29] The implications of insomnia are a reduced quality of life, decreased productivity and increased absenteeism.[30,31] These patients experience significantly more limited activity than those without insomnia and are a greater burden on health services: overall, annual costs attributable to insomnia in the US have been estimated between $92.5 billion and $107.5 billion.[32,33]

As particularly the elderly are affected by sleep disorders, accurate screening and appropriate therapy could improve general health and well-being provided pharmacotherapy is used cautiously and conservatively.[34] It is therefore possible for a physician to be asked to treat such disorders with non-conventional methods such as acupuncture. With auricular diagnosis the therapist may identify some recurrent areas of the ear which can be included in the treatment for improving the patient's quality of sleep. According to DSM IV, primary insomnia must be distinguished from mental disorders that include it as an essential or associated factor, such as depressive disorders.

Sleep disorders can manifest in several ways, ranging from insomnia to sleepiness and from disrupted sleep to lack of restful sleep. Measuring sleep disorders is an area of active research and several patient-reported outcome instruments exist for measuring various aspects of sleep dysfunction. In the systematic review by Devine and colleagues, four essential physical domains were included: (i) sleep initiation; (ii) sleep maintenance; (iii) sleep adequacy; and (iv) sleepiness during the daytime.[35]

For my research, among the instruments measuring these domains, I selected an adapted version of the Basic Nordic Sleep Questionnaire (BNSQ) used in Scandinavian sleep surveys.

I preferred this questionnaire to, for example, the Pittsburgh Sleep Quality Index (PSQI), because the BNSQ allows the patient to record sleep disorders over the previous 3 months while the PSQI is limited to the previous month.

Of the 11 items proposed by BNSQ, seven concern the first three domains listed above and four measure the various aspects of sleepiness during the daytime; the total scoring ranges from 0 to 44.

I examined 153 consecutive patients from my general practice with an average age of 45.6 years using the BNSQ; 16.1% of them were taking more or less regular medication with benzodiazepines or non-benzodiazepines for inducing sleep.

Since insomnia diminishes the quality of life and interferes with general health, I first made a regression line as with the GHQ and found a moderate positive association between the number of tender points and the BNSQ scoring (Fig. 5.19). Afterwards I attempted to identify those auricular areas that more often seemed to be associated with a poor quality of sleep. Since the literature did not report a cut-off line for scoring better and worse sleepers, I chose an arbitrary level of ≤ 21 for the first group and ≥ 22 for the second. The comparison between the mean number of points per sector with paired sample t-test showed a significantly higher concentration of points on sectors 1, 2, 5 and 8 for the worse sleepers (Table 5.3).

As regards the identified clusters of points, we can appreciate the importance of the anterior ear lobe (sector 1), the forehead area (sector 2) and the significance of the cluster on the posterior part of the antitragus, extending from the anthelix–antitragus incisure toward the end of the scaphoid groove (sector 8). The central pivot area (sector 5), possibly related to mood disorders, cyclothymic personality and fear traits, also appears to be associated with sleep disorders (Fig. 5.20).

PHOBIC ANXIETY ON THE AURICLE

Among anxiety disorders, panic attacks with or without agoraphobia are frequent and auricular diagnosis may confirm the existence of or the tendency to develop this mental disorder. There are certain areas that remain tender to pressure even several weeks after a single panic attack; it is possible, however, that such tenderness may reflect the patient's concern about further attacks (on the left of Fig. 5.21). Another possibility regarding this area may be associated with specific phobias brought

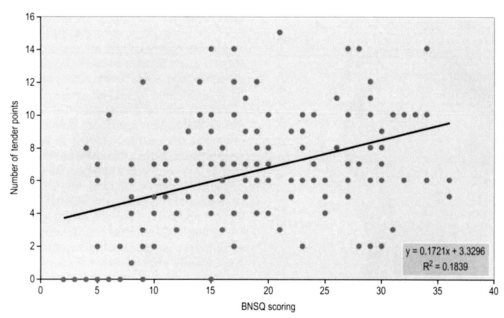

Fig. 5.19 Regression line between the number of auricular tender points and BNSQ scoring in 153 consecutive subjects.

Table 5.3 Paired sample t-test comparing the mean of tender points per sector (right + left ear) in 62 poor sleepers and 91 better sleepers scored with BNSQ

Sectors of the ear	Worse sleepers (BNSQ $\geq$ 22)		Better sleepers (BNSQ $\leq$ 21)		P
	Mean	SD	Mean	SD	
1	0.6	0.78	0.4	0.61	<0.05
2	1.2	1.00	0.5	0.64	<0.001
5	1.0	0.84	0.6	0.70	<0.005
8	1.5	1.13	0.4	0.68	<0.001

on by exposure to a particular feared object or animal, or with phobias provoked by certain types of social situations or performances. From the clinical psychological point of view it is possible to list five types of phobic response: social fears, agoraphobia, fear of physical harm, illness and death, fear of sexual and aggressive scenes and fear of harmless animals. Among the various scales conceived for measuring phobic anxiety with this five-dimensional model is the Fear Survey Schedule III (FSS III) validated by Arrindell[36] and proposed to 11 different countries to determine the cross-national dimensional consistency of self-assessed fears. Subjects were required to indicate the degree of anxiety felt in relation to 52 different stimuli. This was measured on a five-point Likert-type scale ranging from 0 (not at all disturbed) to 4 (very disturbed).

I applied FSS III to 51 consecutive patients in my general practice (31 females, 20 males). Their average age was 41.2 years. None had ever suffered from panic attacks. My aim was to identify the areas that were more often sensitized by the phobic reaction or predisposition of every subject. In addition, their levels of anxiety and depression were measured using the Zung scales for anxiety and depression.[37,38] Comparing the mean distribution of tender points in the two groups with paired sample t-test (respectively with at least 1 and 0 stimuli rated as 'very disturbing'), I identified some areas which were significantly more sensitized on

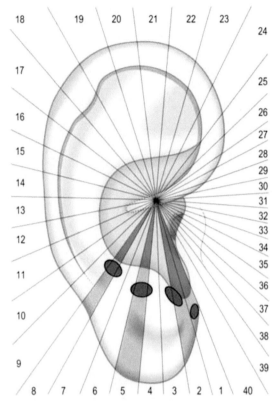

Fig. 5.20 Cluster of tender points in sleeping disorder; the colored sectors are those with a significantly higher concentration of points in the group of worse sleepers compared to better sleepers.

sectors 4, 5, 6, 12 and 39 (on the right of Fig. 5.21). The sensitization of sectors 4, 5 and 6 seems in particular therefore to indicate the possibility of both diagnosing a subject's phobic predisposition and treating patients concerned about a relapse of their panic attacks. It should be noted that subjects with at least one 'very disturbing' phobia were rated as significantly more anxious with the Zung scale for anxiety ($P<0.005$) and more depressed with the Zung scale for depression ($P<0.001$).

THE CO-MORBIDITY OF ANXIETY AND DEPRESSION ON THE AURICLE

Anxiety and depression co-morbidity is quite frequent in epidemiological and clinical settings throughout the world. Patients carrying both diagnoses have the highest utilization of medical services and consequently also incur a higher cost than those with either condition alone, even after

accounting for differences in patient characteristics.[39] There is still no clear evidence that a specific syndrome called 'mixed anxiety and depression' (MAD) exists besides co-morbidity; moreover, this diagnosis may not be stable across time and its utility is questioned by several authors.[40–42]

For the general practitioner it is useful to try to differentiate these conditions and co-morbidity is often found in patients asking to be treated with acupuncture. I tried therefore to make a contribution to this issue and examined the sectors of high value in 90 out of 357 randomly selected patients belonging to two groups of 30, each with self-rated anxiety and depression; the third group was a control group of 30 subjects not declaring any of these symptoms. As reported in Chapter 9, the patients were blindly examined by me after reporting their symptoms on a form and having them checked by an independent assessor.

If we look at the sensitized sites of the auricles in the case of self-rated depression (on the left of Fig. 5.22) and in the case of self-rated anxiety (on the right of Fig. 5.22), at first glance we may have the impression of a simple overlapping of clusters, justifying a diagnosis of anxiety–depression co-morbidity. However, if we consider the relative size of the identified clusters, we may notice that depression presents a threefold sensitization of the areas corresponding to cyclothymic temperament (sectors 4, 5 and 6) and to the external genitals (sectors 25, 26 and 27) according both to Nogier's and the Chinese map. These clusters correspond to two sectors (5 and 26) which are more significantly sensitized in comparison to the control group ($P<0.05$).

The area representing the external genitals seems out of place, but could be associated with difficulties in sexual functioning accompanying mood disorders. In my opinion, however, this area is not only sensitized by the reduction of sexual desire but also by symptoms such as frustration, irritability and increased appetite which develop, for example, in the nicotine withdrawal syndrome after abrupt cessation of cigarette smoking.

If we consider the anxiety group (on the right of Fig. 5.22), we can see a threefold sensitization of an area of the tragus corresponding presumably to the adrenal gland and a remarkable sensitization of the Chinese and French spleen area which seems often involved in anxiety disorders.

These clusters correspond to two sectors (14 and 38) which are more significantly sensitized in

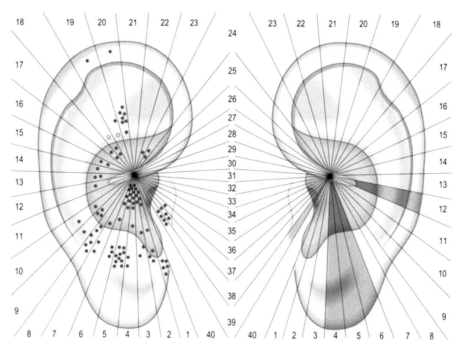

Fig. 5.21 Tender points in 12 patients having experienced at least one panic attack within the previous 6 months (left); colored sectors (right) are the significantly sensitized sectors in 31 subjects with at least one phobic response rated 'very disturbing' at FSS III compared to 20 subjects with no phobic response. Dots = lateral surface; circles = medial surface.

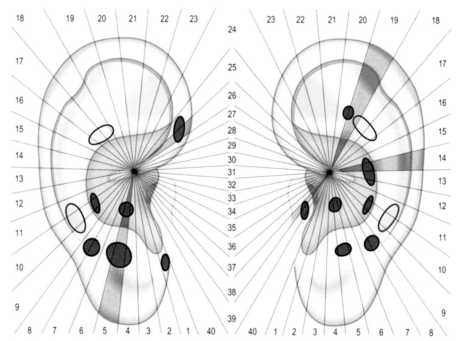

Fig. 5.22 Cluster of tender points and significantly sensitized sectors compared to control group in patients rating themselves 'depressed' on the left; the same for patients rating themselves as 'anxious' on the right.

comparison to the control group ($P<0.05$). Sector 19, moreover, could be related to the stiffness of thoracolumbar muscles or to the activation of the Shen men area which is often associated with somatoform disorders.

I took the opportunity to better differentiate the auricular areas involved with depression and anxiety by a psychometric study on patients in my practice with behavioral eating disorders. Besides the specific scales for this disorder I applied two of the widely used inventories for measuring depression and anxiety, the Beck Depression Inventory (BDI-II)[43] and the State and Trait Anxiety Inventory (STAI-Y) of Spielberger[44] which measures either the state anxiety 'right now, at this moment' (STAI 1) or the trait anxiety which refers more generally to the proneness of the subject to responding to perceived threats in the environment with anxiety (STAI 2). If the reader will permit a brief reminder, possible scores using the BDI-II are: 0–13 for minimal depression; 14–19 for case of mild depression; 20–28 for moderate depression; and 29–63 for severe depression. STAI-Y scores are 0–80 for both inventories.

In a total of 99 patients (80 female and 19 male, average age 41 years) I compared two groups of subjects: those with minimal to mild depression (≤ 19) vs. those with moderate to severe depression (≥ 20). For the scoring of STAI-Y, I carried out a comparison between randomly chosen subjects with a score of ≤ 40 and subjects with ≥ 41.

The paired sample test showed a higher sensitization of sectors 2, 5, 8, 12 and 26 associated with a higher level of depression (on the left of Fig. 5.23) and a higher sensitization of sectors 5, 7 and 8 associated with a higher level of trait anxiety (STAI 2) (on the right of Fig. 5.23).

My group of patients therefore showed an overlapping of areas which corresponds to the clinical evidence of an anxiety–depression co-morbidity or a syndrome with mixed characteristics.

As yet we have not discovered the key for decoding the structures and functions of the brain that could possibly correspond to these auricular

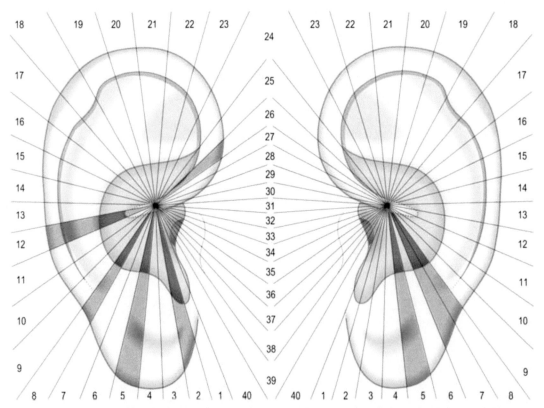

Fig. 5.23 Sectors with a significantly higher number of points in patients rated with BDI-II as moderate-severe vs. minimal-mild depression (left); the same for patients rated with STAI 2 as having higher vs. lower score of anxiety (right).

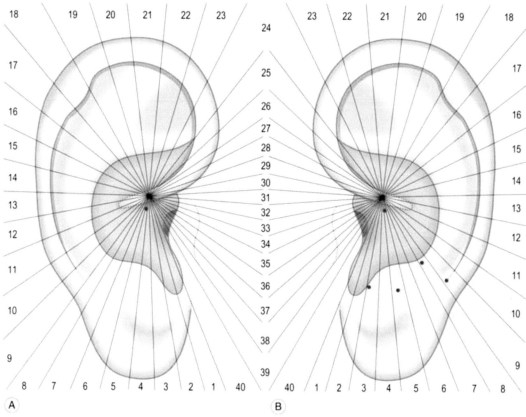

Fig. 5.24 Tender points on the right ear (A) and on the left ear (B) in a 33-year-old female scoring 'very disturbed' to the following fears: crowds, being in an elevator, enclosed places, witnessing surgical operations; scoring 19 (mild depression) at BDI-II and 22 at BNSQ (classified as worse sleeper in this section).

areas and we have to rely upon every tender point we may find in each patient. We need therefore to interpret this syndrome through clinical observation and with the help of some basic psychometric tools, as for example in the following case (Fig. 5.24).

CASE STUDY

The 33-year-old female patient who came to consult me did not show any significant health problem. However, she had lost her father when she was 14 years old and from the ages of 17 to 23 she suffered from panic attacks for which she was treated with psychotherapy. No psychoactive drugs had been prescribed, either during that period or at the time she came for consultation. She felt anxious and tired; moreover her sleep had been disturbed over the last year through nursing her 20-month-old child. PPT revealed a tender point of the mouth–esophagus area on both sides,

which I related to her phobic anxiety. On the left side this point was aligned on sector 5, the same sector with the temple area, representing one of the mood disorder areas. I considered the points on the forehead area (sector 3) and on the brainstem–occiput area (sector 8) in correlation with her poor quality of sleep. I considered the point on sector 9 related to the patient's lack of energy and loss of concentration as the possible expression of a minor depressive disorder. The treatment I applied to these six points, throughout the therapeutic course, reduced her anxiety when she was exposed to particular situations like being in an elevator and significantly improved her quality of sleep. A further positive effect of the treatment was that after the first session the patient was able once again to experience dreaming. This had been impossible during the months of poor quality sleep.

CONCLUSIONS

Summing up this complex subject, I would like to proffer the following conclusions:

1. This is the first study aimed at systematically searching the different auricular areas involved in mental disorders. The identified clusters of points correspond only partially to the areas drawn by the different schools of acupuncture for the treatment of emotional/psychosomatic problems.

2. The identified areas in several cases overlap, indicating a co-morbidity or a common neuro-physiological substrate in the different conditions presented by the patients. However, some areas seem more specific than others in indicating higher levels of anxiety and depression.

3. If we consider the topography of these areas and the relative sectors, we may agree that the posterior part of the ear lobe and the cervical part of the anthelix appear to be important areas for diagnosing anxiety as well as depressive disorders. Another important area seems to be the intertragic incisure and the anterior part of the ear lobe, which may be related to the hypothalamic–pituitary–adrenal axis and to cortical functions such as attention, cognition, appraisal, etc. A further zone between the anterior and posterior part of the ear lobe seems to be related to mood, cyclothymic personality and phobic anxiety. This area is topographically aligned and functionally associated, according to Nogier's principle, with another recurrent area on the inferior concha which seems important for diagnosing the patient's phobic attitude and proneness to panic attacks.

4. Further extensive and systematic study of these areas and their combination is urgently required to find the best therapeutic solutions for our patients with mental disorders. This effort may open up interesting perspectives on a promising application of acupuncture that to date has remained underestimated.

5. In an attempt to find a theoretical model of depression which could possibly fit with the somatotopic mapping reported in this section, we might consider the limbic–cortical dysregulation model proposed by Mayberg.[45] According to this author, across the different PET paradigms searched out in this disorder there is an inverse relationship between the frontal and limbic systems: a decreased activity of the former often corresponds with a relative increase of the latter. The author writes:

the functional state of the depressed brain reflects both the initial insult or functional lesion and the ongoing process of attempted self-correction or adaptation influenced by such factors as heredity, temperament, early-life experiences, and previous depressive disorders. From this perspective, the net regional activity or sum total of various synergistic and competing inputs is what accounts for the observed clinical symptoms. For instance, if frontal hyperactivity is seen, it might be interpreted as an exaggerated and maladaptive compensatory process, manifesting clinically as psychomotor agitation and rumination, whose purpose is to override, at the cortical level, a persistent negative mood generated by abnormal chronic activity of limbic–subcortical structures. In contrast, frontal hypometabolism would be seen as the failure to initiate or maintain such a compensatory state, with resulting apathy, psychomotor slowness and impaired executive functioning as is common in melancholic patients.

HEADACHES AND TRIGEMINAL NEURALGIA ON THE AURICLE

MIGRAINE AND TENSION–TYPE HEADACHE (TTH)

As with mental disorders and DSM classification, the broad spectrum of headaches also needed to be classified with a symptom-oriented classification. The second edition of the International Classification of Headache Disorders (ICHD-2) published in 2004 maintained the three main categories of primary headaches described in the edition of 1988: migraine, TTH, cluster headache and other trigeminal autonomic cephalalgias.

It is important for the practitioner trying to treat these disorders with acupuncture to be familiar with this classification in order to make a differential diagnosis between the first two categories because of their prevalence in the general population. The custom of maintaining the common term 'headache' in acupuncture textbooks is still widespread, even today. This results in auricular charts not reporting different points or areas for treating the two different types of headache. In the Chinese standardized map, for example, the term 'migraine' has been reported only once for the pancreas–gallbladder area (CO11 *yidan*), whereas the indication 'headache' was preferred for other points or areas such as the forehead (AT1 *e*), temple (AT2 *nie*), occiput (AT3 *zhen*), central rim *yuanzhong* and brainstem *naogan*. Moving upwards we find the same indication for Darwin's tubercle (HX8 *jiejie*) and the medial surface of the heart (P1 *erbeixin*), kidney (P5 *erbeishen*) and lower ear root (R3 *xiaergen*). There is no mention on the Chinese map of points to be used for TTH. However,

the neck (AH12 *jing*) and cervical vertebrae (AH13 *jing zhui*) areas, with their indication 'neck stiffness', may be part of the sensitive areas in the case of tension headache, for which previously synonyms such as 'muscle contraction headache', 'psychomyogenic headache', 'stress headache', etc. were used (Fig. 5.25).

Western maps better differentiate between the principal types of primary headaches and several authors report separated sets of points for treating them.[15,46-48]

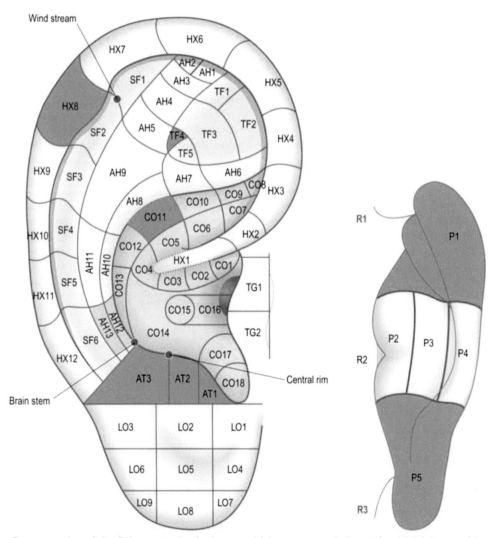

Fig. 5.25 Representation of the Chinese standardized areas which are commonly in use for the treatment of headache (in darker pink); for neck pain and stiffness (in paler pink). AT1 = forehead; AT2 = temple; AT3 = occiput; AH12 = neck; AH13 = cervical vertebrae; CO11 = pancreas/gallbladder; TF4 = Shen men; HX8 = node; P1 = heart of medial surface; P5 = kidney of medial surface; R1 = upper ear root; R3 = lower ear root.

Raphael Nogier[49] reported a specific set of points aimed at diagnosing particular co-factors to be checked in every patient with migraine, such as the oculomotor point pertaining to movements of the eye; the interference of active scars and dental foci according to the principles of neuraltherapy; the irritation due to the so-called 'first rib syndrome' and possible allergy and intolerance to food negatively influencing frequency and intensity of migraine attacks (Fig. 5.26).

My contribution to the issue of differentiating the auricular areas associated with either migraine or TTH was conducted on 90 subjects pertaining to three groups of 30 randomly selected patients; two groups were composed of patients with migraine and TTH; the control group was composed of subjects without these types of headache.

If we look at the sensitized sites of the auricles in the first two groups, at first glance we may have the impression of an overlapping of clusters which is apparently not justified by the different mechanisms on which migraine and TTH are based. If, however, we consider the relative size of the identified clusters, we can see that migraine (on the left of Fig. 5.27) causes a higher sensitization of the antitragus, which is in my opinion the representation of the cerebral vascular system. This area has at least two sectors (3 and 5) which are more significantly sensitized with respect to the control group ($P<0.01$); the first can be correlated with the forehead and the second with the temple area

according to the Chinese map. It is interesting to note the fourfold sensitization of the liver–gallbladder, the threefold sensitization of the elbow and the bigger area of the large intestine compared to the TTH group (on the right of Fig. 5.27). These three areas may be considered correlated, assuming that some of the patients have allergies or food intolerance negatively influencing the normal functions of the liver and the colon.

If we consider the TTH group we can see relatively larger clusters of points on the Chinese occiput, neck and spleen area than in migraine patients; these areas have two sectors in common (8 and 9) which are more significantly sensitized with respect to the control group ($P<0.05$). This sensitization presumably represents the tension of the cervical muscles and, in the observed group, also the tension of the thoracolumbar muscles (on the medial surface of sectors 17–20). It is possible, however, that several factors besides anxiety and depression may cause an increased tension of the cervical muscles, as for example bruxism, dental and sinus foci, after-effects of a whiplash, etc.

TRIGEMINAL NEURALGIA ON THE EAR

As regards the trigeminal system, there is a lack of consensus on the possible representation of this important nerve on the auricle. Durinyan did not report such representation at all whereas Nogier and Bourdiol located the fifth nerve on the border

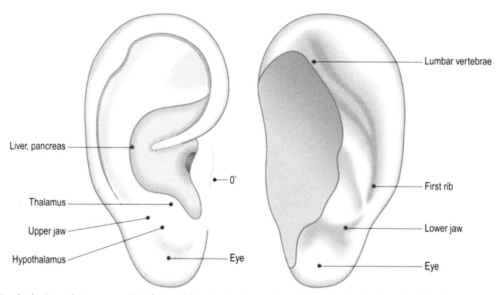

Fig. 5.26   Auricular points proposed by Raphael Nogier for the treatment of migraine *(with permission)*.

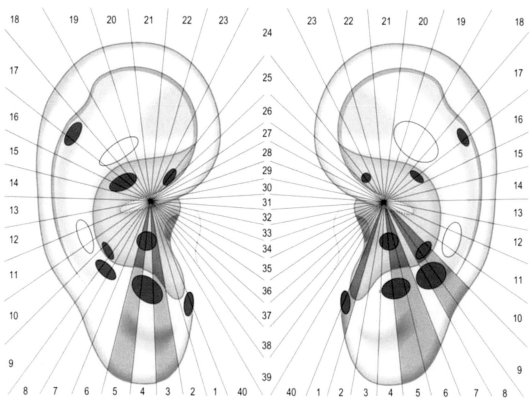

Fig. 5.27 Cluster of tender points and significantly sensitized sectors compared to control group in 30 patients with migraine (left); the same in 30 patients with tension-type headache (right).

of the ear lobe (see Fig. A1.3). The Chinese report only one point/area related to trigeminal neuralgia, the cheek (LO5, 6i *mianjia*) between the eye and the internal ear area. Other areas related to the trigeminal system are the tooth (LO1 *ya*), anterior ear lobe (LO4 *chuiqian*) and jaw (LO3 *he*), which all have toothache as a therapeutic option; interestingly stomach (CO4 *wei*) also has the same indication. The experienced acupuncturist will not be surprised by this indication as he knows that the Stomach meridian starts from the face and with its first seven points covers the neural territory of the second and third trigeminal branch. A further area for treating pain in general is Shen men, which was used extensively in the past in auricular acupuncture hypalgesia for surgical purposes (see Ch. 1).

I was helped by Dr Nicola Brizio in the systematic search for tender points in trigeminal neuralgias of the second and third branch. In his study all atypical facial pain syndromes or any extra-trigeminal pain radiating to the head were excluded. The tender points identified in 21 patients with a

neuralgia of the second branch and in 9 with a neuralgia of the third branch tended to cluster on some areas which were already recognized to be of help in trigeminal pain. The cluster on the lower part of the ear lobe (Fig. 5.28, number 1) tends to overlap with Nogier's trigeminal area, whereas it tends to overlap with the Chinese cheek *mianjia*, eye (LO5 *yan*) and tonsil (LO8 and 9 *biantaoti*); of these points only the cheek point/area holds trigeminal neuralgia as a therapeutic option. The cluster on the antitragus (Fig. 5.28, number 2) can be easily correlated with facial and cephalic pain, and moreover it is aligned with the former on sectors 5–6. What is surprising is the evident sensitization of the auricles on stomach and hand areas (in the same figure, respectively numbers 3 and 4). According to Brizio, who is an experienced acupuncturist in TCM, the sensitization of the stomach area is very common in trigeminal neuralgia as a number of patients suffer commonly with dyspepsia and gastritis. As regards the cluster number 4, we may correlate this concentration of points with

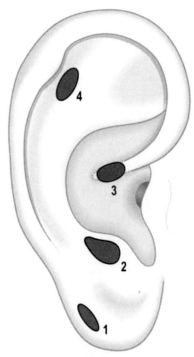

Fig. 5.28 Representation of the sensitized areas of the ear in 30 patients with trigeminal neuralgia (21 of the second branch and 9 of the third branch) according to Brizio.

the Chinese wrist area (SF2 *wan*), which has an indication also for general pain and stomach-ache. A further connection with TCM can be made as tenderness of this area goes in parallel with tenderness at pressure of LI4 (*hegu*), which is an elective point in cases of headache and facial pain.

ALLERGIC CONDITIONS ON THE AURICLE

In the composite world of allergic conditions, the most frequently occurring are rhinoconjunctivitis, asthma, atopic eczema and food allergy, which represent a burden all over the world. In the UK, for example, the rates reported for allergic rhinitis and asthma in the 6th report of the House of Lords were, respectively, 9.4% and 5.5% in an estimated population of 60.6 million. Very close to the rate of asthma was that of atopic eczema and far from negligible was the incidence of infants and adults suffering with food allergy (respectively 5–7% and 1–2%). The incidence of multiple allergies (asthma, eczema and allergic rhinitis together) was also significant (3.7%) and showed an increase of 48.9% between 2001 and 2005.[50]

This affects other countries as well as the UK and there is a worldwide increase, for example in symptoms of allergic rhinoconjunctivitis, especially in the 13–14-year-old age group. This suggests that environmental influences on the development of allergy may not be limited to early childhood.[51,52]

As is known, the main environmental factors associated are exposure to infections and allergens during early childhood, atmospheric pollution and dietary changes. The importance of these factors may explain why 54.3% of the 10 508 US subjects represented in the Third National Health and Nutrition Examination Survey (NHANES III), and undergoing prick-puncture skin tests to 10 allergens, were positive to one or more indoor and outdoor allergens.[53]

Besides the need to individuate the allergens responsible for symptoms as soon as possible, there is also the issue of adequately controlling the disease. For example, according to the Global Initiative for Asthma (GINA) 2006 guidelines,[54] asthma is considered controlled if all the following conditions are fulfilled: diurnal respiratory symptoms less than once a week and no asthma attacks in the last 3 months, no activity limitations (work and other activities) in the last 12 months, no nocturnal symptoms in the last 3 months, short-acting β_2-agonists twice or less per week in the last 3 months and no use of oral steroids in the last 12 months, and a FEV_1 of 80% of predicted value or greater. Although the results of clinical trials demonstrate that asthma control can be reached in most patients, epidemiological evidence suggests poor control of the disease in many subjects: for example 49% of European[55] asthmatic adults using inhaled corticosteroid had uncontrolled asthma and 53% of Canadian[56] patients, despite the effort made in disseminating guidelines, showed suboptimal asthma control and management.

Both sensitization to allergens and poor control of allergic disease are conditions that may be recognized by examining the auricle with PPT. However, the reader should be prepared to find a false-negative auricle as drugs and other remedies may cancel the existing tender points. On the other hand he should not be confounded by a false-positive diagnosis in a patient who is asymptomatic and apparently non-allergic. It is possible in such cases that allergy has still to manifest itself, or more often that the patient is carrying a lifelong contact allergy to nickel or that his organism stores the memory of one or more episodes of urticaria due to the intake of drugs or foods. The diagnostic clues offered by auricular diagnosis are, however, of two types: the sensitization of some recurrent non-specific areas, regardless of the type of allergy, and the sensitization of some specific areas associated with the end organ involved in the allergic mechanism. We may therefore note that in a limited number of cases there is an evident sensitization of sectors 16, 17 and 18 on the scapha and on the aligned points on the helix. What was said in Chapter 4 regarding the possibility of individuating an 'allergic constitution' in patients who have not yet presented allergic symptoms is also applicable to PPT diagnosis.

As already mentioned, the identified areas correspond to the representation of the wrist and elbow, areas which never have been related to allergy before. On the Chinese map, however, the 'Wind stream' point *fengxi*, which carries the whole repertory of indications such as asthma, allergic rhinitis, eczema, urticaria and itching of uncertain origin, is located at the juncture between the hand and the wrist area. It has to be said that before standardization *fengxi* had been drawn by several authors as a larger area called 'urticaria area' (Fig. 5.29). In my opinion the importance given to this area by the Chinese is correct and is moreover confirmed by the indication for cutaneous pruritus given to the whole superior groove of the anthelix.

As regards the specific areas representing the end organs of an allergic reaction, it may be noticed that patients with seasonal rhinoconjunctivitis due to grass pollen, besides the Shen men area, show two further areas tender to pressure (Fig. 5.30A). The first is an area presumably representing the liver; we know about the importance given by TCM to the Liver meridian for treating eye dysfunctions. Another sensitized area is that around the intertragic notch which in my opinion represents the end organ eye–nose of the allergic reaction. According to the Chinese, the anterior and posterior intertragal notches hold indications related to the eye, for example glaucoma and conjunctivitis, but the representation of the nose below the intertragic notch has never been reported by the main schools (see also below).

As regards patients with atopic asthma, in those seen before any intake of oral or inhaled corticosteroids, besides the Shen men area I identified an evident cluster of tender points on the central posterior portion of the antitragus (Fig. 5.30B). This group of points may coincide either with the

occiput area, which holds the indication of asthma, and the apex of the antitragus *duipingjian*, which is indicated for asthma and itching. In my opinion the limited number of aligned points of the concha compared to the antitragus indicates that the most interesting points for diagnosing and treating asthma are probably located out of the commonly accepted representation of the lung. This phenomenon again could be related to the activation of an area belonging to the brainstem as proposed by Durinyan in his representation of 'respiratory centers' of reticular formation (see Fig. 5.16).

As regards contact allergy, the patients in Figure 5.30C show a scattered distribution of points on the whole auricle; this phenomenon may be interpreted with the large extension of the skin as a target organ of the allergic reaction. It is possible, however, that a higher number of patients with dermatitis provoked by contact with metals or other chemical compounds could identify some specific cluster of points.

Generally speaking the set of areas proposed by the Chinese seems exhaustive and fits quite consistently with my data. It is possible that these authors discovered earlier than in the West the antihistamine properties of some points for reducing itching. My experience of this subject has been very positive as the stimulation of some points is indeed able to reduce itching in a few minutes. In my opinion in every allergic reaction releasing histamine and other mediators of inflammation there is a sensitization of the basic areas of allergy belonging to sectors 16–18. The more histamine is released, the more the helix becomes sensitized, extending also to sectors 20 and 21 where Nogier placed his allergy master point (see Fig. A1.17).

Nogier considered further actions of his allergy master point on 'cellular metabolism' and affectivity. He proposed a double location of the point and wrote:

> this point is found at the top of the auricle, almost at the intersection of its internal and external surface. It is therefore accessible from two sides relatively close together, which actually give two points: the first one, hidden, is located under the helix border, and the second one, on the border of the upper part of the auricle.[57]

However, Nogier also proposed, beyond his master point, further points for treating allergic conditions such as the representation of the nose, eye, thymus and ACTH.

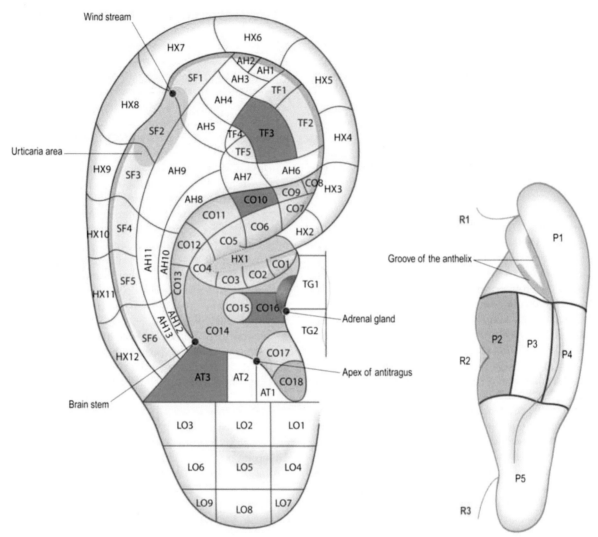

Fig. 5.29 Chinese standardized points/areas indicated for asthma (darker pink): AT3 = occiput; CO16 = trachea; CO10 = kidney; TF3 = middle triangular fossa; apex of antitragus; upper (R1) and lower (R3) ear root on the medial surface. Standardized points/areas for various allergic conditions and/or pruritus (paler pink): CO14 = lung; CO18 = endocrine; HX1 = ear center; urticaria area; Wind stream; adrenal gland; brainstem; P2 = lung and groove of the anthelix.

Summing up this section, it has to be said that we are far from having interpreted the whole range of allergic disorders on the auricle. It would also be interesting to carry out diagnostic research into the various diseases in which autoimmunity is demonstrated or supposed; it is possible that such a systematic study could give us useful information for increasing the therapeutic potentialities of ear acupuncture.

THE PUZZLE OF THE REPRESENTATION OF EAR, NOSE, EYE AND TEETH ON THE EAR LOBE

One of the portions of the outer ear on which no particular consensus has been reached in the last 50 years is the ear lobe. Here, we are not looking for an association with one or more parts of the

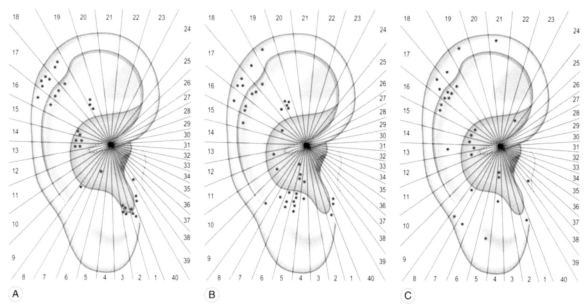

Fig. 5.30   Distribution of tender points in six patients with seasonal rhinoconjunctivitis (A), in six patients with atopic asthma (B), and in six patients with contact allergy (C).

SNC: at the moment this appears to be a step too far. It would seem easier rather to identify the areas associated with some somatic structures represented on the ear lobe such as the ear, nose, eye and teeth, through adequate methodology.

THE REPRESENTATION OF THE EAR ON THE EAR

The representation of the Chinese internal ear (LO6 *neier*) differs greatly in location from Nogier's internal ear, which is represented on the internal portion of the tragus where the Chinese instead locate the pharynx and larynx (TG3 *yanhou*) and internal nose (TG4

neibi) (see Figs A1.1 and A1.2). These confounding interpretations are probably caused by the lack of any of these anatomical structures in Bachmann's historical map. As had happened for the uterus and ovary, every school was forced to make its own interpretation, leading to divergent conclusions.

My contribution to this issue was focused on examining various disorders of the external, middle and internal ear, trying also to identify the areas involved in vestibular dysfunctions.

As is well-known, a hearing impairment may be caused by various factors. The female patient in Figure 5.31 came to my practice presenting a bilateral hearing loss due to two different factors: the

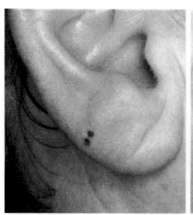

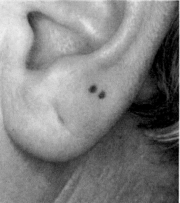

Fig. 5.31   Auricular sensitization in a 51-year-old female patient with bilateral hearing impairment; the tender points on the right ear were related to otitis media (A); the tender points on the left ear were related to a plug of wax (B).

right ear (left side of Fig. 5.31) was affected by otitis media catarrhalis, the left (right side of the same figure) by a plug of earwax. Both ears showed two tender points: those on the left side disappeared soon after removing the plug but those on the right persisted for as long as medication was necessary to free the obstructed Eustachian tube. This case shows that there is consistent overlapping of tender points related to inflammation of the external auditory canal and otitis media, but also an overlapping in hearing loss from exposure to noise for professional reasons.

Dr Pierluigi Mazzini[57] made an interesting evaluation of 189 workers exposed to noise for professional reasons. The recommended exposure limit (REL) proposed by the National Institute for Occupational Safety and Health (NIOSH) is 85 decibels as an 8 hour time-weighted average. By means of audiometric testing Mazzini identified four groups of workers:

a. 57 without hearing loss and without any tender point of the auricle
b. 18 without hearing loss, with at least one tender point
c. 67 with hearing loss, without any tender point
d. 47 with hearing loss, and with at least one tender point.

The workers in group d showed a higher number of tender points than workers in group b ($P<0.05$). In the former group the workers with moderate impairment showed a higher average of tender points vs. the rest of subjects with severe hearing loss (respectively 4.1 to 3.2). Even if the difference was only basically significant ($P=0.057$), we may nevertheless suppose that greater acoustic damage may determine reduced sensitization of the auricle. This phenomenon is in agreement with the hypothesis that an irreversible lesion of an organ or a nerve may interfere with the diagnostic power of PPT and the electrical skin resistance test (ESRT). However, if we examine the distribution of tender points found in group d we can identify some clusters possibly associated with hearing loss. The area with the highest concentration of points is the Chinese internal ear (39%) followed by an area on the antitragus (24.7%) which appears to be aligned on the same sectors 5–7 of the first area (on the left of Fig. 5.32,

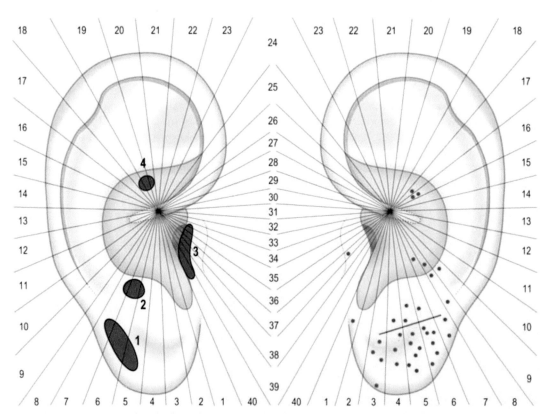

Fig. 5.32 Clusters of tender points in 47 workers with hearing loss due to exposure to noise (left image) *(with permission of Mazzini)*; distribution of tender points in 10 patients (average age 61.8 years) with chronic tinnitus (right image).

numbers 1 and 2). In following order we can find the sensitization of the whole tragus in 16.8% and a concentration of tender points in the superior concha on sectors 18–20 in 10.5% (on the left of Fig. 5.32, numbers 3 and 4). These two minor areas seem to correspond partially to Nogier's internal ear and to Chinese kidney and pancreas–gallbladder areas. The relationship between kidney and ear is well known by practitioners introduced to TCM, but it must be stressed that both areas, according to the Chinese standardization, hold a double indication for hypacusis and tinnitus.

THE REPRESENTATION OF TINNITUS ON THE AURICLE

Tinnitus can have many different causes, but is most commonly associated with hearing loss due to exposure to noise, Ménière's disease, ototoxic medication, etc.

Many people experience chronic tinnitus (at least 10% in the Western world) and it is therefore possible that they might seek remedy through acupuncture when conventional treatment has proven ineffective. Systematic reviews of the literature,[58] however, based on evidence derived from rigorous randomized controlled trials, converge on the equal inefficacy of acupuncture for this complaint. It is therefore important for the practitioner to be cautious about treating a patient with acupuncture alone, and outside a cognitive-behavioral program, even in those cases presenting one or more auricular tender points.

I tried, for example, to treat the tender points located in 10 patients with chronic tinnitus (5 males and 5 females, average age 61.8 years) (on the right of Fig. 5.32). Despite the number of tender points identified (on average 3.7) the result of treatment was deceptive and the only positive effect was that of relaxation, which presumably increased the patient's tolerance of the symptom. The distribution of points, in the hypothesis that they really could be associated with tinnitus, was scattered over the whole ear lobe. This dispersion, in my opinion, indicates a multiple-site dysfunction and confirms the existence of multifactorial causes which should be managed only with an interdisciplinary approach aimed at improving this condition.

THE REPRESENTATION OF THE SYMPTOM OF DIZZINESS ON THE AURICLE

Dizziness and vertigo are not well-defined entities, but rather symptoms of a multisensory syndrome. This may be induced by stimulation of the intact sensori-motor system through motion (i.e. motion sickness) or by pathologic dysfunction of any of the stabilizing sensory systems, for example the peripheral vestibular in the case of neuritis or Ménière's disease and the central vestibular in the case of vertebral–basilar ischemia. As differential diagnosis is not customary for a physician, an empirical approach is usually followed in which the symptom rather than the underlying disorder is treated. This uneasiness may be one of the reasons why acupuncturists limit themselves to treating only the symptom. The lack of differential diagnosis is also reflected on the auricle where we are at a loss to understand if central disorders have a different representation from peripheral dysfunctions.

Chinese standardization reports three points/areas carrying the indication of Ménière's disease: the internal ear, the occiput and the brainstem. The whole antitragus (forehead, temple, occiput) with the central rim point are furthermore recommended for treating dizziness.

On Western maps the points indicated for dizziness and vertigo are really scanty: Nogier proposed a point on the lower end of the scapha coinciding with the maxillary point and several German authors reported a motion sickness point near the Chinese brainstem point. Two otologists from Munich, Rolf and Detlef Pildner von Steinburg,[59] however, carried out an interesting study on 100 patients with vestibular dysfunctions. With the help of a Punctoscope, the device produced by Sedatelec before the Agiscop, they identified an almost vertical line of points which could efficiently reduce lateral nystagmus and the accompanying dizziness (on the left of Fig. 5.33, line A). Another line starting from the anthelix–antitragus notch and extending forward along the rim of the antitragus (on the same figure, line B) was moreover effective in reducing purely vertical nystagmus which is usually central in origin. What is interesting in this study is the convergence of these lines on the brainstem point which the authors defined as the 'mesencephalic point of the fasciculus longitudinalis medialis' (on the same figure, M).

Together with the otologist Fabio Caporiccio, we tried to make our contribution to the issue of vestibular representation on the auricle. We examined a series of consecutive patients undergoing caloric reflex test for dizziness and vertigo. The Fitzgerald–Hallpike test (FHT) consists of introducing

250 cc of warm water (44°C) into the ear canal in 40 s, one ear after the other, and counting the number of eye movements at the culminating moment between the 60th and 90th second after the beginning of the FHT. We made the following observations on 30 consecutive subjects:

1. In healthy subjects, approximately 2 minutes after the caloric reflex test the ipsilateral ear became sensitive in one or two points. Sensitization lasted for about 3–5 minutes and then disappeared entirely. The sensitized area corresponded partially to the Chinese internal ear but frequently shifted toward the border of the ear lobe and the helix on sectors 7–9 (on the right of Fig. 5.33).
2. In the case of asymmetric vestibular activity, the auricle with a number of eye movements exceeding 2.5–3/s was basically also tender before performing the FHT, whereas the auricle on the hypoactive side never became sensitized if the beats/sec were less than 1.

3. In those cases in which the nystagmus gave a stronger indication of a central disorder, we identified further tender points corresponding not only to the brainstem but also to the internal border of the antitragus and the anthelix. It is on these that the Chinese locate the most caudal portion of the spleen (CO13 *pi*) and where Bourdiol[1] located the vertebral artery. He said about its representation: 'it passes forwards to reach, as in macrosopic anatomy, the cervical vertebrae from C6 to C1, at the level of the claustrum, running alongside the paravertebral sympathetic chain. At the level of the post-antitragal sulcus, it penetrates behind the posterior pole of the antitragus to attain the mastoid face, where it gives off the basilar trunk' (Fig. 5.34). My observations on patients with vertigo caused by central vestibular disorders are basically in agreement with Bourdiol's hypothesis, but further research is urgently required to unveil the potentialities of ear acupuncture in this field.

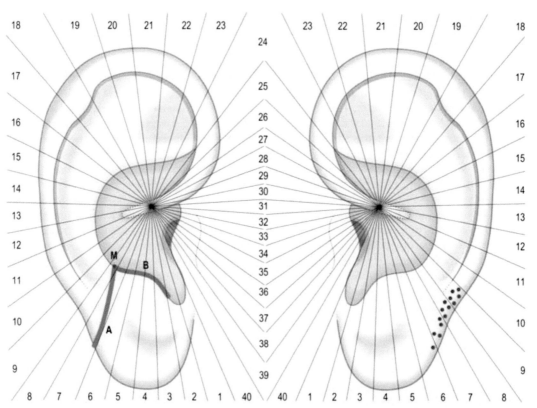

Fig. 5.33 The most effective points for reducing nystagmus in vestibular dysfunctions according to R. and D. Pildner von Steinburg (left image); sensitized area during caloric test in nine healthy subjects (right image).

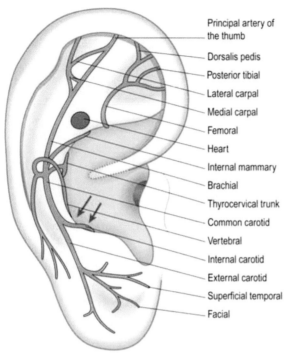

Principal artery of
the thumb

Dorsalis pedis

Posterior tibial

Lateral carpal

Medial carpal

Femoral

Heart

Internal mammary

Brachial

Thyrocervical trunk

Common carotid

Vertebral

Internal carotid

External carotid

Superficial temporal

Facial

Fig. 5.34 Representation of the cardiovascular system according to Bourdiol *(with permission)*. The arrows indicate the possible sites of sensitization in cases of central vestibular disorders.

THE REPRESENTATION OF THE NOSE ON THE EAR

Another divergent location according to Nogier's and Chinese cartography is the representation of the nose. The main reason for this divergence may be related to the lack of any representation of this anatomical part on Bachmann's drawing of 1957. The olfactive point was added later by Nogier[21] on the anterior part of the lobule approximately 1 mm behind the auricular insertion line on the lateral side, half way up the lobule (see Fig. A1.1).

The Chinese, on the other hand, differentiated between the representation of the external nose (*waibi*) and that of the internal nose (*neibi*) (see Fig. A1.2). The first is located between tragus areas 1 and 2, carrying indications such as nasal vestibular inflammation and rhinitis; the second is located on the internal wall of the inferior part of the tragus and has the indications rhinitis, sinusitis and nose bleeds.

My contribution on this issue was made by making observations of two groups of patients, the first with facial injury and fracture of the nasal

bones, the second much more frequent group with acute coryza of possible viral origin. In both cases the same area became sensitized (on the left of Fig. 5.35, area number 1), overlapping with Nogier's olfactive point but with some differences: in cases of nasal trauma both ears were usually sensitized, whereas in rhinitis the lobe was more often unilaterally tender on the same side as the more obstructed nostril. In this case even massage of the tender point could relieve the symptom through a presumed anti-inflammatory and decongesting effect on nasal mucosa. A third group with a similar representation is the above-mentioned group of patients with allergic rhinoconjunctivitis (see Fig. 5.30A).

When the catarrhal condition of the nose extends itself to the frontal sinuses, the process of sensitization shifts toward the Chinese forehead area (on the left of Fig. 5.35, area number 3). Between these areas it is possible to find a few very tender points in the case of ethmoid sinusitis (same figure, area number 2). If the inflammatory process primarily or secondarily involves the maxillary sinuses, a further area becomes sensitized which may overlap with the Chinese temple area (same figure, area number 4).

All these areas are the expression of local inflammation; in the case of accompanying neuralgic pain the distribution of tender points may, however, vary and shift toward the border of the ear lobe, as happens in toothache (see next section).

It is interesting to note that vasomotor (non-allergic) rhinitis probably has a different distribution of tender points than allergic rhinitis. This is in agreement with the hypothesis concerning this disorder which is supposed to be caused either by a hyperactive parasympathetic nervous system or by an imbalance between the latter and the sympathetic nervous system. Even if recent reviews state that both allergic and vasomotor rhinitis respond to the same drugs, such as azelastine and fluticasone nasal spray, the pathophysiology of the two disorders seems rather different. It may be remembered that vasomotor rhinitis is characterized by prominent symptoms of nasal obstruction, rhinorrea, and congestion exacerbated by certain odors, alcohol, spicy foods, emotions and environmental factors such as temperature, barometric pressure changes and bright lights.[60]

In three patients (2 females, 1 male, average age 34.3 years) with non-allergic rhinitis and symptoms such as frequent sneezing and runny nose, the tender points tended to overlap with both the Chinese

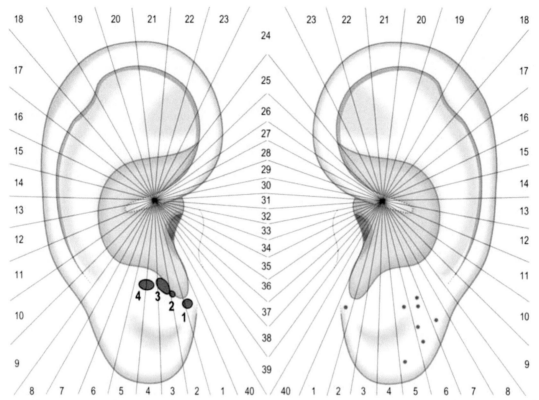

Fig. 5.35 Sensitized areas in patients with coryza (1), ethmoidal sinusitis (2), frontal sinusitis (3) and maxillary sinusitis (4) (left image); sensitization of the auricle in three patients with vasomotor rhinitis (right image).

occiput and internal ear, whereas the anterior part of the ear lobe seemed much less sensitive (on the right of Fig. 5.35). The treatment of these points with semi-permanent needles for a period of 2–3 months significantly reduced the vasomotor non-allergic symptoms which previously had responded hardly at all to medication with antihistamines.

THE REPRESENTATION OF THE EYE ON THE EAR

One of the most puzzling representations on the ear is that of the eye. Nogier[21] wrote:

it is the point we think of stimulating when earrings are put on to improve the sight or strengthen the eye itself in a conjunctivitis case. ... the localization of the eye point is imprecise. It is in the center of a round arch formed by the lower curve of the lobule, often on the transversal and oblique fold descending from the front towards the back of the lobule.

Despite the imprecise localization there is a consistent overlapping with the Chinese eye area (LO5 *yan*) which holds the generic indication 'inflammation of the eye' with reference especially to conjunctivitis and stye. The tradition in folk medicine to apply moxibustion on the ear apex for treating acute conjunctivitis has been maintained as an indication for this point also in the current standardization.

However, the most interesting evolution in the identification of points/areas related to eye disorders concerns two points reported in 1959 by Dr Xu Zuo-Lin of Beijing in the first Chinese clinical validation on ear acupuncture (see Fig. 1.11). The points were located on the posterior–lateral and anterior–internal edge of the intertragic notch and called by the author respectively astigmatism and glaucoma. The points were then placed definitely on the external border of the intertragic notch and renamed Eye 1 and 2 by the Chinese Academy of Traditional Medicine. Their common and unique indication was 'pseudomyopia', intending by this perhaps a defect in sight simulating myopia. The points were included in the standardization process and renamed as anterior and posterior intertragic points with the respective Pinyin of *pingjianqian* and *pingjianhou*. Their main indication was changed to 'ametropia' but further disorders were added too such as glaucoma and conjunctivitis. A further indication for glaucoma was proposed for the liver area (CO12 *gan*) in accordance with the importance given to the Liver meridian by TCM.

I did not feel at all satisfied with this scanty representation and I thought that an important organ such as the eye could perhaps have a much larger representation following the *homunculus* principle. The only possible way to find an answer to this issue was again to carry out systematic checking of auricular tenderness in patients with various eye disorders.

I began by observing 132 consecutive patients consulting the local emergency ophthalmology clinic. The subjects generally came for assistance

because they had corneal abrasions or corneal foreign bodies. Since the patients showed 80% clustering of tender points around the intertragic notch, my first hypothesis was that the points identified at this level by Chinese authors could represent the external part of the eye (on the left of Fig. 5.36). This impression was strengthened by the observation of 17 patients before and after cataract surgery: during the few hours following surgery, in 13 of these patients I could identify a temporary sensitization of the same area (on the right of Fig. 5.36).

I realized then that the more the internal part of the eye was involved in the disease, the more the tender points moved caudally and behind toward the classical representation of the eye. The disorder which seemed best to overlap with the representation of the eye was undoubtedly glaucoma. In a further group of 12 patients with glaucoma the cluster coincided with Nogier's and the Chinese eye (on the left of Fig. 5.37), despite the fact that intraocular pressure was kept under control by

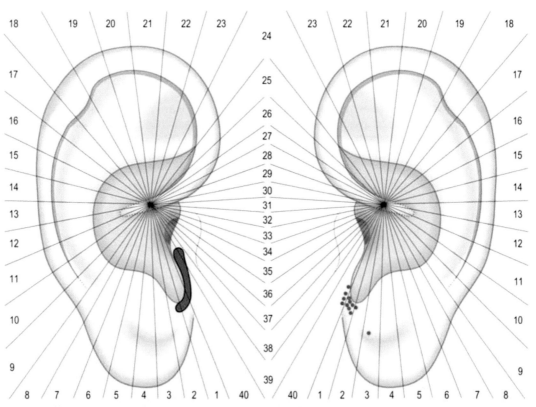

Fig. 5.36 Sensitized area in 18 patients with corneal abrasion (left image); tender points in 13 patients after surgery for cataract (right image).

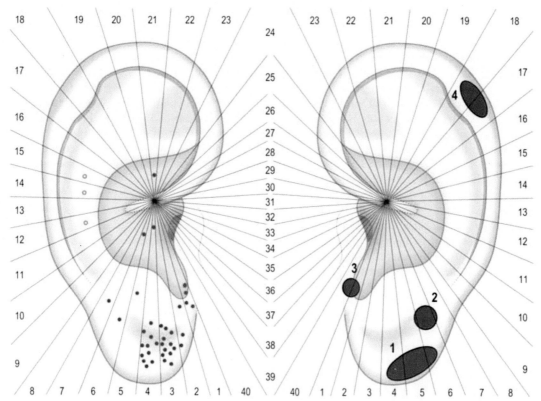

Fig. 5.37 Sensitization of the ear lobe in 12 patients with glaucoma (left); cluster of tender points in 20 patients with hypertensive retinopathy (right) *(unpublished data, with permission of Berteramo)*. Dots = lateral surface; circles = medial surface.

timolol and other drugs. This phenomenon could be interpreted, in the absence of hypertension, as the persistence of the pathologic mechanism provoking this symptom, indicating the need in these patients to face their metabolic disorders, style of life, etc. more incisively. On the other hand this persistence could be transformed into a possible complementary treatment of glaucoma with ear acupuncture, a treatment which has not yet been studied.

As regards the extreme posterior part of the eye and diseases such as hypertension and diabetes possibly affecting the retina, we can observe a further shift of tender points toward the border of the ear lobe, covering also sectors positioned further back. The ophthalmologist Luigi Berteramo carried out a preliminary diagnostic study in 20 patients (15 males and 5 females, average age 71.5 years) with retinopathy due to sustained hypertension over a prolonged period of time. The retinal arterial narrowing was evaluated grade II and III at the optic fundus examination. More than 50% of

the tender points were located in the peripheral part of the ear lobe (sectors 4–6) and on a further area of uncertain meaning located upwards (on the right of Fig. 5.37, areas 1 and 2). Other involved areas, on the intertragic incisure and on the upper part of the helix, were presumably correlated to high blood pressure and to metabolic disorders which are so frequent in patients with retinopathy (same figure, areas 3 and 4).

Summing up, the representation of the eye and the function of sight on the ear appears much more extended than supposed and tends, in proportion, to cover larger parts of the ear lobe compared to other particular senses such as hearing, taste and smell.

THE REPRESENTATION OF THE TEETH AND THE TEMPOROMANDIBULAR JOINT

Bachmann in his historical map drew a clear representation of the upper and lower jaw located further forward with respect to the cheek. On the

Chinese maps, however, the jaw area has always been located behind the cheek area. This divergence has become more evident over time as Nogier later shifted both jaws and the temporomandibular joint (TMJ) toward the junction of the ear lobe with the scapha, whereas the Chinese separated the tooth area (LO1 *ya*) from the jaw (LO3 *he*), interposing the tongue (LO2 *she*) between these two areas (see Figs A1.1 and A1.2). Both LO1 and LO3 share the same indication for toothache together with the neighboring anterior ear lobe and occiput, but the jaw area carries the indication also for TMJ disorders. This puzzling and somewhat confusing distance between the teeth and the jaw was probably caused by the importance which has been given by Chinese authors, since the 1970s, to some specific points of the anterior ear lobe for 'anesthesia for extraction of teeth' of the upper and lower jaw.[61,62]

I have always been intrigued by this question and have not been helped by auriculomedicine which claims to find the corresponding points with the help of the vascular autonomic signal (VAS) and Nogier's frequencies. My hypothesis was that such an important sensory cranial nerve as the fifth should have a much larger representation on the auricle according to the *homunculus* principle. The only way I had for clarifying this was by attempting to identify the corresponding tender points with PPT, one tooth after the other. Every time I visited patients with toothache or who had undergone minor operations such as tooth extraction or implantation, I checked the ear lobe systematically and made the following observations:

1. When pain was local I found in general only one point: needle contact test (NCT) and acupuncture on the identified point were generally able to reduce the pain in a few minutes.
2. When the pain was more intense or diffused the number of points increased and tended to shift cranially toward the antitragus or caudally toward the border of the ear lobe, overlapping with the points of trigeminal neuralgia (see section above). In these cases a multiple NCT and needle insertion generally controlled the pain syndrome.
3. Clusters of points related to the teeth of the upper jaw (Fig. 5.38A, areas a, b and c) tended to be located more cranially with respect to the lower jaw (a1, b1) but this difference appeared less evident in considering single cases.

4. The posterior teeth (7 and 8) tended to overlap with both Nogier's and the Chinese representation of the upper and lower jaw (Fig. 5.38A, areas a and a1). As the corresponding clusters of points tend to project themselves on sectors 7 and 8, the Sectogram could be a helpful guide to locate the representation of the other points. The premolar and the first molar (4, 5, 6) could therefore be found on sectors 4, 5 and 6 (in the same figure, areas b and b1), whereas the anterior teeth tend to cover sectors 2 and 3 (in the same figure, area c for the upper incisors and canine).

One should not to be surprised to find the representation also of other structures such as the lips in this area (Fig. 5.38B).

As regards the TMJ, especially in the Chinese occiput area, we may find one or more sensitive points related to bruxism and craniomandibular disorders. As discussed in Chapter 8, this point has an important diagnostic value in every case of recurrent myofascial pain of the neck area related to problems of mastication.

In summary, the representation of the teeth is much more expanded than might be supposed and covers large parts of the ear lobe.

THE MAJOR DIVERGENCES BETWEEN NOGIER'S AND THE CHINESE AURICULAR REPRESENTATION OF INTERNAL ORGANS

THE CARDIOVASCULAR SYSTEM

One of the major differences between the different schools concerns the auricular representation of the cardiovascular system. It is still a mystery why the heart area, drawn in 1957 by Bachmann in the lower concha and coinciding perfectly with the current Chinese heart (CO15 *xin*), was moved afterwards by Nogier and Bourdiol. The heart area was shifted finally to the anthelix where the Chinese locate the chest (AH10 *xiong*) (see Fig. 5.34). Regarding the new location Bourdiol[1] wrote:

it projects on the D4–D5 radius, onto the body of the anthelix, in the middle of the thoracic territory ... under normal physiological conditions, its largest surface-area occupies the left mastoid face, being the left ventricular area the most developed.

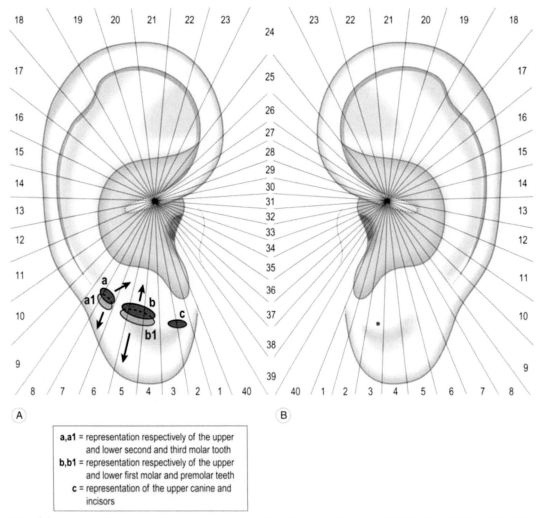

a,a1 = representation respectively of the upper
       and lower second and third molar tooth
b,b1 = representation respectively of the upper
       and lower first molar and premolar teeth
   c = representation of the upper canine and
       incisors

Fig. 5.38 (A) Areas of recurrent sensitization in patients with toothache; the arrows indicate the shifting of tender points in case of more intense/diffuse pain. (B) Sensitization of the ear lobe in a 22-year-old male patient stung by a bee on the upper lip.

In my opinion it is possible that this divergence of representation depends on a different interpretation that in the first version represents the organ of the heart beneath the lung in the inferior concha, and in the second version perhaps the typical cardiac pain referred to the chest and the arms.

It is true, however, that both schools extended their research to other complementary points: Nogier proposed at least two related to cardiac functions on the internal border of the anthelix where the sympathetic ganglia, the 'circulatory system' evidently related to the heart area and the 'marvelous point' belonging to the middle cervical ganglion are represented (see Figs A1.7 and A1.17). The Chinese on the other hand proposed a further cardiac point, *xinzangdian* (named heart 2 by Oleson), which was located on the tragus between the external ear *waier* and the apex of tragus *pingjian*. The point had the indications atrial fibrillation and tachycardia, but was omitted in the standardization process (see Fig. A1.8).

In my opinion the most interesting interpretation of the auricular areas related to heart function was that proposed by Durinyan.[22,23] For these he considered a large area covering the whole inferior concha and the antitragus. Within this area he identified at least seven points influencing the contractility of cardiac muscle, its electrical activity and the perfusion of coronary arteries (Fig. 5.39). Durinyan's interpretation seems to me to be more realistic and could offer a sound basis for further research aimed at combining ear acupuncture with the commonly used medications in cardiac patients.

An interesting pilot study was conducted by two Swedish authors during their several years of research on the treatment of severe angina pectoris with either TENS or epidural spinal electrical stimulation.[63,64] They were interested especially in helping patients refractory to therapy waiting for coronary bypass intervention; therefore they tried to stimulate the Chinese heart point *xin* (named heart 1 by Oleson) bilaterally with a current of low frequency. The authors were impressed by the results and reported the case of a patient aged 70 who was relieved from acute pain in 2–5 seconds; this benefit lasted for about 24 hours after each treatment.[65]

The heart deserves a systematic diagnostic study of the auricle in larger groups of patients to identify the recurrent areas involved in specific heart disorders.

My contribution to the topic is represented by two single cases which I was able to follow up over time.

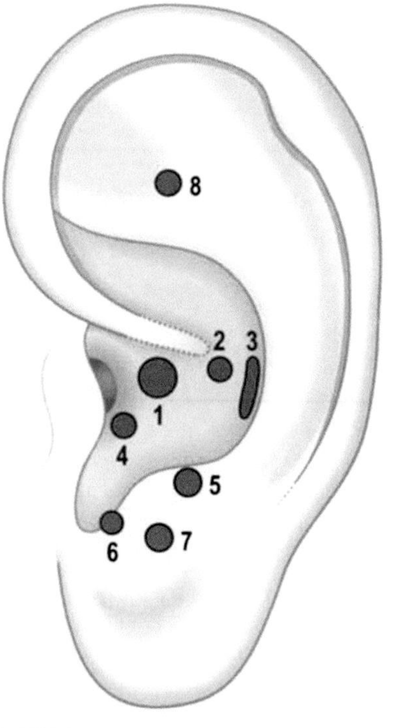

1 = basic zone for heart and coronary circulation
2 = chronotropic point
3 = area for stroke volume and contractility of the heart
4 = circulatory point
5 = hypothalamic regulatory center
6 = hypothalamic point of neurohypophysis
7 = circulatory center of reticular formation
8 = antistress point (Shen men)

Fig. 5.39 Representation of the cardiovascular system according to Durinyan.

CASE STUDY 1

A female patient aged 44 was affected by severe mitral stenosis. This was confirmed by Doppler test, the valve area being less than 1 cm^2; the pressure gradient was 18 mmHg and moderate pulmonary hypertension was therefore presumable. The patient often suffered quickly from fatigue when doing housework and going upstairs and she had been admitted to hospital for lung edema 3 weeks previously. When I performed PPT on her auricles for the first time I found two tender points on the left concha and one on the right concha, presumably related to her previous heart failure and lung edema (Fig. 5.40, red points).

After 3 months she underwent mitral commisurotomy; 1 year later the result was still considered acceptable as the valve area was rated 2.2 cm^2 with only very limited regurgitation evidenced at the Doppler control test. The patient nevertheless complained of dyspnea on making slight efforts and an ECG recorded atrial fibrillation with high ventricular frequency. On this occasion I had the opportunity of checking the patient's auricles again: the tender point on the right auricle had disappeared whereas the left concha still had two tender points but in a different position: one was shifted further upwards to the 'basic zone for heart and coronary circulation' (area 1); the other was shifted backwards toward Durinyan's area 3 shown in Figure 5.39 (Fig. 5.40, gray points).

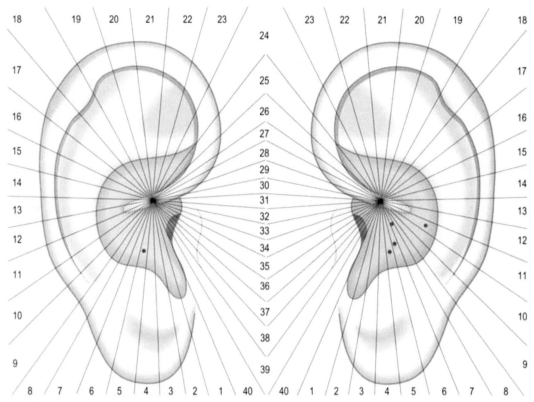

Fig. 5.40 Tender points detected with PPT in a 44-year-old female patient with stenotic mitral valve before commisurotomy (red); the same patient 1 year after surgery (gray).

CASE STUDY 2

The second case was a male patient aged 57 who drove on average 4–5000 km a month, smoked cigarettes and had a persistently disorderly lifestyle. One month before I saw him he started to suffer from moderate neck pain with some radiation to both arms. A first ECG was negative and the patient's family doctor prescribed nimesulide and benzodiazepines. With the analgesic medication the remission of pain lasted only 6 hours. Examining the patient's neck I found a stiffness which he also associated with a whiplash he had suffered a few years before. On inspection of the left ear I noticed an incisure of the anthelix and with PPT I found three tender points which could be associated with a cervical–brachial syndrome (Fig. 5.41, red points); however, ear acupuncture and manipulation of the cervical–thoracic tract of the spine did not yield satisfactory

results. Checking the patient's auricles again I found a very sensitive point close to Durinyan's 'basic zone for heart and coronary circulation' (Fig. 5.41, gray point). An ECG was repeated (1 month after the first) and this time signs of inferior necrosis were evident, even though myocardial enzymes were negative. The Bruce stress test with increasing loads confirmed signs of transmural ischemia with ST-segment elevation in D2, D3 and aVF until the seventh minute of recovery. Medication based on nitrates, calcioantagonists and heparin eliminated the neck pain as well and I could not find any of the tender points on the anthelix identified during the first examination.

Hypertension-related points/areas on the ear

In order to have a clear picture of the representation of the cardiovascular system on the ear, we also need to know the auricular patterns of

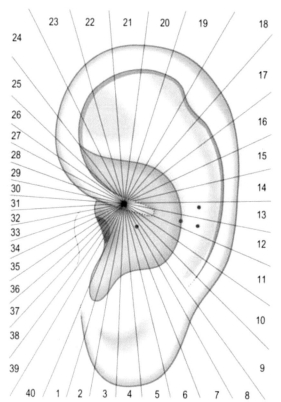

Fig. 5.41 Tender points detected with PPT in a male patient aged 57, associated at first with a cervical-brachial syndrome (red), afterwards with myocardial ischemia (gray).

sensitization in subjects with hypertension and on medication for lowering blood pressure. The set of areas proposed by Chinese authors for treating hypertension represents another puzzle of difficult interpretation (see Fig. A1.8). Beyond the obvious heart area of the medial surface and the nearby groove for lowering blood pressure, we may also find related to hypertension the liver (CO12 *gan*): the expert in TCM will probably cite on this subject some typical syndromes such as 'Liver raising *Yang*' or 'Liver fire'.

A further area associated with this kind of dysfunction to remember is 'Liver *Yang*' of the early Chinese ear acupuncture authors, carrying the indications hypertension, headache and dizziness, which was located on Darwin's tubercle. These indications were left unchanged in the standardized version but the area was renamed node (HX8 *jiejie*). Moreover, the indication for high blood pressure was also summed to tonsillitis for the whole portion of the helix including areas

1–4. The other areas to mention are the superior triangular fossa (TF1 *jiaowoshang*), the ear apex and the antitragus apex; another point which has been left out of the standardized version is the point for lowering blood pressure *gaoxueyadian*, within area TG2, which is curiously very near to the adrenal gland *shenshangxian* carrying the opposite indication for increasing blood pressure (see Fig. A1.6). These apparently discordant indications, already cited in Chapter 4, may perhaps indicate one of the important sites related to the complex mechanisms regulating blood pressure.

I tried to make my contribution to the identification of some recurrent areas associated with hypertension by examining a group of 26 patients (17 females and 9 males, average age 53.2 years) in whom a hypertensive condition was found incidentally: none were taking drugs for lowering blood pressure or other medications such as analgesics or benzodiazepines which could affect correct identification of the points (see Ch. 9). I made two measurements at least 5 minutes apart and if there was a discrepancy of more than 10 mmHg I performed a third reading: systolic pressure averaged 182 mmHg and diastolic 99 mmHg. An ECG and blood tests including creatinine, electrolytes, glucose and cholesterol were then carried out on each patient, as well as PPT: four subjects did not show any tender point whereas the others showed an average of 5.9 points which were mainly concentrated on sectors 1, 2, 39 and 40. Indeed, 60% of the tender points were concentrated on the rim of the lower part of the tragus and on the hidden part of the intertragic notch, at the junction with the floor of the external auditory canal (Fig. 5.42). Other minor areas were the heart area, especially in those patients who showed an initial cardiac overload, and a further area, of uncertain significance, aligned with the former on the ear lobe. I found a minor concentration of points (only 8.5% of the total) on the Chinese groove for lowering blood pressure, therefore I am not able to confirm the importance of this area. I made a regression line for each patient between the number of tender points and the respective level of systolic and diastolic pressure. I was surprised to obtain quite different results as the coefficient R was very low in the case of systolic pressure and P was not significant; instead, in the case of diastolic pressure I obtained an $R = 0.582$ and a $P < 0.005$. These findings have in my opinion a double value for the practitioner: first that especially higher levels of diastolic pressure tend

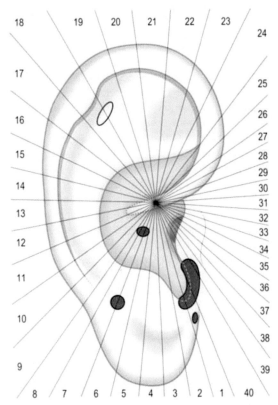

Fig. 5.42 Sensitized areas in 26 new, still untreated, hypertensive patients. Red areas = lateral surface; blank area = medial surface.

to sensitize the auricles; second that the persistent tenderness of some auricular points, despite the intake of antihypertensive drugs, is a possible sign of a non-optimal strategy for lowering blood pressure.

Convergent results have been obtained in a pilot study still in progress conducted by general practitioners Rosaria Di Noia and Giuseppina Facendola, examining the auricles of two groups of 20 subjects each: one with hypertension already in treatment with various classes of drugs; the other without hypertension representing the control group. The first physician records heart rate and blood pressure three times 5 minutes apart in all subjects; the second physician blindly identifies their active points with ESRT and PPT. The first results show that systolic and diastolic pressure do not present significant differences between the two groups (average 131 and 76.1 mmHg in the hypertension group vs. 123 and 72.6 in the control group). This is of course a good result for the general practitioner, indicating an effective control of the

patient's hypertension with the medication prescribed. The groups, however, are not homogeneous with regard to the number of points identified with ESRT and PPT: there are no differences between them in the total number of tender points; with ESRT, however, sectors 1, 2 and 40 show a significantly higher number of points with a relative low electrical skin resistance (ESR) ($P<0.05$) in the hypertension group (on the left of Fig. 5.43) than in the control group (on the right of Fig. 5.43).

In addition, sector 23, which apparently seems correlated with the colon, bladder and sciatic nerve, shows a higher number of points. However, if we check the Chinese standardized map we find, within this sector, the area TF1 *jiaowoshang* on the superior triangular fossa, with the main indication for hypertension.

The convergent results of these observations may point to the importance of the tragus and the intertragic notch representing at least one of the possible mechanisms of primary/essential hypertension which in 90–95% of adults does not show an identifiable cause according to the American Heart Association. It has been estimated that as many as 30% of essential hypertensive patients have a primary neurogenic stimulus contributing to their hypertension.[66] In particular, the role of sympathetic neural mechanisms in the pathogenesis of hypertension has been an issue of enduring interest and productive investigation for several years.

Recent studies on humans evaluating sympathetic activity with sophisticated techniques such as the radiolabeled noradrenaline (norepinephrine) technique and the microneurographic quantification of sympathetic nerve traffic have demonstrated the participation of adrenergic mechanisms in the early and late phases of the hypertensive process. Evidence has been provided also that the activation of the sympathetic nervous system is peculiar to the essential hypertensive state, parallels the degree of blood pressure elevation, is triggered by reflex and humoral mechanisms, and may exert deleterious metabolic and cardiovascular effects, accelerating the progression of the end organ damage accompanying hypertension. According to Grassi:[67]

these findings explain why non-pharmacological and pharmacological approaches to the treatment of hypertension should be aimed not only at lowering elevated blood pressure values but also at exerting sympathetic-inhibitory effects.

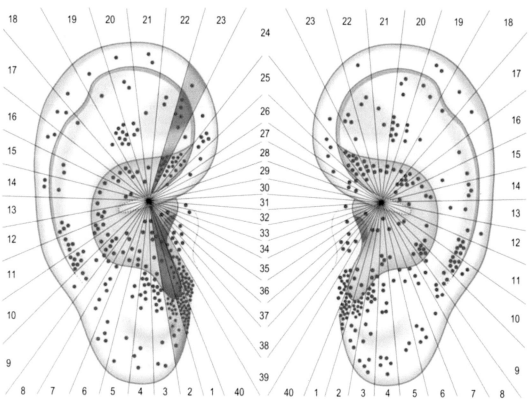

Fig. 5.43 Sectors with significantly higher concentration of points with lower ESR in a group of 20 hypertensive patients under treatment (on the left) compared to a control group of subjects with normal blood pressure (on the right) (unpublished data, with permission of Facendola and Di Noia).

It is possible, therefore, that the repeated/lasting stimulation of the tragus–intertragic area could have such a regulating effect, provided that the patient is sufficiently motivated to change his lifestyle in terms of losing weight, restricting salt intake and exercising.

THE REPRESENTATION OF THE URINARY SYSTEM

The representation of the kidney

One of the better known divergences between Nogier's and the Chinese auricular map is the representation of the kidney.

It is unclear why Nogier felt it was necessary to move the representation of this organ from the upper concha to the upper part of the helix. Nogier described its location in the following way:

it is situated on the triangular fossa axis, under the rim edge. This localisation is linear and extends in front, under the helix knee, and in the back, up to the Darwin point, under the auricle rim.

This unusually long somatotopic representation of the kidney was probably the result of collaboration with Bourdiol (Fig. 5.44). This author said 'it is thought that this whole zone represents a relic of the metanephros'. Beyond this embryological hypothesis, however, it is difficult to imagine the kidney far from the representation of the bladder and the urethra which maintained the same position in both maps.

My own experience concerning the representation of the kidney is limited to 14 cases with ureterolithiasis in which the progress of calculi in the ureter was troublesome despite medication. Only in 11 of the 14 cases did ultrasound demonstrate the presence of calculi; in all cases PPT detected tender points on the same side as the pain which were not in a fixed position but tended to shift forward along a line passing through the Chinese ureter point *shuniaoguan* located at the junction of the

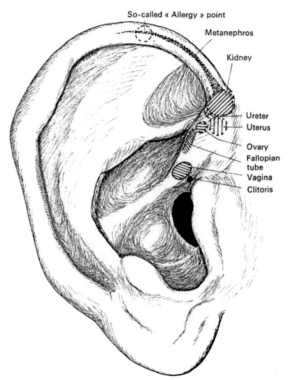

So-called « Allergy » point
Metanephros
Kidney
Ureter
Uterus
Ovary
Fallopian tube
Vagina
Clitoris

Fig. 5.44 Representation of the genitourinary system according to Bourdiol (with permission).

kidney and bladder area. The application on average of 2.8 single-use steel implants (ASP) reduced pain by 70–80% in eight cases and by 40–70% in four cases; in two cases this had no effect at all. The reduction of colic and the presumed relaxation of the smooth muscle of the ureter favored the expulsion of calculi in the following hours/days; however, this was demonstrated in only eight out of 14 cases. The diameter of the calculi in no case exceeded 5–6 mm; on examination six calculi were found to be of calcium oxalate, two of uric acid. In only one of these cases did I find tenderness on Nogier's kidney and ureter point.

THE REPRESENTATION OF THE GENITAL SYSTEM ON THE EAR

Regarding the representation of the genital system, the main reason for the great differences in the representation of the uterus and ovary is, in my opinion, due to the fact that Nogier 'forgot' to draw the somatotopy of these organs in either 1957 or in 1969, when his *Traité d'Auriculothérapie* was published. Only in 1977, in the French edition of his

Handbook to Auriculotherapy, did he describe the point of gonads related to ovary and testicle 'hidden under the rising branch of the helix' at a short distance from point 0. Nogier and Bourdiol both represented the uterus on the internal part of the ascending helix on the axis to the lower branch of the anthelix. As Bachmann's drawing did not indicate any somatotopic area to be associated with internal genitals, the Chinese were forced to discover their own representations. The uterus was definitely located in the triangular fossa which thus became one important reference zone of the ear for every disease or dysfunction regarding the reproductive system. The anterior third of the triangular fossa, in its lower part, was indeed named the internal genital area (TF2 *neishengzhiqi*), carrying the indications for dysmenorrhea, irregular menstruation and dysfunctional uterine bleeding. Another area related to the reproductive system is the pelvis (TF5 *pengqiang*), with the indications for adnexitis and irregular menstruation.

What has been intriguing for me and several other practitioners has been the representation of the ovary *luanchao* and testicle *gaowan* on the medial side of the antitragus. The indications for both points were hypogonadism, and epididymitis for the first and abnormal menstruation for the second. The indications for both points were extended by Li Su Huai to dwarfism, hypofunction of the anterior pituitary, hypothalamic amenorrhea, sexual disorders, etc.[68]

The testicle and ovary areas were, however, removed during the standardization process and only the endocrine area still maintained indications related to the female genital system such as dysmenorrhea, irregular menstruation and climacteric syndrome. We are at a loss to understand why part of the reproductive system has been located on the antitragus, but it can be presumed that, according to Bossy's *homunculus* principle, the anterior part of the antitragus may be associated with dysfunctions of the pituitary–gonadotropic axis. On this subject we need to mention Nogier's 'genital master point' located at the anterior extremity of the antitragus, on its external surface, carrying indications such as disorders of the external genital organs and climacteric syndrome (see Fig. A1.17).

The possibility that the Chinese have mismatched the representation of the gonads with the pituitary–gonadotropic axis fits very well with Durinyan's hypothesis of an enlarged surface of the endocrine area, extending itself from the antitragus to the tragus. The fascinating hypothesis still to be proved is that this area could carry a sort of topographic specialization according to the different corresponding axis. In this case we would have the corticotropic axis represented on the tragus and the gonadotropic axis represented on the anterior part of the antitragus; in the middle, as indicated by both Nogier and Durinyan, a third axis could be imagined such as the thyrotropic axis influencing the thyroid gland (see Fig. A1.5). Even if this hypothesis is appealing, only a long series of observations focused on hypo/hyperactivity of a specific gland, during time and with medication aimed at regulating its functions, could give further elements for diagnostic purposes.

Regarding the male genital system, indications such as orchitis and epididymitis were conferred to the external genital area (HX4 *waishengzhiqi*) on the axis to the lower branch of the anthelix, overlapping therefore with the French uterus/prostate.

My contribution to this complex issue firstly concerns the external genitals. In the case shown on the left of Figure 5.45, the 44-year-old female patient had a very painful abscess of the excretory duct of Bartholin's gland. Treatment with semi-permanent needle on one of the two identified points reduced her pain. On the right of Figure 5.45 is a 26-year-old male patient with venous ectasia of the pampiniform plexus (>3 mm diameter) diagnosed as a varicocele of 2–3°. Before varicocelectomy two points were identified with PPT; they maintained a constant position and disappeared immediately after surgery.

We tried to find more reliable information on the localization of parts of the genital system with the collaboration of gynecologists Daniela Bellu and Biagina De Ramundo.[69] Our observational study originated from the knowledge that

hysteroscopy is still considered a painful procedure by most gynecologists and patients and that ear acupuncture could in theory be used to reduce the pain experienced by patients undergoing this examination, provided that stimulation could be applied on reliable points/areas. Since there was no consensus between the French and Chinese schools, we worked on the hypothesis that the insertion of the optic fiber into the cervix could perhaps briefly activate the corresponding area on the ear. Both diagnostic techniques, PPT and ESRT with Agiscop (−), were thus applied before (T0) and immediately after (T1) hysteroscopy in 52 consecutive patients (average age 51.5 years, SD 11.8, range 30–79) with various gynecological disorders such as suspected intrauterine outgrowth (endometrial polyps, submucosal myomas), abnormal uterine bleeding, endometrial hyperplasia, etc. At ~10 min after hysteroscopy, patients were asked by another operator, who was not directly involved with the procedures, to rate the pain experienced on a numeric verbal scale (NVS) scoring from 0 (absence of pain) to 10 (extreme pain). Using an innovative technique called 'addition–subtraction' we identified all the 'appearing' (new) and 'disappearing' points at T1 by means of PPT and ESRT and transcribed them on the Sectogram. If we look at Figure 5.46 we can see that there is a great difference in the number of sensitized sectors before and after hysteroscopy. The new points tend to cluster mainly on sector 24, especially on the ascending branch of the helix but partially also on the internal genital area (TF2 = *neishengzhiqi*) (on the left of Fig. 5.46). The vanishing points seem to be scattered at random over the whole auricle (on the right of Fig. 5.46). However, if we examine the clusters of points we may suppose that the mental and muscular relaxation following hysteroscopy may be immediately

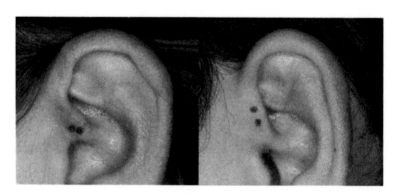

Fig. 5.45 Sensitized area in a 44-year-old female patient with an abscess of the excretory duct of Bartholin's gland (left image); sensitized area in a male patient aged 26 with varicocele of 2–3° (right image).

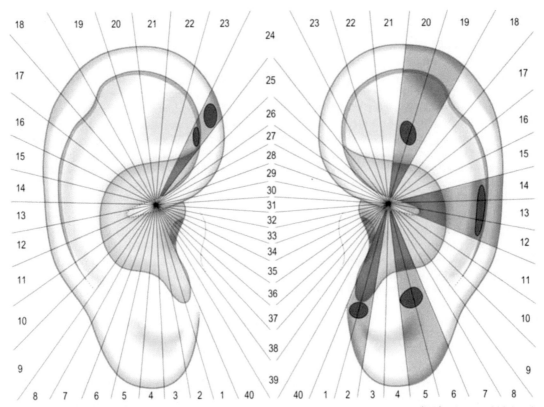

Fig. 5.46 Cluster of high value in the distribution of 'new' tender points after hysteroscopy (left); cluster of high value in the distribution of 'vanishing' tender points after hysteroscopy (right).

succeeded by a loss in sensitization of several correlated areas. The same phenomenon was observed with ESRT (–): the new points tended to cluster on sectors 23, 24 and 25 and the vanishing points lost their lower electrical resistance in several sectors.

As regards the aim of our study, we could conclude that both PPT and ESRT had identified an area which corresponded only partially to the Chinese representation of the external genitals and seemed positioned rather far from Nogier's analogous somatotopic area.

The representation of the uterus on the ear

My contribution to this topic mainly concerned patients observed in my practice who were affected by hypermenorrhea.

For example, a 44-year-old female patient showed this symptom because she had multiple uterine leiomyomas of about 1–2 cm diameter. She also suffered with recurrent lumbar pain, perhaps because she had uterine retroversion. Treatment on the anthelix points gave good results

regarding her backache; moreover, after the first sessions her excessive menstrual bleeding, as measured by the number of sanitary towels necessary, was reduced to less than half (Fig. 5.47). I was satisfied with the clinical result, but after 4 months ultrasound showed a further increase in size of some of the leiomyomas and the patient could not avoid hysterectomy 6 months later. This case led me to think about the mere symptomatic effect obtained on uterine bleeding by stimulating this area. I questioned myself whether there could have been a better outcome by slowing down the growth of leiomyoma, perhaps adding points in the endocrinal area.

The representation of the ovary on the ear

A possible somatotopy of the ovary was researched by the gynecologist Dr Ilaria Cavaliere on a group of 21 women undergoing in vitro fertilization and embryo transfer. The patients, mainly affected by idiopathic infertility, followed the same protocol of treatment which was aimed at stimulating the

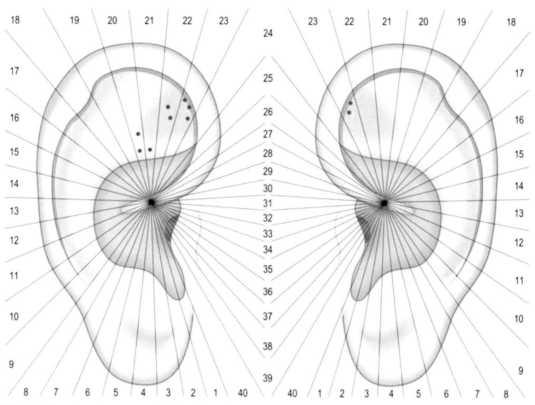

Fig. 5.47 Tender points in a 44-year-old female patient with excessive menstrual bleeding in multiple uterine leiomyomas.

ovaries with purified gonadotropin for 10–16 days. Follicular growth was checked every day or every 2 days until an approximate diameter of 18–20 mm was reached. PPT was performed in all patients before starting hormonal treatment (T0) and at the end of it (T1); nine out of the 21 patients showed a cluster of 13 new points on the upper part of the triangular fossa (on the left of Fig. 5.48). Afterwards ovulation was induced by 10 000 U of chorionic gonadotropin and 36 hours later the oocytes were aspirated from the follicles. Before this operation the tenderness of the auricles was tested again (T2): three patients showed no sensitivity whereas in the other six a threefold number of tender points appeared on the triangular fossa and, in a minor ratio, on the ascending part of the helix also (on the right of Fig. 5.48). The following day PPT was carried out a third time (T3), showing the same number of points but with an average increase in tenderness for each.

Dr Cavaliere made the following observations regarding her pilot study:

1. It is possible that the representation of the ovary needs to be searched out in the upper part of the triangular fossa.
2. Pharmacological induction of ovulation, when effective, sensitizes this area to a much greater extent in responders than in non-responders.
3. There is also a minor area of sensitization of the ascending branch of the helix which seems to correspond to the Chinese external genital area and/or to the French uterus on the internal border.

As frequently happens on the auricle, the reflex points of different anatomical structures may stratify on the same area. This is the case, for example, with thrombophlebitis of the right vena poplitea which generally sensitizes an area overlapping the representation of the ovary. This area, however, corresponds also to an important acupuncture point for gynecological disorders, such as SP6 *sanyinjiao* whose tenderness at pressure may be reduced by the needle contact test (NCT) (see Ch. 8).

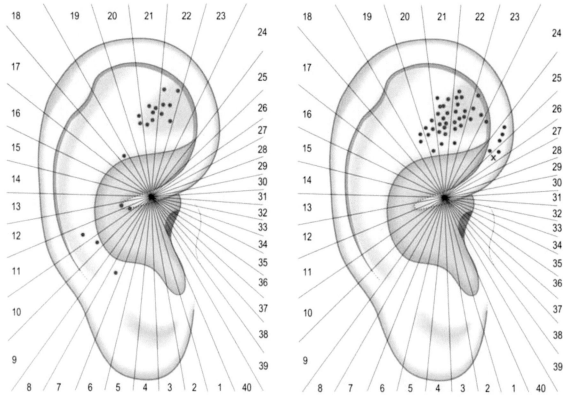

Fig. 5.48 'New' tender points in nine women undergoing in vitro fertilization and embryo transfer; at the end of pharmacological treatment with purified gonadotropin (T1) (left); after inducing ovulation with 10 000 U of chorionic gonadotropin (T2) (right). Dots = lateral surface; cross on sector 26 (right image) = internal border of the helix.

References

[1] Bourdiol RJ. Elements of auriculotherapy. Moulins-les-Metz: Maisonneuve; 1982.

[2] Alimi D, Geissmann A, Gardeur D. Auricular acupuncture stimulation measured on fMRI. Med Acup 2002;2:18–21.

[3] Liboni W, Romoli M, Allais G et al. La fMRI nella validazione dell'agopuntura auricolare: un protocollo sperimentale. Asti: XXII Congresso Nazionale Società Italiana Riflessoterapia, Agopuntura, Auricoloterapia (SIRAA); 16–17 November 2007.

[4] Taubert K. Diagnostik über das Ohr? Z Arztl Fortbild 1992;86:945–6.

[5] Goldberg DP. Manual of the General Health Questionnaire. Windsor: NFER; 1978.

[6] Bellantuono C, Fiorio R, Zanotelli R et al. Psychiatric screening in general practice in Italy. A validity study of the GHQ. Soc Psych 1987;22:113–7.

[7] Maigne R. Diagnostic et traitement des douleurs communes d'origine rachidienne

[8] Maigne R. Le syndrome de la charnière dorso-lombaire. Sem Hop Paris 1981;11–12:545–54.

[9] Maigne R. Low back pain of thoracolumbar origin. Arch Phys Med Rehabil 1980;61:389–95.

[10] Wolfe F, Smythe HA, Yunus MB et al. The American College of Rheumatology 1990 criteria for the classification of fibromyalgia: report of the multicenter criteria committee. Arthritis Rheum 1990; 33:160–72.

[11] Lawrence RC, Felson DT, Helmick CG et al. Estimates of the prevalence of arthritis and other rheumatic conditions in the United States. Part II. Arthritis Rheum 2008;1:26–35.

[12] Gur A, Oktayoglu P. Central nervous system abnormalities in fibromyalgia and chronic fatigue syndrome: new concepts in treatment. Curr Pharm Des 2008;13:1274–94.

(fig. 358). Paris: Expansion Scientifique Française; 1989.

[13] Mayhew E, Ernst E. Acupuncture for fibromyalgia – a systematic review of randomized clinical trials. Rheumatology 2007;5:801–4.

[14] Finckh A, Morabia A, Deluze C et al. Validation of questionnaire-based response criteria of treatment efficacy in the fibromyalgia syndrome. Arthritis Care Res 1998;2:116–23.

[15] Lange G. Akupunktur der Ohrmuschel. Schorndorf: WBV; 1987.

[16] Ablin JN, Shoenfeld Y, Buskila D. Fibromyalgia, infection and vaccination: two more parts in the etiological puzzle. J Immunol 2006;27:145–52.

[17] Chen P. Modern Chinese ear acupuncture. Brookline: Paradigm; 2004.

[18] Abbate S. Chinese auricular acupuncture. Boca Raton: CRC Press; 2004.

[19] Huang L. Auriculotherapy diagnosis and treatment. Bellaire: Longevity Press; 1996.

[20] Nogier PFM. Traité d'auriculothérapie. Moulins-les-Metz: Maisonneuve; 1969.

[21] Nogier PFM. Handbook to auriculotherapy. 2nd ed. Brussels: SATAS; 1998.

[22] Durinyan RA. Physiologic bases of auricular reflexotherapy (in Russian). Erivan: Ayastan; 1983.

[23] Durinyan RA. Anatomy and physiology of auricular reflex therapy. Scand J Acup Electrother 1986; 3–4:83–91.

[24] Paykel ES. Methodological aspects of life events research. J Psychosom Res 1983;5:341–52.

[25] Kellner R, Sheffield BF. A self-rating scale of distress. Psychol Med 1973;1:88–100.

[26] Romoli M, Giommi A. Ear acupuncture in psychosomatic medicine: the importance of the *Sanjiao* (Triple Heater) area. Acup Electrother Res 1993;18:185–94.

[27] Wang SM, Kain ZN. Auricular acupuncture: a potential treatment for anxiety. Anesth Analg 2001;92:548–53.

[28] Wang SM, Peloquin C, Kain ZN. The use of auricular acupuncture to reduce preoperative anxiety. Anesth Analg 2001;93:1178–80.

[29] Léger D, Poursain B, Neubauer D et al. An international survey of sleeping problems in the general population. Curr Med Res Opin 2008; 1:307–17.

[30] Kuppermann M, Lubeck DP, Mazonson PD et al. Sleep problems and their correlates in a working population. J Gen Intern Med 1995;10:25–32.

[31] Zammit GK, Weinger J, Damato N et al. Quality of life in people with insomnia. Sleep 1999;Suppl. 2: S379–85.

[32] Reeder CE, Franklin M, Bramley TJ. Current landscape of insomnia in managed care. Am J Manag Care 2007;13(Suppl. 5):S112–6.

[33] Stoller MK. Economic effects of insomnia. Clin Ther 1994;16:873–97.

[34] Subramanian S, Surani S. Sleep disorders in the elderly. Geriatrics 2007;12:10–32.

[35] Devine EB, Hakim Z, Green J. A systematic review of patient-reported outcome instruments measuring sleep dysfunction in adults. Pharmacoeconomics 2005;9:889–912.

[36] Arrindell WA, Eisemann M, Richter J et al. Phobic anxiety in 11 nations. Part I: dimensional constancy of the five-factor model. Behav Res Ther 2003;41:461–79.

[37] Zung WWK. A self-rating depression scale. Arch Gen Psych 1965;12:63–70.

[38] Zung WWK. A rating instrument for anxiety disorders. Psychosom 1971;12:371–9.

[39] McLaughlin TP, Khandker RK, Kruzikas DT et al. Overlap of anxiety and depression in a managed care population: prevalence and association with resource utilization. J Clin Psych 2006;8:1187–93.

[40] Wittchen HU, Schuster P, Lieb R. Comorbidity and mixed anxiety-depressive disorder: clinical curiosity or pathophysiological need? Hum Psychopharm 2001;16(Suppl. 1):21–30.

[41] Weisberg RB, Maki KM, Culpepper L et al. Is anyone really M.A.D.?: the occurrence and course of mixed anxiety-depressive disorders in a sample of primary care patients. J Nerv Ment Dis 2005;4:223–30.

[42] Means-Christensen AJ, Sherbourne CD, Roy-Byrne PP et al. In search of mixed anxiety-depressive disorder: a primary care study. Depress Anxiety 2006;4:183–9.

[43] Beck AT, Steer RA, Ball R et al. Comparison of Beck depression inventories -IA and -II in psychiatric outpatients. J Pers Ass 1996;3:588–97.

[44] Spielberger CD, Gorusch RL, Lushene RE. Manual for the state-trait anxiety inventory. Palo Alto: Consulting Psychologist Press; 1970.

[45] Mayberg HS. Depression: a neuropsychiatric perspective. In: Panksepp J, editor. Textbook of biological psychiatry. Chichester: John Wiley; 2004. 197–229.

[46] Linde N. Ohrakupunktur: ein Leitfaden für Theorie und Praxis. 3rd ed. Stuttgart: Sonntag; 2000.

[47] Rouxeville Y, Meas Y, Bossy J. Auriculothérapie-Acupuncture auriculaire. Paris: Springer; 2007.

[48] Oleson TD. Auriculotherapy manual. Chinese and Western systems of ear acupuncture. 3rd ed. Edinburgh: Churchill Livingstone; 2003.

[49] Nogier R. Auriculothérapie personnalisée – 1er degré. Montpellier: Sauramps; 2000.

[50] The extent and burden of allergy in the United Kingdom. House of Lords – Science and Technology, 6th report; 24 July 2007.

[51] Asher MI, Montefort S, Bjorkstén B et al. Worldwide time trends in the prevalence of symptoms of asthma, allergic rhinoconjunctivitis, and eczema in childhood: ISAAC phases one and three repeat multicountry cross-sectional surveys. Lancet 2006;368:733–43.

[52] Bjorkstén B, Clayton T, Ellwood P et al. Worldwide time trends for symptoms of rhinitis and conjunctivitis: phase III of the International Study of Asthma and Allergies in Childhood (ISAAC). Pediatr Allergy Immunology 2008;2:110–24.

[53] Arbes SJ, Gergen PJ, Elliott L et al. Prevalences of positive skin test responses to 10 common allergens in the US population: results from the Third National Health and Nutrition Examination Survey. J Allergy Clin Immunol 2005;2:377–83.

[54] National Heart Lung and Blood Institute. Global Initiative for Asthma. Global strategy for asthma management and prevention. NHLBI/WHO workshop report. Bethesda: National Institutes of Health; NHLBI publication no. 02–3659. 2006.

[55] Cazzoletti L, Marcon A, Janson C et al. Asthma control in Europe: a real-world evaluation based on an international population-based study. J Allergy Clin Immunol 2007;6:1360–7.

[56] McIvor RA, Boulet LP, Fitzgerald JM et al. Asthma control in Canada. Can Fam Phys 2007;53:672–7.

[57] Mazzini, PL. Deficit uditivi da rumore e auricolopuntura: proposta di una mappa. Tesi Associazione Italiana Ricerca Aggiornamento Scientifico (AIRAS), Padova; 1993.

[58] Park J, White AR, Ernst E. Efficacy of acupuncture as a treatment for tinnitus: a systematic review. Arch Otolaryngol Head Neck Surg 2000;4:489–92.

[59] Pildner von Steinburg R, Pildner von Steinburg D. Die Behandlung der zentralen vestibulären Dysfunktion mittels Akupunktur (Reflextherapie). HNO Praxis Heute 1983;3:161–7.

[60] Wheeler PW, Wheeler SF. Vasomotor rhinitis. Am Fam Phys 2005;6:1057–62.

[61] Nanjing Ear Acupuncture Compiling group of Nanjing Military Headquarters. Shanghai: People's Publishing House; 1973.

[62] An outline of Chinese acupuncture. Bejing: Foreign Languages Press; 1975.

[63] Mannheimer C, Carlsson CA, Emanuelsson H et al. The effects of TENS in patients with severe angina pectoris. Circulation 1985;71:308–16.

[64] Mannheimer C, Augustinsson LE, Carlsson CA et al. Epidural spinal electrical stimulation in severe angina pectoris. Br Heart J 1988;59:56–61.

[65] Hansson SO, Mannheimer C. Treatment with ear acupuncture in patients with severe angina pectoris. Pain Clin 1991;1:53–6.

[66] Rahn KH, Barenbrock M, Hausberg M. The sympathetic nervous system in the pathogenesis of hypertension. J Hypertens 1999;17(Suppl. 3):11–14.

[67] Grassi G. Role of the sympathetic nervous system in human hypertension. J Hypertens 1998;16:1979–87.

[68] Li Su Huai. Points 2001. Taipei: China Acupuncture and Moxibustion Supplies; 1976.

[69] Romoli M, Allais G, Bellu D et al. Can hysteroscopy clarify the somatotopic representation of the uterus on the outer ear? (submitted for publication).

Chapter 6

Measuring electrical skin resistance on acupuncture points

Filadelfio Puglisi

INTRODUCTION

For many decades, practitioners have used electrical devices to locate specific points for acupuncture, both in association with, or to replace, manual methods such as the pain pressure test (PPT). The main assumption underlying such electrical devices is that an acupuncture point is characterized by its different electrical resistance (or its reciprocal, conductance) compared to that of the skin surrounding it. This statement derives mainly from the work of some researchers in the 1950s, for example Voll[1] and Nakatani and Yamashita.[2] They found that a lower skin resistance value often coincided with spots that traditional Chinese medicine indicated as effective for acupuncture treatment. Although Niboyet[3] meticulously re-examined the method, it was only in 1975 that experiments by Reichmanis[4] and colleagues truly awakened interest in the topic. This author employed a rod electrode for roughly locating higher electrical conduction points on the skin, and then a roller-type electrode for tracing conductance curves along lines passing through those points.

More than 30 years of episodic research has produced no consensus on the effectiveness of measuring electrical resistance for identifying acupuncture points. The work up to the late 1970s has been reviewed by Mannheimer and Lampe[5] and, more recently, a comprehensive review was presented by Ahn and Martinsen.[6]

Over the last decades many devices for locating acupuncture points based on resistance measurement have become commercially available. Their very simple electronics and low cost have made them widely accessible. However, acupuncturists rarely know more about them than that when an LED lights up or a beep is heard the machine has detected a variation in resistance. This is because very few commercial makers describe their devices or the principles behind them in depth.

It is the aim of this chapter to examine the physical principles on which such devices are based, and explain the structure of a simple machine for measuring ear skin electrical resistance, together with its clinical validation.

Is is suggested that the reader keep in mind that the acupuncturist can also derive many useful data from the work of other researchers, since electrical resistance of the skin is important in several fields of application. Broadly speaking these applications are of two different types. In the first, an endogenous generator establishes a flow of current through the body. This flow of current originates an electric potential that can be measured on the skin. In the second, an electrical generator outside the body applies a potential to two points of the skin and establishes current inside the body. Electromyography, electrocardiography and electroencephalography belong to the first category, and to the second impedance tomography, body composition scanners, psychogalvanic reflex, acupuncture point location and percutaneous transport in iontophoresis.

Also relevant are all electrostimulation techniques in which a current is applied for therapeutic reasons, such as transcutaneous nerve stimulation, therapeutical nerve stimulation and functional electrostimulation. Moreover, dermatological applications such as cosmetology, wound healing and percutaneous gas monitoring all have some interest in assessing the physical properties of the epidermis.

Research in the above fields has focused on some aspects of skin resistance and its controlling parameters, and is therefore worth studying for getting different angles of view on the subject.

ELECTRICAL SKIN RESISTANCE (ESR)

Electrically speaking, the resistance R denotes the ratio of the voltage V applied to a conductor to the current I flowing in it: $R = V/I$.

When taking measurements, it must be kept in mind that resistance may be a non-linear parameter which depends on the value of applied voltage (i.e. doubling the voltage, the current does not double) and on the type of tissue. If the voltage varies with time, as in the case of the commonly used alternating current, the parameter R is substituted by a complex parameter termed 'impedance' (which is a function of frequency). The situation is often confusing when trying to compare literature data, some obtained with constant, some with alternating currents of different frequencies. But even restricting the definition to the case of a constant voltage, when measuring skin resistance the current flows through a complex path, and which resistance is measured is not so clear.

Normal commercial devices for locating low skin resistance spots have a large common 'reference' or 'indifferent' electrode held by the subject in one hand, generally a cylinder of 2–3 cm diameter or a similar contrivance (Fig. 6.1).

A 'probe' consisting of a narrow electrode is put into contact with the skin at the location to be investigated, usually with the help of a small spring to keep the contact pressure within a known range. The main prerequisite is for the area of skin contact at the reference electrode to be much larger than that at the measuring probe, so that the resistance at the reference electrode compared with that

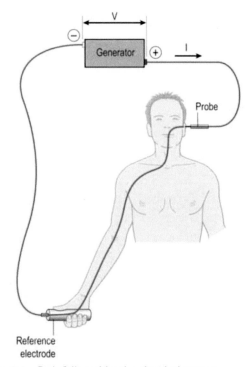

Fig. 6.1 Path followed by the electrical current.

at the measuring probe can be disregarded. The current flows from the large to the small electrode, passing through a number of biological tissues and two skin/electrode interfaces. The usual approximation is to consider the electrical skin resistance (ESR) as V/I where V is known because it is pre-set by the generator, while I is measured.

The measured value of ESR includes contributions from several elements, but the most determining arises from the stratum corneum of the skin. On the derma lies a complex of tissues which constitute the epidermis, whose thickness is on average about 50–150 µm but can be as high as 1500 µm on the plantar aspect of the foot.[7] It is made up of several superimposed specialized cell strata, of which the external is the corneum, consisting of regular rows of dead flat cells filled with keratin, a fibrous protein.

This stratum corneum continuously loses dead cells at its surface, which are replaced by new cells originating from the lower stratum. Its thickness (both absolute and as a fraction of the epidermis) depends on location. For instance, Sandby-Møller et al[8] found a thickness from 11 µm on the shoulder to 18.3 µm at the dorsal aspect of the forearm, while Jacobi and Kaiser[9] give 17 µm to 28 µm for the stratum corneum for porcine ear skin which they judge to give similar results in humans. The stratum corneum is characterized by very low water permeability, low ion mobility and high electrical resistance. Its interest here lies in the fact that, from experiments where the stratum corneum is removed and the decrease of resistance monitored, it is evident that skin resistance is produced mainly in the stratum corneum.

There are several well documented methods of skin ablation. The commonest, probably because it does not require any special equipment, consists of stripping the dead cells by successive applications of adhesive tape. Examples of this technique are described in Yamamoto and Yamamoto,[10] Kalia and Guy,[11] Kalia et al[12] and Bashir et al.[13] Another method consists of laser ablation,[14] while the most recent method uses a flow of abrasive particles, as described in Gill et al.[15]

The removal of the stratum corneum is commonly used in esthetic applications for skin remodeling, and in methods of preparing the skin for drug conveyance, such as iontophoresis. They interest us only for the electrical measurements taken to correlate quantity and thickness of removed material and skin resistance.

Tape stripping seems to increase ion mobility by two orders of magnitude (that is a hundredfold increase).[12] This correlates very well with the findings on microdermabrasion, which decreases resistance from thousands of kΩ to tens of kΩ.[15] Gill and colleagues[15] give a value of about 20–80 kΩ for skin resistance after complete stratum removal.

To give an order of magnitude for skin resistance, in an earlier work Inada et al[16] had given 12–120 kΩ/cm², while Kalia and Guy[11] found a value of 187 kΩ for the real part of the complex skin impedance in hydrated skin with intact stratum corneum at 1 Hz, with electrodes of 3.14 cm². Oleson et al[17] give, instead of resistance, the amount of current flowing through the skin under a voltage of 9 V. They found spots of low resistance allowing the passage of 300 µA, but unfortunately they do not specify the internal electrical resistance of the device used.

In fact, the very strong influence of the stratum corneum had been noted extremely early in articles seeking to locate acupuncture points by electrical methods. McCarrol and Rowley[18] deliberately damaged the stratum corneum by applying a very high pressure (2 kg/mm²) at the tip of the searching electrode, observing a dramatic drop in skin impedance, which, in one case, amounted to 94% of the impedance measured previously using a tip loaded with 0.1 kg/mm². Their experiment was conducted at 1000 Hz, but no details of the tip's dimension are given. Their conclusion was that when trying to locate an acupuncture point by measuring skin conductance with a small electrode, the chances are that we are simply measuring the integrity of the stratum corneum. Therefore, we can suspect that any macroscopic variations are probably due to accidental stratum corneum abrasions.

As an alternative assumption, acupuncture points may be associated with areas of thinner or more hydrated stratum corneum.

This takes us to the definition of a 'gold standard' for an 'acupuncture point', or at least to some kind of specific histological findings for acupuncture loci.

There is almost nothing in the literature on this subject. A valuable contribution is the experiment by Terral and Rabischong.[19] They made histological sections of the skin of rabbits on the spots where they had located acupoints and found that at locations with lower electrical resistance the connective tissue was more lax, and contained a number of nerve fibres and other structures. It is, however, to be noted that rabbits had been carefully shaved, therefore it is not possible to know how the stratum corneum had been altered.

ESR SOURCES OF VARIABILITY

Even if the resistance of the path through the body were constant, a number of external factors introduce a large amount of variability on the reading. Some are under control by setting the measuring device, others by conditioning the measuring technique. This means that before taking a measurement, decisions must be made regarding a number of choices:

1. whether to use direct current or variable current
2. in the case of direct current, its absolute value and polarity; in the case of variable current its shape, frequency and absolute value
3. whether to use constant current or constant voltage generators
4. the material and shape of the electrode itself.

In addition, the measuring technique must take into consideration the following problems:

1. how to maintain a constant pressure and angle of the electrode with respect to skin surface
2. how to keep the influence of sweating under control (by constant room temperature, or taking into account seasonal variations or other methods).

Keeping in mind that from the innumerable combinations among all the possible parameters listed above each researcher has made his or her own particular choice, it is not surprising that it is almost impossible to reconcile 50 years of literature on the subject!

And that is not all. Once a pair of electrodes has been applied to the human body, the resistance measured is not constant, but varies over time in a manner which is not easy to define. This is very well known to those who make that variation their specific field of investigation, such as researchers on the psychogalvanic effect, but not so well known to acupuncture practitioners, who usually take only one measurement for any specific spot, and several measurements in rapid succession.

In the late 1940s there were attempts at classifying different types of time variations, for example by Van Der Valk and Groen.[20] Almost 50 years later Terral and Rabischong[19] were tackling the same puzzling problem, trying to understand why in one subject the resistance seemed to go up, and in another to go down, and in both cases in different ways (for instance a sudden increase followed by slow stabilization, or a simple slow steady decrease, and so on), for no apparent reason.

With such premises it is clear that a measurement instrument must also show time variations of the resistance, and some guidelines or at least a reasonable decision must be agreed upon as to how many seconds have to elapse before the ESR can be measured. An attempt to harmonize all these requirements is described in the rest of this chapter.

DESIGN OF AN INSTRUMENT FOR ESR

A research program was designed to answer the following questions:

1. Can a simple instrument for clinical use be built on the indications arising from the preliminary results highlighted above?
2. Are measurements of ESR repeatable intra- and inter-rater?

To answer these questions a measuring device for clinical use was built with the following specifications:

- A probe with a 1 mm diameter steel tip, loaded with a spring to ensure a contact force of about 20 g.
- A hand-held reference electrode made from a 30 mm diameter steel cylinder.
- A range of measurement with 20% accuracy from 10 kΩ to 100 MΩ.
- A computer displayed a resistance vs. time diagram with a logarithmic scale, with the possibility of displaying numerical value of resistance every second and the average of the last 10 s.

The block diagram is shown in Figure 6.2.

In such a circuit the measurements of low values of ESR are taken at practically constant current, if the reference resistance (RR) is much higher than the tested resistance. The high values are measured practically at constant voltage, since RR in this case is much smaller than the measured resistance. The former situation is obtained when RR is a few MΩ and skin resistance value is a few tens of kΩ and the latter when ESR is several tens of MΩ. So there are controlled conditions (constant current or voltage respectively) in the high and low ranges where

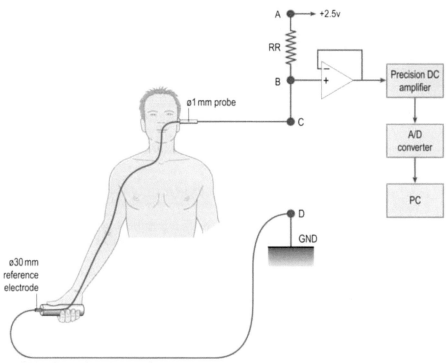

Fig. 6.2 Block diagram of the device for measuring resistance at steady contact pressure. RR is a reference resistance in series with ESR.

ESR tends to cluster, and more uncertain conditions (both current and voltage change) in the middle range.

The probe design is shown in Figure 6.3 and its physical aspect in Figure 6.4.

This hardware is connected with a laptop through a National Instrument acquisition A/D converter, the USB8000, which provides also the 2.5 V supply. The laptop must be used disconnected from the mains and operated only by its internal 12 V battery for safety reasons.

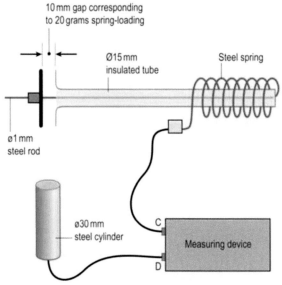

Fig. 6.3 Measuring system, showing the hand-held electrode and the probe design.

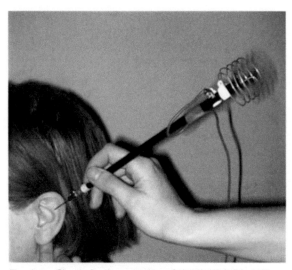

Fig. 6.4 Simple implementation of the hand-held probe, with an external spring to keep constant pressure on skin.

A switch button on the box of the device allows the operator to trigger a series of 10 resistance readings, at 1 s intervals. At the end of the 10 readings the software calculates the average and shows it on the computer monitor. An averaged value of resistance over a time range seems more reliable than a single reading, especially when an unsteady hand can cause continuous small slips of the probe tip on the skin.

In this research we did not investigate the possible optimization of the time interval, but adopted 10 s as a compromise between an excessively long measurement time in a clinical setting and the desire of extending measurements until an acceptable stabilization of the resistance value.

For the same reason it was decided to wait 5 s before triggering the series of 10 measurements, for avoiding transient effects of ESR at its first generally rapid descent when the probe is applied to the skin. The value so obtained may not be a true stabilized value of ESR, but at least it is measured under controlled conditions and gives an overall idea of the speed at which the resistance is dropping.

A typical diagram obtained with this device is shown in Figure 6.5. In this figure it is possible to appreciate the instant of probe tip application and withdrawal, at about 185 s and 200 s. Initially the resistance does not seem to drop in any significant

way, due to some hesitation of the operator's hand. Then good contact is established, at about 188 s, and resistance drops suddenly. Two changes in inclinations are visible within the first 4 s. For the remaining time of contact there is not a true stabilization, but the resistance continues to fall at a slow pace. The 10 measurements are indicated, together with the final average, concluding the test at about 199 s. The average is what will be called the ESR of the specific skin spot.

CLINICAL VALIDATION

In the experiment, 11 asymptomatic subjects (4 males and 7 females) aged 20–63 (average 41.9 years) were examined.

A total of five bilateral points were randomly chosen on different anatomical locations (helix, anthelix, triangular fossa, tragus, antitragus) (Fig. 6.6). This pattern was the same for all the 11 subjects for a total of 110 points. Further points to test were identified with the commercial device Agiscop which has been used for all the clinical investigations in this book and will be described in some detail in Appendix 2. The ears of all subjects were examined thoroughly with Agiscop (modality −) and a total of 118 points were found. The total number of points suitable for the experiment was therefore 228.

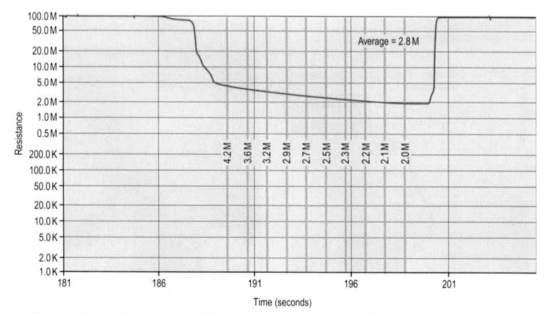

Fig. 6.5 Typical diagram of resistance as a function of time, measured on a logarithmic scale. Ten measurements are taken at 1 s intervals after the initial transient. The final average is shown.

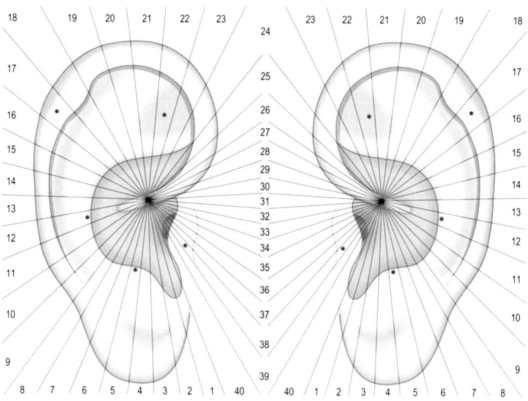

Fig. 6.6 Location of five random points on each ear. The pattern is symmetrical.

The clinical validation was designed by Dr Romoli, who had a special interest in comparing these results with the performance of commercially available devices such as the Agiscop, described in Appendix 2.

There were two operators taking the ESR measurements: (A) a trained operator with 10 years experience in ear acupuncture diagnosis and (B) a professional medical operator with no previous experience in acupuncture. The computer was operated by a third independent researcher, who observed the contact time between the probe tip and the skin then waited 5 s and triggered the 10 measurement series. Neither operator A nor operator B had access to any results of any measurement during the session.

At each point two measurements were taken by rater A, and the same number by rater B. The succession of measurements was A, B, A, B. The time lag between each measurement was 5–10 minutes. Neither A nor B knew what their own first measurement of a given point was. All measurements were taken during the months of May, June and July, with an indoor temperature varying from 22 to 27 degrees Celsius.

A histogram of all 912 measurements by rater A and B, related to a total of 228 points, is given in Figure 6.7.

It will be appreciated that the frequency is not distributed uniformly across the range, but is clustered around very high and very low values, with a difference of four orders of magnitude. A similar behavior was also found in the second session by rater A and in both sessions by rater B.

The histograms of the random points and the points identified with the Agiscop are represented in Figures 6.8 and 6.9. It is possible to appreciate that Agiscop points tend to cluster around lower values in comparison with the random points.

It is difficult to treat these data using parametric statistical analysis, since a few points acting differently from their neighbors can cause mean and standard deviations to vary wildly. For instance, following 10 points grouping together in the hundredths of kΩ range, one point around 100 MΩ is enough to shift the mean to around 10 MΩ and cause the standard deviation to shoot up. In such a case the mean and standard deviation retain their mathematical meaning,

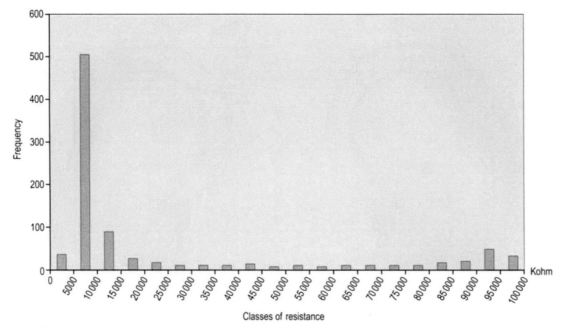

Fig. 6.7 Histogram of all points measured in this experiment from 0 to 100 000 Kohm.

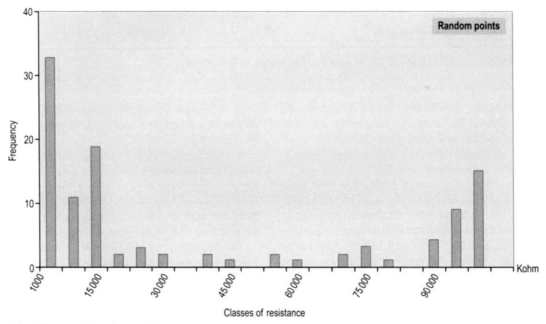

Fig. 6.8 Histogram of random points.

but no longer give a good idea of the data distribution.

It is thus opportune to adopt a threshold type of differentiation. In order to establish the threshold, a more refined histogram is traced for only the values below 10 000 kΩ. It is possible to see that most values lie below 1500 kΩ (Fig. 6.10). Therefore

a value of 2 MΩ can be considered a reasonable separation point between points to be classified as either low or high resistance. In addition, it is relevant to observe that of the 118 points which were identified with the Agiscop, most were under the 2 MΩ threshold (109 for rater A and 105 for rater B).

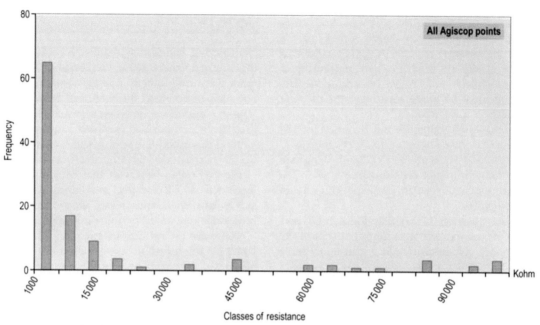

Fig. 6.9 Histogram of points identified with the Agiscop.

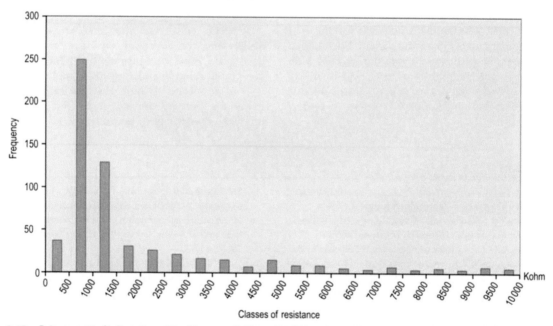

Fig. 6.10 Enlargement of left section of the histogram in Figure 6.7. Only points with resistance lower than 10 000 KΩ are included.

INTRA-RATER REPEATABILITY

Using this 2 MΩ threshold intra-rater repeatability is checked. That is to say, how many times a point that a rater classifies as belonging to one of the two classes (above or below 2 MΩ) in the first measurement is confirmed by the same rater as belonging to the same class in the second measurement.

Rater A successfully repeated 82.0% of his own measurements on the 228 points. For rater B the percentage of success was 81.1%.

INTER-RATER RELIABILITY

Inter-rater reliability is how many times rater B confirms the finding of rater A (point below or above the $2\,M\Omega$ threshold) when measuring a point immediately after A has measured it. The comparison must be made separately for the first and the second measurement.

In the first measurement A and B agreed for 182 points over 228, corresponding to 79.8% success.

In the second measurement A and B agreed again for 182 points (not the same points as in the first measurement) over 228, corresponding again to 79.8% success.

Now the question is whether these high percentages of success are meaningful, or partially due to chance. To answer such a question I have adopted Cohen's kappa coefficient, which is easily adaptable to the case of data belonging to two classes.[21] But it must be underlined that Cohen's kappa coefficient is normally judged as not comparable with other studies.

In our case rater A had a kappa = 0.506 and rater B a kappa = 0.585 in the intra-rater tests, while in the inter-rater tests kappa was 0.580 for the first measurement and 0.535 for the second. Such kappa values seem to indicate a moderate success both of the intra- and the inter-rater tests, slightly above midway between the case of kappa = 0 (results due to chance alone) and kappa = 1 (raters in perfect agreement).

CONCLUSIONS

Considering the above results, we can conclude that the extremely wide variations in skin resistance from one spot to another nearby, and from one measurement to the next, call for a threshold type of comparison between measurements, rather than for a comparison between ranges. With the method described, the spot resistance can be classified in two categories: either high or low.

We have also observed that by considering as 'high' values of electrical resistance above $2\,M\Omega$, and as 'low' the values below, we get an acceptable intra-rater repeatability and inter-rater reliability.

There are no indications as to why this value of $2\,M\Omega$ for the threshold is so successful. It is possible that it corresponds to some physiological fact, keeping in mind that this holds true only for our specific device's geometry, setting and ambiance parameters (in particular overall temperature and sweating conditions). It may be that some value around $2\,M\Omega$ is even better, but we did not investigate this possibility.

It seems confirmed that with the geometrical design and the electrical specifications that have been used here, measurement of ESR can be an acceptably reliable and repeatable method.

It is important to note that the causes of ESR variations were not investigated. This is the scope for further work yet to be undertaken.

References

[1] Voll R. Messbare Akupunktur-Diagnostik und Therapie für den Praktiker. Erfahrungsheilkunde 1955;4.

[2] Nakatani Y, Yamashita K. Ryodoraku acupuncture. Tokyo: Royodoraku Research Institute; 1977.

[3] Niboyet JEH. La moindre résistance à l'électricité de surfaces punctiformes et de trajets cutanés concordant avec les points et les méridiens, bases de l'acupuncture. Marseille: Thèse Sciences; 1963.

[4] Reichmanis M, Marino AA, Becker RO. Electrical correlates of acupuncture points. IEEE Trans Biomed Eng 1975;22:533–5.

[5] Mannheimer JS, Lampe GN. Clinical transcutaneous electrical nerve stimulation. Philadelphia: FA Davis; 1984.

[6] Ahn AC, Martinsen OG. Electrical characterization of acupuncture points: technical issues and challenges. J Altern Complement Med 2007;8:817–24.

[7] Olivo GM, Toni G. Atlante di anatomia microscopica. Milano: Vallardi; 1965.

[8] Sandby-Møller J, Poulsen T, Wulf HC. Epidermal thickness at different body sites: relationship to age, gender, pigmentation, blood content, skin type and smoking habits. Acta Derm Venereol 2003;6:410–3.

[9] Jacobi U, Kaiser RM. Porcine ear skin: an in vitro model for human skin. Skin Res Technol 2007;1:19–24.

[10] Yamamoto Y, Yamamoto T. Measurement of electrical bio-impedance and its applications. Med Prog Technol 1987;3–4:171–83.

[11] Kalia YN, Guy RH. The electrical characteristics of human skin in vivo. Pharm Res 1995;11:1605–13.

[12] Kalia YN, Pirot F, Potts RO et al. Ion mobility across human stratum corneum in vivo. J Pharm Sci 1998;12:1508–11.

[13] Bashir SJ, Chew AL, Anigbogu A et al. Physical and physiological effects of stratum corneum tape stripping. Skin Res Technol 2001;1:40–8.

[14] Jacques SL, McAuliffe DJ, Blank IH et al. Controlled removal of human stratum corneum by pulsed laser. J Invest Dermatol 1987;1:88–93.

[15] Gill HS, Andrews S, Fedanov A et al. Microdermabrasion of skin for drug and vaccine delivery. American Institute of Chemical Engineers Annual Meeting 2006;#184, 14 November 2006.

[16] Inada H, Ghanem AH, Hiquchi WI. Studies on the effects of applied voltage and duration on human epiderma membrane alteration/recovery and the resultant effects upon iontophoresis. Pharm Res 1994;5:687–97.

[17] Oleson TD, Kroening RG, Bresler DE. An experimental evaluation of auricular diagnosis: the somatotopic mapping of musculoskeletal pain at ear acupuncture points. Pain 1980;2:217–29.

[18] McCarroll GD, Rowley BA. An investigation of the existence of electrically located acupuncture points. IEEE Trans Biomed Eng 1979;3:177–81.

[19] Terral C, Rabischong P. A scientific basis for acupuncture? J Altern Complement Med 1997; 3(Suppl. 1):S55–65.

[20] Van Der Valk JM, Groen J. Electrical resistance of the skin during induced emotional stress. Psychosom Med 1950;5:303–14.

[21] Bakemann R, Gottman JM. Observing interactions: an introduction to sequence analysis. New York: Cambridge University Press; 1997.

Chapter 7

The electrical skin resistance test

Following Puglisi's introduction to the issue of electrical skin resistance (ESR) and the instruments needed to measure it in Chapter 6, we need now to examine the diagnostic possibilities offered by the electrical skin resistance test (ESRT).

There is a major difference between body and ear acupuncture as regards the purpose of detecting points with reduced ESR. In body acupuncture the exact location of points may be necessary for basic research aimed at differentiating the resistance of a true meridian point from that of nearby chosen points for comparison. The exact identification of a meridian point by means of an electronic device may be useful for a beginner or for a physician wishing to identify the points with the lowest ESR in the belief that such points are also the most effective. In parallel with this strategy there is the custom followed by several practitioners who palpate the anatomical area corresponding to a specific meridian point, selecting for treatment the most sensitive spot.

The localization of points with reduced ESR on the auricle has, however, a true diagnostic purpose, since the practitioner is blind as regards the points he will find and which moreover will probably correspond only partially to the expected representation of the suffering organ or apparatus.

ADVANTAGES AND LIMITS OF AURICULAR DIAGNOSIS WITH ESRT

The advantage of using an electronic device is essentially to be able to explore the auricle systematically without the collaboration of the patient, needed for example in PPT for identifying those points most tender at pressure. Also, a beginner can easily identify the points, mark them with ink and transcribe their location onto the Sectogram.

The limit of ESRT is the fact that commercial devices are able to measure only one point at a time. This makes the procedure time-consuming as several points have to be tested within the area representing the suffering part of the body; moreover commercial devices usually do not store data which could be accessed over time, for example during a therapeutic course or in the follow-up period.

There are at least two further time-consuming factors which need to be borne in mind:

1. As illustrated in Chapter 6, the ESR is a time-dependent factor and the practitioner has to wait several seconds before ESR values stabilize. It should be noted that in some cases this stabilization does not occur at all and the resistance value goes down practically to zero if enough time elapses. This is why we chose to average the ESR value over a reasonable period of time (10 seconds).
2. The necessity to attribute hierarchical importance to the identified points is also time-consuming, supposing, as mentioned above, that points with the lowest ESR are also those with higher therapeutic value. As proposed by some manufacturers, each point should be measured in respect to baseline, readjusting it each time against a so-called 'zero' value of a part of the ear believed to be free of acupuncture points.[1] This strategy may be misleading, however, as no part of the ear, in my opinion, can with any safety be considered free of somatotopic representations.

REASONS FOR CHOOSING AGISCOP AND ADOPTING A FIXED ESR THRESHOLD IN THE VALIDATION PROCESS

The first problem I had to face when I started with my project of validation of auricular diagnosis was the choice of the most reliable electric device. As there had been no report in the literature comparing the characteristics of the devices commercially available, I chose the French Agiscop manufactured by Sedatelec, for which I declare the absence of any conflict of interest.

The ancestor of Agiscop was the Punctoscope, developed in the 1960s by Nogier himself on the basis of the pioneering research of Niboyet who dedicated his doctoral thesis in 1963 to the issue of the lower ESR of acupuncture points and meridians.[2]

As Agiscop is sold without an adequate technical description, we decided with F. Puglisi to carry out research aimed at answering the following basic questions:

1. Are the values obtained with this device to be referred to absolute levels of ESR or to differences of resistance between neighboring tissues or points?
2. Which are the values of ESR measured corresponding to the different positions (1 to 6) of the 'sensitivity knob'? (See Fig. A2.3.)
3. What is the significance of the knob changing – to the + position?

To answer these questions it was necessary first to create an instrument which could measure ESR according to the basic principles of electrology aside from its clinical applications. The device developed and its characteristics have been described in Chapter 6.

We compared Agiscop with our device measuring the skin resistance of a number of points under controlled conditions (see the section on Clinical validation in Ch. 6). The results show that Agiscop has the best intra- and inter-reliability performance when the ESR threshold is about $2\,M\Omega$, corresponding to position 3 of the above mentioned knob.

From the empirical point of view the threshold of $1\,M\Omega$, corresponding to position 4 of the knob, seems more convenient for the majority of the examined subjects allowing the identification of a sufficient number of points for diagnosis. This threshold was maintained constantly throughout the whole validation process on 506 patients.

As shown in Chapter 6, the choice of 1 or $2\,M\Omega$ does not invalidate the classification of points in two categories, one with high and the other with low ESR values, since the former includes points with ESR $2 \div 100\,M\Omega$ and the latter includes points with ESR $0 \div 2\,M\Omega$.

All patients were measured with the – polarity of the knob which corresponds to a difference of ESR due to a lower resistance of the surrounding coaxial electrode with respect to the central electrode (see Fig. A2.1). This modality was chosen because the average number of points identified with the – polarity was 2.3 times greater than the + polarity; indeed this difference allowed a higher diagnostic success of the first modality (see Table 9.3).

One of the reasons for the higher number of points identified with the (−) modality has been explained in Appendix 2 as being due to the possible indentation of the skin under the measuring probe, causing greater contact with the coaxial rather than with the central electrode (Fig. A2.4).

It should be noted that another commercial device (Pointoselect by Schwa-medico) utilizes a similar differential technique and a similar coaxial electrode. However, it is able to recognize automatically if the coaxial electrode has a higher or lower ESR in comparison with the central one.

Whatever commercial device is chosen for auricular diagnosis, it should be underlined that the information offered to professionals by the various manufacturers is incomplete at best and in the majority of cases it is really unsatisfactory. Practitioners are apparently considered incapable of developing any knowledge whatsoever in technical matters.

In my opinion it is unethical for a practitioner to use a device on his patients when he is ignorant of its elementary functions and the meaning of the measurements.

THE GENERAL DISTRIBUTION OF POINTS WITH LOWER ESR ON THE AURICLE

If we examine the general distribution of points with lower ESR (∼1 MΩ) on the outer ear in 325 patients with the − modality, we get an average of 5.24 on the right side compared to 5.98 on the left. This non-significant difference of distribution may appear to indicate a homogeneous and symmetrical distribution of points but that is not the case. If we analyze the clusters per sector we may notice that the left ear shows a higher number of sectors of high value compared to the right (Fig. 7.1). This phenomenon, similarly to what happens with PPT (see Fig. 5.5), is not easily explainable: we have to assume that the asymmetry of distribution may be intrinsic to the ear or may be the result of an asymmetrical activation of the auricles which manifests itself physiologically in the majority of patients. Our hypothesis, also expressed in Chapter 9, is that this phenomenon could be related to the asymmetrical lateralization of some functions in our brain such as language, handedness, etc.

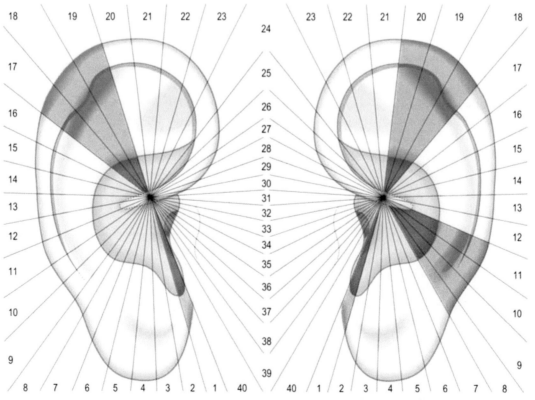

Fig. 7.1   Sectors of high value identified by cluster analysis of points with low ESR in 325 patients.

DIFFERENCES IN THE DIAGNOSTIC PERFORMANCES OF ESRT AND PPT

Both these methods show a similar performance on the total of symptoms (32.9% for ESRT and 34.6% for PPT) but their combination provides a better outcome (52.3%), which is significantly higher compared to either ESRT or PPT considered on its own ($P<0.001$). However, if we compare the success rates in the identification of the symptoms of various bodily systems, we may notice that there are some significant differences. For example, PPT shows a better outcome with musculoskeletal, teeth–temporomandibular joint (TMJ) and nervous system disorders, whereas ESRT seems to be more suitable for detecting mental and gastrointestinal problems.

The reasons for these differences may be attributed to various factors, as for example the different ability in detecting points on the various parts of the auricle and/or the intrinsic specificity of each method in diagnosing symptoms belonging to different apparatus.

I tried to find an answer to these issues by first comparing the distribution of points identified with ESRT and PPT on the auricle. We can see that ESRT identified points principally on the medial surface, followed by the lower and upper concha, whereas PPT identified a higher percentage of points on the ear lobe followed by the anthelix and the medial surface (Table 7.1). However, in my opinion these slight differences may be related at least partially to the differing anatomical composition of the tissues on which diagnosis is performed. For example, the higher number of points detected by ESRT on the medial surface may depend on the reduced thickness of the skin covering this part of the auricle. For the concha (in total 25.6% to 20.3% of PPT) we may also suppose an anatomical factor represented by the particular density of sebaceous glands in this area. We are however not sure that the ducts of sebaceous glands may favor the electrical shunt as has been supposed for sweat glands; in effect sebum seems not to be an ion conducting material such as sweat.

As regards PPT and the higher number of tender points on the ear lobe, I have suggested in Chapter 5 that this higher sensitization may result from the lack of cartilaginous support leading the practitioner inadvertently to exert a higher pressure than intended on this zone. The higher number of tender points on the anthelix could nevertheless be associated with the bias, typical in

Table 7.1 Concentration of identified points on the different zones of the ear in 325 patients. (a) % of points with low ESR; (b) % of tender points

ESRT (a)		PPT (b)	
Auricular zone	%	Auricular zone	%
Medial surface	19.0%	Ear lobe	15.2%
Lower concha	13.3%	Anthelix	14.6%
Upper concha	12.3%	Medial surface	14.4%
Ear lobe	11.7%	Lower concha	12.0%
Scapha	10.6%	Helix	9.8%
Helix	8.2%	Antitragus	8.8%
Anthelix	7.8%	Upper concha	8.3%
Triangular fossa	5.9%	Triangular fossa	5.7%
Tragus	4.7%	Scapha	5.2%
Intertragic notch	3.9%	Tragus	3.8%
Antitragus	2.6%	Intertragic notch	2.2%
Total	100%	Total	100%

the West, towards starting auricular exploration from this part, representing as it does the spine and other structures of the musculoskeletal system.

LOOKING FOR A SUITABLE METHODOLOGY TO COMPARE THE INTRINSIC DIAGNOSTIC SPECIFICITY OF ESRT AND PPT

Systematic research has never been carried out on this subject. Nevertheless I think it is of particular interest for all practitioners who wish to combine both methods to obtain maximum information on their patients.

Table 7.2 compares the diagnostic abilities of ESRT and PPT in identifying symptoms of some systems and disorders:

a. musculoskeletal apparatus
b. teeth and TMJ dysfunction
c. nervous system
d. mental disorders
e. metabolic disorders
f. gastrointestinal tract
g. cardiovascular system
h. skin disorders
i. genitourinary tract.

Table 7.2 Diagnostic success rates obtained on various apparatus and disorders in 325 patients with two methods, ERST (−) and PPT, and comparison with paired samples *t*-test

a) Musculoskeletal apparatus

Diagnostic success rate	ESRT (−) = 35.89%	PPT = 43.82%	Two methods combined = 55.84%
Comparison (paired samples *t*-test)	Mean difference	CI 95% for mean	P
ESRT (−) vs. PPT	−7.93%	(−11.10% ; −4.76%)	<0.001
ESRT (−) + PPT vs. ESRT (−)	19.95%	(17.68% ; 22.22%)	<0.001
ESRT (−) + PPT vs. PPT	12.02%	(10.18% ; 13.86%)	<0.001

b) Teeth and TMJ dysfunction

Diagnostic success rate	ESRT = 14.02%	PPT = 54.21%	Two methods combined = 59.81%
Comparison (paired samples *t*-test)	Mean difference	CI 95% for mean	P
ESRT (−) vs. PPT	−40.19%	(−51.62% ; −28.5%)	<0.001
ESRT (−) + PPT vs. ESRT (−)	3.28%	(36.20% ; 55.39%)	<0.05
ESRT (−) + PPT vs. PPT	45.79%	(1.18% ; 10.04%)	<0.001

c) Nervous system

Diagnostic success rate	ESRT = 19.30%	PPT = 47.95%	Two methods combined = 53.22%
Comparison (paired samples *t*-test)	Mean difference	CI 95% for mean	P
ESRT (−) vs. PPT	−28.65%	(−37.08% ; −20.23%)	<0.001
ESRT (−) + PPT vs. ESRT (−)	33.92	(26.75% ; 41.09%)	<0.005
ESRT (−) + PPT vs. PPT	5.26	(1.88% ; 8.64%)	<0.001

d) Mental disorders

Diagnostic success rate	ESRT = 50.51%	PPT = 44.95%	Two methods combined = 74.46%
Comparison (paired samples *t*-test)	Mean difference	CI 95% for mean	P
ESRT (−) vs. PPT	5.56%	(0.74% ; 10.39%)	<0.05
ESRT (−) + PPT vs. ESRT (−)	23.95%	(21.13% ; 26.77%)	<0.001
ESRT (−) + PPT vs. PPT	29.51%	(26.49% ; 32.53%)	<0.001

e) Metabolic disorders

Diagnostic success rate	ESRT = 13.68%	PPT = 8.42%	Two methods combined = 18.95%
Comparison (paired samples *t*-test)	Mean difference	CI 95% for mean	P
ESRT (−) vs. PPT	5.26%	(−2.80% ; 13.30%)	NS
ESRT (−) + PPT vs. ESRT (−)	5.26%	(0.69% ; 9.84%)	<0.001
ESRT (−) + PPT vs. PPT	10.43%	(4.24% ; 16.81%)	<0.05

Continued

Table 7.2 Diagnostic success rates obtained on various apparatus and disorders in 325 patients with two methods, ERST (−) and PPT, and comparison with paired samples t-test—cont'd

f) Gastrointestinal tract

Diagnostic success rate	ESRT = 26.69%	PPT = 19.93%	Two methods combined = 40.88%
Comparison (paired samples t-test)	Mean difference	CI 95% for mean	P
ESRT (−) vs. PPT	6.76%	(2.00% ; 11.51%)	<0.01
ESRT (−) + PPT vs. ESRT (−)	14.19%	(11.37% ; 17.01%)	<0.001
ESRT (−) + PPT vs. PPT	20.95%	(17.66% ; 24.23%)	<0.001

g) Cardiovascular system

Diagnostic success rate	ESRT = 29.29%	PPT = 27.27%	Two methods combined = 47.81%
Comparison (paired samples t-test)	Mean difference	CI 95% for mean	P
ESRT (−) vs. PPT	2.05%	(−5.12% ; 9.17%)	NS
ESRT (−) + PPT vs. ESRT (−)	18.52%	(15.92% ; 25.16%)	<0.001
ESRT (−) + PPT vs. PPT	20.54%	(14.08% ; 22.96%)	<0.001

h) Skin disorders

Diagnostic success rate	ESRT = 28.57%	PPT = 26.79%	Two methods combined = 45.24%
Comparison (paired samples t-test)	Mean difference	CI 95% for mean	P
ESRT (−) vs. PPT	1.79%	(−7.26% ; 10.84%)	NS
ESRT (−) + PPT vs. ESRT (−)	16.67%	(12.53% ; 24.38%)	<0.001
ESRT (−) + PPT vs. PPT	18.45%	(10.97% ; 22.36%)	<0.001

i) Genitourinary tract

Diagnostic success rate	ESRT = 24.50%	PPT = 19.21%	Two methods combined = 37.09%
Comparison (paired samples t-test)	Mean difference	CI 95% for mean	P
ESRT (−) vs. PPT	5.30%	(−3.57% ; 14.16%)	NS
ESRT (−) + PPT vs. ESRT (−)	12.58%	(7.23% ; 17.93%)	<0.001
ESRT (−) + PPT vs. PPT	17.88%	(11.70% ; 24.60%)	<0.001

Practitioners should, however, be aware that the clusters of points they are going to identify with both methods often represent a puzzle which can be solved only through sufficient medical knowledge.

To compare the diagnostic abilities of ESRT and PPT, I applied the following methodology. An independent assessor randomly chose 20–40 patients with the same symptom and a sex- and age-matched control group containing the same number of subjects without this symptom. The number of tender points or reduced ESR sector by sector was first analyzed in the group with a given symptom and in the control group by means of paired samples t-test. The second analysis was then made in the first group comparing the concentration of points identified in each sector with ESRT and PPT. The clusters of points were graphically reproduced on the Sectogram with a size which was directly proportionate to the percentage of the total; clusters with a percentage below 5% were not included in the figures in this chapter.

Let us consider, for example, the case of irritable bowel syndrome (IBS).

Two randomly selected groups were chosen for the first analysis: the first was composed of 40 patients with diarrhea- or constipation-predominant discomfort; the second group consisted of 40 subjects without this disorder. Only two sectors (15 and 16, related to liver and pancreas–gallbladder) showed a significantly higher number of points with PPT in the IBS group compared to the control group, whereas for ESRT no differences were found. Much more interesting was the comparison between ESRT and PPT: the first showed a significant concentration of points with lower ESR on the colon area represented in sectors 23–25 (on the left in Fig. 7.2), whereas PPT showed a significantly higher number of tender points on sectors 16–19 and 4–8 (on the right of Fig. 7.2). The interpretation of these areas is not immediate but becomes easier when circumscribing the clusters of points located on these sectors. With regard to the first group of sectors identified with

PPT, the significant sensitization comes from the sum of clusters belonging to the liver–pancreas–gallbladder area with the Chinese abdomen area (AH8 *fu*) and the elbow–wrist area. In trying to solve this puzzle we may be reassured by the fact that the area of the abdomen also has indications, for example, for diarrhea with abdominal distension and pain, which are typical symptoms of IBS. Also the sensitization of the elbow–wrist area, which I consider related to allergy and food intolerance, should not be considered out of place since, for example, a lactose intolerance could mimic the symptoms of IBS.

As regards the lower group of sectors, a significant difference of sensitization was found for sectors 4–6 ($P<0.05$) and for sectors 7–8 ($P<0.01$). One cluster was found on the antitragus, on the Chinese forehead area, representing the tendency to sinusitis or migraine in these patients; another cluster was found on the posterior part of the ear lobe representing depressed mood. It is noteworthy that headache, depression and fibromyalgia have been

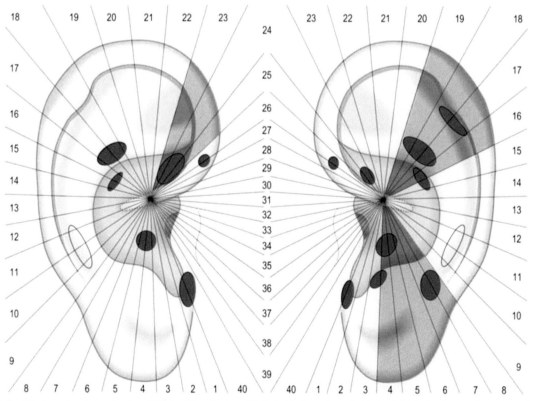

Fig. 7.2 Cluster of points with low ESR in 40 patients with irritable bowel syndrome on the left; cluster of tender points with PPT of the same patients on the right. The colored sectors correspond to a significantly higher concentration of points, respectively, for ESRT vs. PPT on the left side or for PPT vs. ESRT on the right side of the figure. Colored areas = lateral surface; blank areas = medial surface.

identified by several authors as co-morbidities or medical conditions accompanying IBS.[3,4]

This methodological approach, as appealing as it may appear, is, however, not free from limitations:

1. The patients of my group were middle-aged (on average 53.2 years) and their auricles showed the representation of somatic and functional symptoms related to several bodily systems.
2. The patients of the control group, randomly selected among those without IBS, nevertheless belonged to the main group itself and therefore could not be regarded as truly healthy or asymptomatic subjects. In my opinion this is a frequent limitation of current clinical research which does not take into consideration a sufficient number of clinical and instrumental parameters in the control group, to exclude co-morbidity or a possible medical condition associated to the disorder which is the object of the study.

THE CLUSTERS OF POINTS IDENTIFIED WITH ESRT AND PPT FOR SOME SYSTEMS AND DISORDERS

THE MUSCULOSKELETAL APPARATUS

Despite the above-mentioned limitations, it is nevertheless possible to weigh up the distribution of points detected with ESRT and PPT on the different sectors with paired samples *t*-test.

Concerning the musculoskeletal apparatus, for example, among the symptoms determining the diagnostic superiority of PPT to ESRT (Table 7.2a) we may take for comparison lumbar–sciatic pain and knee pain.

Lumbar–sciatic pain

Sectors 17–21, on the right of Figure 7.3, show a significantly higher concentration of tender points which is the sum of two main clusters: one

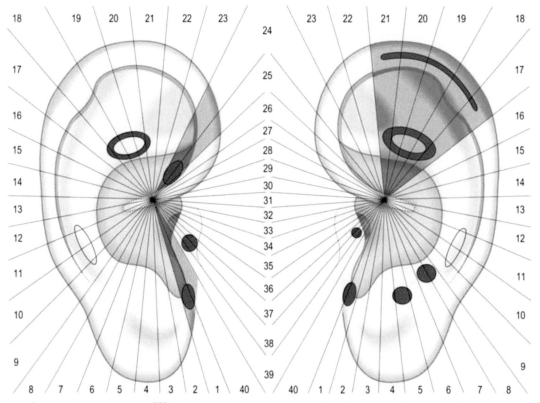

Fig. 7.3 Cluster of points with low ESR in 30 patients with lumbar–sciatic pain on the left; cluster of tender points with PPT of the same patients on the right. The colored sectors correspond to a significantly higher concentration of points, respectively, for ESRT vs. PPT on the left side or for PPT vs. ESRT on the right side of the figure. Colored areas = lateral surface; blank areas = medial surface.

corresponds roughly to both Nogier's and the Chinese representation of lumbosacral vertebrae; the other is aligned on the helix and presumably represents the neuropathic part of lumbar–sciatic pain. It is interesting to note that the first cluster shows an overlapping of tender points of the lateral and medial surface: the former presumably represents the rate of pain related to structures of the spine such as ligaments, articular facets etc., whereas the latter may represent the muscular contracture of the lumbar muscles accompanying the sciatic pain.

As regards ESRT we can find, on the left of Figure 7.3, a significantly larger colon area compared to PPT. This seems to be a recurrent nonspecific phenomenon, possibly related to the technique itself. Also the significantly larger cluster of points in the pituitary–adrenal area (sectors 1 and 40) are characteristic of ESRT and could indicate that this technique is more efficient for identifying function-related points than PPT.

Knee pain

A similar distribution of points to that for lumbar–sciatic pain may be observed in 20 patients with knee pain: but it is interesting to note that the large cluster of tender points on the upper part of the anthelix tends to split into two minor clusters which seem to hold different meanings (on the right of Fig. 7.4). The clusters on sectors 19–21, which are significantly larger with PPT than ESRT ($P<0.05$), correspond presumably to the hip and the knee, being at mid distance between Nogier's and the Chinese representations. This cluster is composed almost entirely of tender points on the lateral surface whereas the significantly larger cluster of tender points on sectors 16–18 is almost exclusively located on the medial side and is presumably related to muscles of the thoracolumbar tract of the spine. It can be questioned, of course, whether this tenderness is a consequence of postural changes in a patient with chronic knee pain or represents a co-morbidity. Also the sensitization

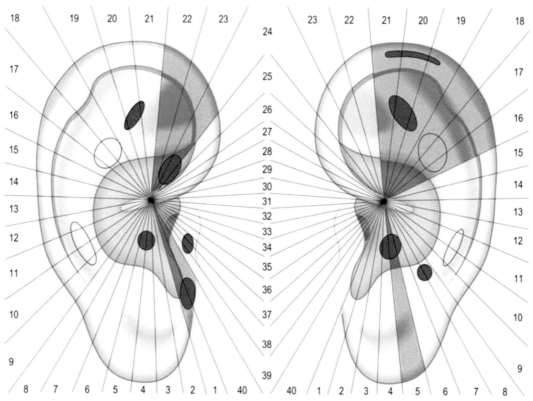

Fig. 7.4 Cluster of points with low ESR in 20 patients with knee pain on the left; cluster of tender points with PPT of the same patients on the right. The colored sectors correspond to a significantly higher concentration of points, respectively, for ESRT vs. PPT on the left side or for PPT vs. ESRT on the right side of the figure. Colored areas = lateral surface; blank areas = medial surface.

of the occiput–TMJ area, even if not reaching a significant difference compared to ESRT, may be considered concomitant or a consequence of postural changes in patients with lumbar–sciatic and knee pain. The particular concentration of points on the lung area moreover could be related to metabolic disorders accompanying osteoarthritis of the knee.

TEETH AND TEMPOROMANDIBULAR JOINT DYSFUNCTION

As regards the teeth and the TMJ, PPT had a better diagnostic outcome than ESRT, especially in the search for the exact location of tender points for reducing toothache (Table 7.2b). Another frequent application of auricular diagnosis, as will be shown in the next chapter, is for bruxism and TMJ disorders.

Comparing PPT with ESRT, we can see that sectors 7 and 8 have a significantly higher number of tender points (on the right of Fig. 7.5). This large cluster of points coincides mainly with the Chinese occiput area; it is noteworthy that the

Chinese author Li Su Huai also listed for it indications such as trismus, TMJ locking and cervical syndrome. This combination of symptoms indicates that this part of the ear probably represents an overlapping of the representation of trigeminal and cervical nerves and may be useful also for diagnosing postural disorders of the spine associated with malocclusion disorders.

THE NERVOUS SYSTEM

Starting from the superiority of PPT over ESRT in diagnosing neurological disorders (Table 7.2c), we should reconsider the topic of migraine since so many patients seek relief for this symptom through acupuncture.

In Chapter 5 we compared the sensitization of the ear in migraine and tension-type headache (TTH) (see Fig. 5.27). Applying ESRT to both groups of patients we can see that patients with migraine show the already well known cluster of points on the colon area (on the left of Fig. 7.6) whereas

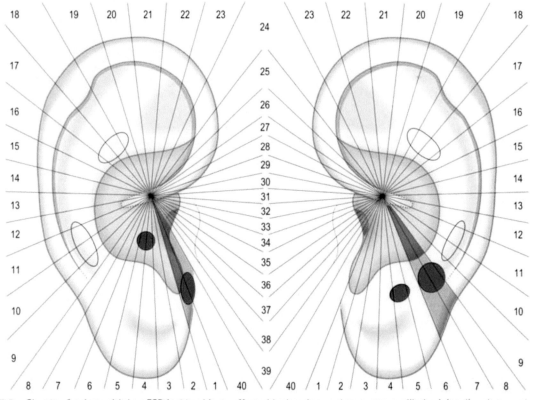

Fig. 7.5 Cluster of points with low ESR in 20 subjects affected by bruxism and temporomandibular joint disorders on the left; cluster of tender points with PPT of the same subjects on the right. The colored sectors correspond to a significantly higher concentration of points, respectively, for ESRT vs. PPT on the left side or for PPT vs. ESRT on the right side of the figure. Colored areas = lateral surface; blank areas = medial surface.

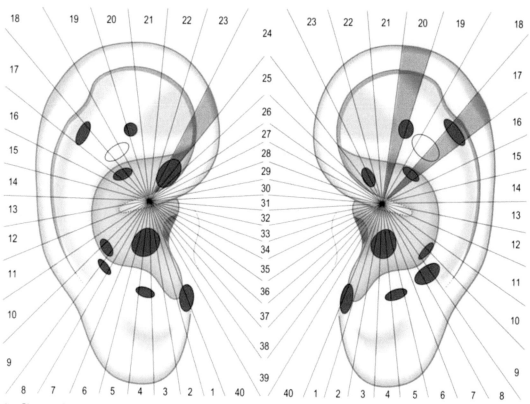

Fig. 7.6 Cluster of points with low ESR in 30 patients suffering with migraine on the left; cluster of points with low ESR in 30 patients suffering with tension-type headache on the right. The colored sectors correspond to a significantly higher concentration of points, respectively, for migraine vs. TTH on the left side or for TTH vs. migraine on the right side of the figure. Colored areas = lateral surface; blank areas = medial surface.

patients with TTH show a significantly higher number of points with reduced ESR on sector 20 (Shen men area) and 17 (muscles of the lumbothoracic tract) (on the right of Fig. 7.6). In addition, sectors 7, 8 and 9, comprehending both the brainstem area and part of the Chinese spleen on the inferior concha, show a higher concentration of points in patients with TTH: the difference with the migraine group is only just below significance ($P = 0.065$).

The parallel comparisons of PPT and ESRT may also offer us indications for treatment: migraine could be preferentially treated with points of the antitragus, and the upper concha, whereas TTH could be controlled using points of the Shen men area, the lower concha and the brainstem.

MENTAL DISORDERS

The symptoms of psychological disorders deserve particular attention since in my group of patients they ranked second only to those of the musculoskeletal

apparatus with 22.5% of the total. Psychological/psychiatric problems were declared by patients to be the main reason for their visit or were identified among other symptoms during the diagnostic procedure. As Table 7.2d reports, in 325 patients mental disorders were identified more frequently through ESRT than PPT ($P<0.05$).

If we wanted to outline and clearly differentiate anxiety disorders from depressive conditions on the auricle, we would probably be disappointed to find only minor differences between these two major fields of psychiatry. In a first analysis we compared two groups of 30 randomly chosen patients declaring only anxiety or depression with a third group of 30 control patients without these symptoms. Compared to the control group, the anxiety group showed at least five sectors which had a significantly higher concentration of points, whereas the depression group showed not a single one. This phenomenon could be interpreted as a better recognition of anxiety by the practitioner and the patient himself, especially when excessive anxiety and worry are accompanied by additional symptoms such as restlessness, difficulty in concentrating, muscle tension, trembling, sweating, frequent urination, etc.

It can be more difficult to diagnose depression because some depressed subjects suffer from increased irritability or persistent anger which could be misinterpreted as anxiety. Other individuals emphasize somatic complaints (for example pain syndromes) rather than reporting feelings of sadness. As is well known, culture can influence the experience and communication of symptoms of depression which can be expressed widely in somatic terms. According to DSM IV:

complaints of 'nerves' and headaches in Latino and Mediterranean cultures; weakness, tiredness or 'imbalance' in Chinese and Asian cultures; problems of the 'heart' in Middle Eastern cultures may all express the depressive experience. Such presentations combine features of the depressive, anxiety and somatoform disorders.[5]

The frequent combination of symptoms and possible co-morbidity are in my opinion the main reason why in my patients only sectors 9–11 of the anxiety group (on the right of Fig. 7.7) showed a significantly higher number of points with low ESR compared to depression. Only the clusters of points corresponding to the Chinese spleen area or to Nogier's cervical sympathetic ganglia seem therefore to mark anxiety disorders. The expert in traditional Chinese medicine (TCM) is well aware that a deficiency of *qi* of Spleen and Heart are at the basis of worry, which is an essential feature of anxiety disorders. The treatment of this area is indeed very suitable for anxiety symptoms such as difficulty in swallowing or 'a lump in the throat', aphonia, etc.

There are, however, further minor clusters of points which can orient diagnosis more toward depressive disorders (on the left of Fig. 7.7), such

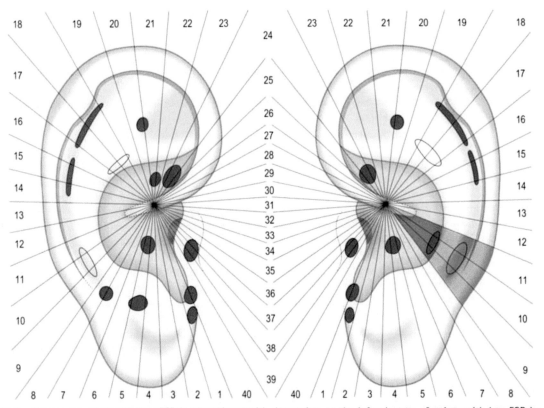

Fig. 7.7 Clusters of points with low ESR in 30 patients with depression on the left; clusters of points with low ESR in 30 patients with anxiety on the right. The colored sectors correspond to a significantly higher concentration of points, respectively, for depression vs. anxiety on the left side or for anxiety vs. depression on the right side of the figure. Colored areas = lateral surface; blank areas = medial surface.

as the two areas related to mood located on sectors 7–8 and 4–6. The pituitary–adrenal gland area is slightly enlarged and there is also a small cluster observable on the kidney area. Both disorders show a similar activation of the Shen men area and an interesting distribution of points on the scapha, in proximity to the internal border of the helix.

This distribution corresponds partially to the 'vegetative groove' of Lange and to the concentration of points observed in patients with fibromyalgia (see Fig. 5.15).

ASTHENIA AND FAMILIAL HYPERTENSION AND DIABETES

Asthenia (Greek *asthenēs*, without strength) is a very common symptom and several patients from my group complained of symptoms such as tiredness or fatigue. As we know, asthenia may have different causes but is commonly associated with chronic pain, depression, sleep disorders, fibromyalgia and of course with infectious diseases or chronic disorders of the heart, lung or kidney.

If we simply compare ESRT and PPT in a group with this symptom we can see that the first diagnostic method shows several groups with significant concentrations of points. The richest cluster of points in proportion to the total (25%) corresponds to the pituitary–adrenal gland area. Next is the cervical muscle area on the medial side and in third place we have a broad area covering both the Chinese kidney and bladder area (on the left of Fig. 7.8). TCM could also be cited for this area because asthenia with depression and chronic pain, often reported by my middle-aged patients, particularly females, could imply a deficiency of *Yin/Yang* Kidney. Regarding PPT, there is a major sensitization of one of the depressive mood areas which nevertheless does not reach a significant difference compared to ESRT (on the right of Fig. 7.8).

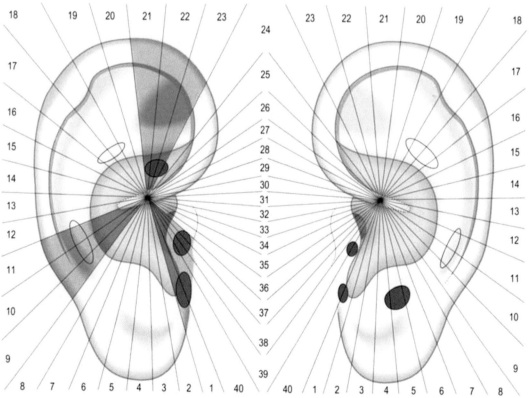

Fig. 7.8 Cluster of points with low ESR in 30 subjects suffering from asthenia on the left; cluster of tender points with PPT of the same subjects on the right. The colored sectors correspond to a significantly higher concentration of points, respectively, for ESRT vs. PPT on the left side or for PPT vs. ESRT on the right side of the figure. Colored areas = lateral surface; blank areas = medial surface.

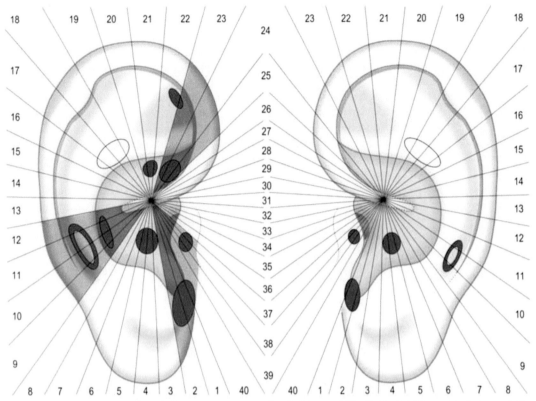

Fig. 7.9 Clusters of points with low ESR in 26 patients with familial hypertension but who themselves have normal blood pressure values on the left; cluster of tender points with PPT of the same subjects on the right. The colored sectors correspond to a significantly higher concentration of points, respectively, for ESRT vs. PPT on the left side or for PPT vs. ESRT on the right side of the figure. Colored areas = lateral surface; blank areas = medial surface.

It is interesting, in my opinion, to see how these patterns of distribution of sectors can also be observed in other patients who, for example, have familial hypertension and diabetes but who are not affected by these disorders themselves (Figs 7.9, 7.10).

It is noteworthy that co-morbidity of these diseases is particularly manifest in the metabolic syndrome which seems to affect an increasing number of people. According to the American Heart Association,[6] for this syndrome to be diagnosed at least three of the following should be present:

- Elevated waist circumference: men – equal to or greater than 40 inches (102 cm); women – equal to or greater than 35 inches (88 cm).
- Elevated triglycerides: equal to or greater than 150 mg/dL.
- Reduced HDL ('good') cholesterol: men – less than 40 mg/dL; women – less than 50 mg/dL.

- Elevated blood pressure: equal to or greater than 130/85 mmHg or use of medication for hypertension.
- Elevated fasting glucose: equal to or greater than 100 mg/dL (5.6 mmol/L) or use of medication for hyperglycemia.

For the comparison shown in Figure 7.9 I considered a group of subjects without hypertension but who had at least one close relative with high blood pressure. An exclusion criterion in this group was that no subject should be diabetic or have familial diabetes.

For the comparison shown in Figure 7.10 I considered a group of subjects without diabetes but who had at least one member in their family who was being treated for hyperglycemia. In this group an exclusion criterion was that no subject should be treated for high blood pressure or have familial hypertension.

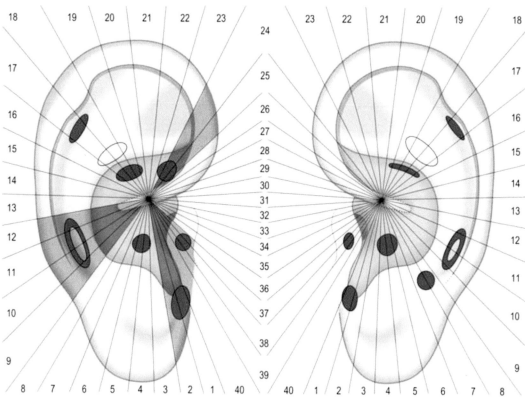

Fig. 7.10 Cluster of points with low ESR in 22 patients with family history of diabetes but who themselves have normal glucose levels on the left; cluster of tender points with PPT of the same subjects on the right. The colored sectors correspond to a significantly higher concentration of points, respectively, for ESRT vs. PPT on the left side or for PPT vs. ESRT on the right side of the figure. Colored areas = lateral surface; blank areas = medial surface.

Both groups showed a similar trend as regards the significantly higher concentration of points with reduced ESR in several sectors compared to PPT (on the left of Figs 7.9 and 7.10); on the other side not a single sector reached significance when comparing PPT with ESRT (on the right of Figs 7.9 and 7.10). The highest concentration of points with low ESR was on the pituitary–adrenal gland area; in second place were sectors 9–12 which contain clusters of points possibly corresponding to various structures: the cluster on the medial side corresponds to the cervical muscles, the cluster on the lateral side seems to be related to other structures such as the shoulder or the thyroid gland. In third place were sectors 23–25 related to the colon area, but in the group with familial hypertension we also find a cluster on the upper part of the triangular fossa overlapping with TF1 *jiaowoshang* area which has the main indication for hypertension (on the left of Fig. 7.9).

In the group with familial diabetes we can see at least three aligned clusters on sectors 16–19 which, summed up, do not show any significant difference between ESRT and PPT. If we exclude the cluster related to the back muscles we can note a higher concentration of points on the other two clusters which may be related to the pancreas–gallbladder area in the concha and to the area of allergy represented on the elbow–wrist zone. This coupled activation, in my opinion, could be the representation of a subliminal glucose intolerance. This condition may be considered a transitional state from normoglycemia to frank diabetes and current knowledge suggests that development of this disease may be initiated by insulin resistance and worsened by the compensatory hyperinsulinemia.

An interesting phenomenon has been the observation, over time, in patients without metabolic syndrome of the loss of tenderness of these areas only when replacing white sugar with other sweeteners.

SMOKING HABIT AND EATING DISORDERS

Two of the fields in which ear acupuncture has often been applied are those of tobacco addiction and obesity. In this paragraph they will be considered together because they have some common features such as depressive mood, compulsory behavior and craving which have often been the object of treatment with acupuncture. Even if the systematic reviews on both subjects are inconclusive as regards their efficacy over time, it is nevertheless noteworthy that auricular stimulation on one or more points has been added to almost every smoking cessation and weight loss program.

For addiction to tobacco, 25 smokers were compared to 25 sex- and age-matched non-smokers: ESRT showed at least eight sectors with a higher concentration of points than PPT (on the left of Fig. 7.11). Some of them contained clusters of points which have often been found in different medical conditions and should therefore be considered non-specific and perhaps related to the electrical detection itself. There is another cluster on sectors 25–27, both with ESRT and PPT, which on the contrary is original and has never been found in other symptoms. This cluster is located on the ascending branch of the helix and overlaps both with the Chinese external genital (HX4 *waishengzhiqi*) and urethra (HX3 *niaodao*) areas.

This area belongs to the so-called 'libido' areas proposed by Durinyan for the treatment of sexual disorders. It is possible that this area represents a craving area particularly for those smokers who stop smoking but who continue for some days/weeks to have a pronounced desire for cigarettes. What is surprising is that the craving for pleasures other than sex, such as sweets, ice cream, chocolate, etc., may also cause a concentration of points in this area.

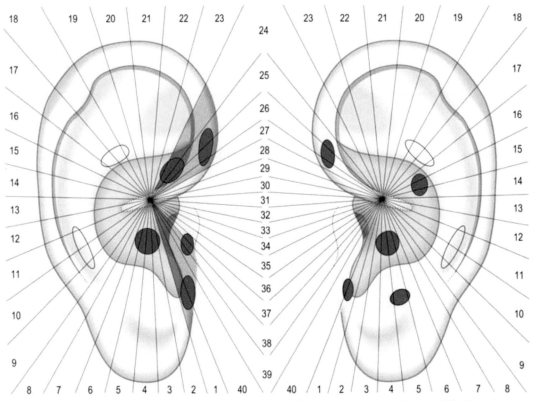

Fig. 7.11 Clusters of points with low ESR in 25 smokers on the left; cluster of tender points with PPT of the same subjects on the right. The colored sectors correspond to a significantly higher concentration of points, respectively, for ESRT vs. PPT on the left side or for PPT vs. ESRT on the right side of the figure. Colored areas = lateral surface; blank areas = medial surface.

As regards the liver area (sectors 14–16) and the cyclothymic area (sectors 4, 5 and 6), these show a slightly larger cluster with PPT than with ESRT (on the right of Fig. 7.11). The lung area, which is a classical zone of the ear used for the treatment of abstinence syndromes (see Ch. 1), is symmetrically observable both with ESRT and PPT.

The distribution of points in 25 subjects with obesity and eating disorders is quite different from that in smokers. ESRT shows three groups of sectors with significant differences: two are the colon and the pituitary area, the third, on sectors 20 and 21, corresponds to the representation of the Chinese kidney (on the left of Fig. 7.12). It may be questioned whether the activation of the kidney area is concomitant with the low metabolism of these subjects or may depend, according to TCM, on a deficiency of *Yin* of Kidney which is accompanied by asthenia and psychologically by a loss of will.

Another important area carrying a larger amount of low ESR corresponds to the mouth–esophagus area: according to the standardization process, in fact this area carries the same indication (withdrawal syndrome) as the lung area.

PPT shows only one group of sectors (7–10) with a significant concentration of points compared to ESRT (on the right of Fig. 7.12). This cluster is located mainly on the helix area 4 which has indications for tonsillitis, fever and hypertension. In several obese patients this area often looks swollen, reddish and is moreover tender to thumb–index palpation. We are at loss to interpret this phenomenon: perhaps the representation of the thyroid gland on these sectors may activate a series of aligned points on this part of the helix which could therefore also be called the 'metabolism-related area'. Another impression, however, emerges in considering that this area becomes sensitized especially

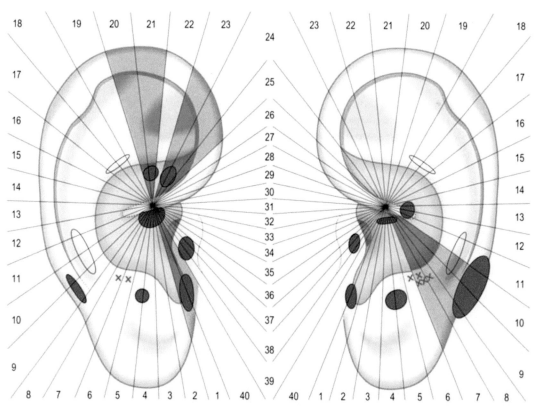

Fig. 7.12 Clusters of points with low ESR in 25 patients affected by obesity and eating disorders on the left; cluster of tender points with PPT of the same patients on the right. The colored sectors correspond to a significantly higher concentration of points, respectively, for ESRT vs. PPT on the left side or for PPT vs. ESRT on the right side of the figure. Colored areas = lateral surface; blank areas = medial surface; areas with crosses = internal border of the antitragus.

in subjects inclined to binge eating and that treatment here seems to reduce the number of uncontrolled eating episodes and also seems to control the night eating syndrome.

Two further areas seem moreover to be related to eating: the first corresponds to the cyclothymic temperament, whereas the second, on the internal surface of the antitragus (see the area with the crosses on Fig. 7.12), seems to overlap with Nogier's hypothalamus on the lateral surface of the antitragus. In my opinion this area becomes sensitized when a delay in feeling satiety is prevailing; stimulating these points and at the same time inviting the subject to slow down food intake may help in restoring physiological appetite.

CONCLUSIONS

As already discussed in Chapter 6 and in the first part of this chapter, in my opinion there are some factors limiting the wide application of auricular diagnosis with ESRT.

The first limitation is that practitioners do not really know exactly what is happening when the display of the device begins to flash or a sound is heard when the measuring probe is applied on one point rather than on another.

The second limitation is, as already discussed in the first paragraph, that the search for points with lower ESR is much more time-consuming than the identification of tender points with the pressure-probe.

A further limitation is made up of the artifacts related to the technique which cannot always be avoided, such as skin humidity, the more or less full contact of the probe tip with the skin and the possible rupture of the stratum corneum due to an unskillful application of the probe tip on the skin.

According to Ahn and Martinsen:[7]

the susceptibility of electrodermal measurements to factors associated with skin clarifies why rigorous attention should be paid to the testing conditions of the skin. The investigator should pay particular attention to skin hydration, stratum corneum thickness, skin structural integrity, and sweat-gland density.

According to my observations it is not clear enough whether one method is superior to the other in detecting individual symptoms or the whole range of disorders belonging to the same apparatus. My clinical impression is that the search for auricular points related to pain syndromes is more precise with PPT than ESRT. On the other hand psychological/psychiatric disorders appear to be more correctly identified with ESRT; the same happens with addiction and eating disorders. Also, dysfunctions of the autonomic nervous system causing hypo- or hyperactivity in internal organs or in systems such as the gastrointestinal tract appear to be more precisely identified with ESRT.

References

[1] Usichenko TI, Lysenyuk VP, Groth MH et al. Detection of ear acupuncture points by measuring the electrical skin resistance before, during and after orthopaedic surgery performed under general anesthesia. Acup Electrother Res 2003;3–4:167–73.

[2] Niboyet JEH. La moindre résistance à l'électricité de surfaces punctiformes et de trajets cutanés concordant avec les points et les méridiens, bases de l'acupuncture. Marseilles: Thèse Sciences; 1963.

[3] Cole JA, Rothman KJ, Cabral HJ et al. Migraine, fibromyalgia, and depression among people with IBS: a prevalence study. BMC Gastroenterol 2006;6:26.

[4] Kurland JE, Coyle WJ, Winkler A et al. Prevalence of irritable bowel syndrome and depression in fibromyalgia. Dig Dis Sci 2006;3:454–60.

[5] Diagnostic and statistical manual of mental disorders (DSM IV) (p. 324). 4th ed. Washington: American Psychiatric Association; 1994.

[6] Grundy SM, Brewer Jr HB, Cleeman JI et al. Definition of metabolic syndrome: report of the National Heart, Lung, and Blood Institute/American Heart Association conference on scientific issues related to definition. Circulation 2004;3:433–8.

[7] Ahn AC, Martinsen OG. Electrical characterization of acupuncture points: technical issues and challenges. J Altern Complement Med 2007;8:817–24.

Chapter 8

The needle contact test

INTRODUCTION

In 1995 the physician Stefano Marcelli proposed the 'active point test' ('Il test dei punti attivi').[1] His intention was to introduce a diagnostic method which could quickly and accurately identify the most effective points for therapy. The test was used by Marcelli in the case of painful syndromes and required the collaboration of the patient, who was asked to keep his attention fully focused on his perception of pain throughout the test. Among the meridian acupuncture points suitable in the treatment of a given painful condition Marcelli was able, through his test, to identify the point/s which succeeded in reducing the intensity of symptoms. The test was proposed to doctors and physiotherapists and the author recommended several kinds of stimulation, among them acupressure. A needle was to be applied to the acupuncture point for a few seconds, touching the skin without penetration. The sensation that should be felt by the patient was that of a superficial puncture of such light intensity that it should not cause any bother at all. The best diameter for the testing needle was between 0.25 and 0.35 mm. Especially in the case of more widespread pain syndromes, different points were tested following the concepts of harmonization and redistribution of energy in the meridians which typify traditional Chinese medicine (TCM). Once the meridian point effective in reducing pain was identified, the same needle was inserted into the skin for starting treatment. According to Marcelli, the result of the test could be rated as indifferent, negative, moderately and strongly positive. An indifferent answer corresponded to no variations, negative to a worsening of pain and positive to more or less rapid and widespread reduction of pain.

THE NEEDLE CONTACT TEST ON THE AURICLE

I applied this test extensively on the outer ear, renaming it the 'needle contact test' (NCT). The main difference between NCT and Marcelli's procedure is that it is first necessary to detect the auricular points with other diagnostic systems such as the pressure pain test (PPT) or the electrical skin resistance test (ESRT). Once the different points have been identified and marked with ink one can start gently passing the tip of the needle from one point to the other; 5–10 seconds of contact are sufficient for obtaining an answer. In my experience the auricle requires only a negative or positive binary rating; this means that after contact of a maximum of 10 seconds, aided by the patient's collaboration, one should be able to recognize which points do or do not react to NCT.

It is probable that the sensitivity of the test may be related to the remarkable nervous supply of the outer ear and its particular connections with the CNS which allow a shortened reflex circuit. Among the advantages of this original and appealing diagnostic method are its simplicity and the short time needed for carrying it out. Patients are usually very glad to feel their pain is going to diminish or even disappear and the acupuncturist reaps much satisfaction from the appreciation of his treatment.

Of interest for both clinicians and researchers are the different applications of NCT and the methodology used for measuring the response to needle contact over time.

APPLICATIONS OF THE NEEDLE CONTACT TEST

NCT may be helpful in various conditions. For each of them there is a diagnostic phase which is then completed by therapeutic intervention.

The main applications are for pain conditions of whatever origin and for symptoms related to the locomotor system such as myofascial pain and stiffness with reduced range of motion. A particular

section is dedicated to NCT and muscular hypertonus in bruxism.

The different applications examined to date are:

1. for current pain
2. for migraine attack
3. for pain on palpation of tender points/areas
4. for pain provoked by movement
5. for deactivating myofascial trigger points (MTPs) and improving the range of motion
6. for muscular hypertonus: our experiences with craniomandibular disorders.

FOR CURRENT PAIN

The test can be applied in any case of spontaneous pain provided the patient has a full perception of it and is able to measure its variations over time.

The best results of NCT are in acute pain due to trauma (for example bruising, sprains, fractures, etc., visceral disorders or postoperative pain). After the needle has been applied for 5–10 seconds one must wait for the effect, which usually manifests in the following minute. If the reduction of pain is rated by the patient to be at least 25–30%, one can wait for a further 2–3 minutes to verify if the effect is going to pass rapidly or remain stable in time. There is of course great anticipation on the part of the patient and this initial variation of pain can be considered a placebo effect. Other neighboring points can therefore be tested, with the aim of obtaining an analgesic effect beyond the threshold of the placebo effect (commonly rated as being about 35–40% of the total). For example, the lady in Figure 8.1 suffered with acute pain of her sixth upper right tooth which was rated about 7 on a verbal numeric scale (VNS). She had undergone devitalization of the tooth the day before and at the time of auricular diagnosis had not taken any painkillers. Two different points were located with PPT on the central area of the lobe, which does not correspond either to the French or to the Chinese representation of the jaw (LO3 *He*) (see the representation of the teeth described in Ch. 5). The points were very close to each other, the distance between them no greater than 1 mm (Fig. 8.1). They were consecutively tested; the pain was rated as 5 in severity 1 minute after needle contact of the lower point, but 3 minutes later had again reached 6–7; however, NCT on the upper point lowered the pain steadily to 3 and this level remained stable for

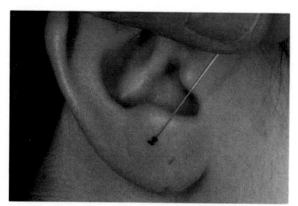

Fig. 8.1 Two close tender points identified with PPT in a case of pain of the 6th upper right tooth: NCT performed for 10 seconds on the upper point reduced pain significantly.

the next 5 minutes. A temporary sterile disposable steel implant was placed in this point and the patient had no relapse of pain.

FOR MIGRAINE

My reasons for distinguishing this pain from musculoskeletal pain is that migraine is a neurovascular pain which manifests itself on the trigeminal territory and tends to relapse over time. Migraine is a disabling disorder with a high social and economical impact which requires a careful strategy of prophylaxis for reducing the number of attacks and preventing the chronic abuse of painkillers. Here acupuncture can gain ground with honor as an alternative treatment or for use in combination with pharmacological therapy.[2–8]

Besides body acupuncture, using formulae or personalized sets of points, ear acupuncture also seems to have an interesting role. Its main difference is that at every ear acupuncture session it is necessary to make a diagnosis and to find out which points to treat. Migraine requires a very accurate localization of the points; especially in the case of an attack, the algometer should be used with a light hand in order not to overly bother the patient.

In 15 patients with migraine attacks (13 female, 2 male) pain scoring with a VNS was repeated 1, 5, 15 and 30 minutes after NCT. Pain decreased about 26.4% after 1 minute and 47.4% after 5 minutes; in the succeeding time intervals the pain level remained unchanged (Fig. 8.2). The points identified with NCT were mainly distributed in the area of the forehead (AT1 *e*) and the temple (AT2 *nie*) on

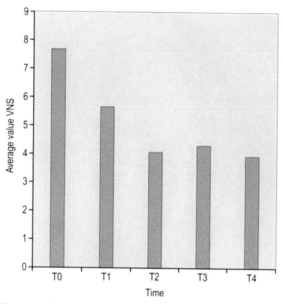

Fig. 8.2 Reduction of pain in 15 patients with migraine attack in T1 (1 minute after NCT for 10 seconds); in T2 (5 minutes after); in T3 (15 minutes after) and in T4 (30 minutes after).

the Chinese map and frequently also on the supero-internal surface of the antitragus overlapping partially with the Chinese subcortex area (AT4 *pizhixia*) (Fig. 8.3).

It has to be stressed that AT4 extends itself to the bottom of the medial wall of the antitragus and carries the generic indication 'painful symptoms'. The first documented application of NCT in a case of migraine attack was performed on one of these patients and a steady level of analgesia was maintained up to the 60th minute.[9]

In a still ongoing study with the collaboration of Dr Gianni Allais of the Women's Headache Center at Turin University, we treated a group of 40 females with an average age of 42.4 years affected by acute migraine pain. Our aim was to record the intensity of pain beyond the above-mentioned interval, adding a further recording at 120 minutes and 24 hours. The preliminary data show that the pain level drops from an average of 5.1 to 2.1 after 10 minutes and remains unchanged to the next day.

The application of NCT during a migraine attack is, however, a little different to that of musculoskeletal pain for the following reasons:

1. Pain relief is slower the greater the time lapse from the onset of pain. The patient often feels tired and weak and this may delay appreciation of any variation in pain intensity. To overcome

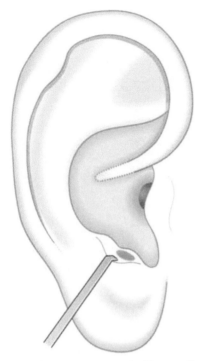

Fig. 8.3 The area of the antitragus which was effective with NCT for reducing pain in 15 patients with migraine attack.

this the duration of needle contact can be protracted up to 30 seconds and the first measurement of pain level postponed to 3–4 minutes after NCT.

2. In the case of bilateral migraine it must be remembered that each half of the head is controlled by the auricle of that side. Therefore if NCT is begun on the right ear the patient needs to be instructed to consider, a few minutes after NCT, any difference of pain between the right and left side of his head. It is always surprising to witness how patients can be aware of the pain diminishing on the same side as the stimulated auricle and compare that sensation with the unchanged intensity in the pain on the opposite, as yet untreated, side. Obviously, once diagnosis and treatment have been accomplished on one side, the same operation has to be performed on the opposite side.

FOR PAIN PROVOKED BY PALPATION

Any part of the body, if painful at palpation, can be challenged with NCT.

The locomotor apparatus is the favorite for this kind of test, and inflammation of the joints, bursitis

and tenosynovitis are often successfully treated. For example, in Figure 8.4 the 45-year-old male patient had been suffering with tennis elbow for 3 months. In the previous 2 weeks the pain had increased and he was limited in his daily activities. He felt acute pain on palpation and pressure on his right lateral epicondyle. Also movements of pronation of the arm and dorsiflexion of the wrist were very painful.

The patient asked for treatment with steroids but I convinced him to try ear acupuncture first. Performing PPT, I found a sensitive point on the scapha corresponding to the representation of the elbow. NCT on this point lowered pain at palpation of the lateral epicondyle (Fig. 8.4A) and a temporary sterile single-use steel implant (ASP) was placed there. Two more ASPs immediately beneath improved pain at pronation of the arm and dorsiflexion of the wrist (Fig. 8.4B). This treatment with three grouped implants in all was efficacious enough to make steroid treatment unnecessary. The patient received similar therapy 15 days later with lasting results.

As regards the issue of the different representation of the lower limb in the French and Chinese maps, see the section on the musculoskeletal system in Chapter 5 (p. 115). The hypothesis that different parts of the knee and the ankle may have a different representation on the ear was forwarded by Dr Caterina Fresi. She examined 34 patients with knee pain caused by current injury of the lateral

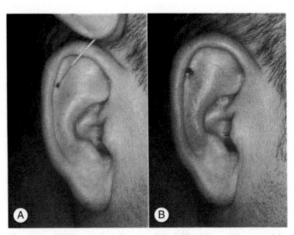

Fig. 8.4 NCT on a tender area identified in a 45-year-old male suffering with tennis elbow (A); three single-use steel implants (ASP-Sedatelec) for reducing pain at palpation and pain at movements of arm and wrist (B).

capsule–ligament complex (14 patients) or of the medial complex (20 patients). In the first group the pain syndrome evoked a sensitization of an extended oval area covering the Chinese hip and knee area (area 1 in Fig. 8.5), whereas in the second group the sensitized area was rather rounded and corresponded to the French thigh and knee area (area 2 in Fig. 8.5). Dr Fresi also examined 15 patients with ankle pain caused by current injury of the capsule–ligament complex of the malleolus lateralis (8 patients) or of the complex of the malleolus medialis (7 patients). In the first group the sensitized area corresponded to the Chinese ankle and toe/heel area (area 3 in Fig. 8.5) whereas in the second group the sensitized area corresponded to the French foot area (area 4 in Fig. 8.5).

The following procedure was applied by Dr Fresi in all these patients: pain was rated at palpation by means of the VNS. The most tender point was identified and marked with ink on the knee

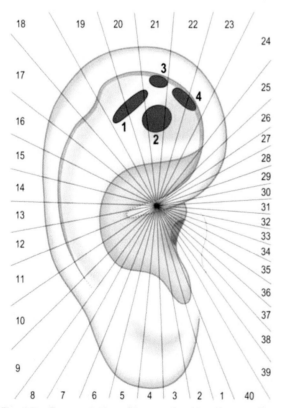

Fig. 8.5 Representation of knee and ankle pain according to Dr Caterina Fresi *(unpublished data, with permission).* 1 and 2 = lateral and medial capsule–ligament complex of the knee; 3 and 4 = capsule–ligament complex respectively of lateral and medial malleolus.

or the ankle as well as on the auricle of the same side, with PPT identifying the most sensitive point. A second pain score was obtained after 15 seconds of NCT followed by a further interval of 45 seconds. The average pain dropped from 7.4 to 3.8 in the whole group of patients with knee pain, and from 7.6 to 3.5 in those with ankle pain. Four patients with chronic and widespread musculoskeletal pain were excluded from this evaluation, as these symptoms were a possible sign of fibromyalgia. The advice of Dr Fresi is therefore to exclude fibromyalgic patients from this kind of experimentation.

FOR PAIN PROVOKED BY MOVEMENT

If the patient does not manifest spontaneous pain, NCT is best performed adopting the position in which the symptom presents most severely. A painful shoulder may be examined better in a sitting position and the movements of passive and active flexion challenged from behind; a lumbar pain, on the other hand, may be challenged better in a standing position, inviting the patient to flex or extend his back.

All these maneuvers which increase the sensation of pain usually sensitize the corresponding zone of the ear, but we do not know at the start which point will be the most effective for performing NCT. Therefore all the identified points should be marked and subsequently tested. It is always useful to check the effect of the pressure test itself. For example, some patients react very well to this stimulation, especially in the case of recent pain.

In the case of backache it is very interesting to observe how NCT on the medial surface of the auricle improves forward flexion.

If patients are suffering with chronic lumbar pain, the points to test frequently lie on the bottom of the groove of the anthelix which may be particularly pronounced (see Plates XIVC and D).

In such cases the parameter for recording improvement may be to measure the distance between the fingertips and the ground.

FOR DEACTIVATING MYOFASCIAL TRIGGER POINTS AND IMPROVING RANGE OF MOTION

Myofascial pain is a major cause of morbidity and has a considerable economical impact causing much absence from work and a large number of consultations in primary care and at pain clinics.

According to the authors who first introduced the basic concept of the myofascial trigger point (MTP), Janet Travell (1901–1996) and David Simons, several clinical features can be observed.[10] The reader will permit me to list some of the most important:

1. MTP is a hyperirritable locus or a point of maximal tenderness located within a taut or palpable band of skeletal muscle.
2. Its compression may elicit local pain and/or referred pain that is similar to the patient's usual clinical complaint (pain recognition). Dr Travell said 'the more hypersensitive the MTP, the more intense and constant is the referred pain and the more extensive is its distribution'.
3. The pattern of referred pain from MTPs is predictable because it is specific for each individual muscle in the body.
4. The compression across the muscle fibers or snapping palpation may elicit a local twitch response which consists of a brisk contraction of the muscle fibers in or around the taut band.
5. Patients with MTPs may have associated localized autonomic phenomena, including vasoconstriction, pilomotor response, hypersecretion, etc.
6. Active MTPs show spontaneous pain or pain in response to movement. Latent MTPs show pain or discomfort only if elicited by compression. According to Dr Travell, a latent MTP can be activated directly by overload of the muscle, overwork, fatigue, chilling; or indirectly by other factors, for example visceral diseases and emotional distress.
7. Both active and latent MTPs may cause stiffness, weakness of the muscle and limited range of movement.

The treatment and subsequent disappearance of a majority of active and latent MTPs seems of great importance in a rehabilitation program. Among the different techniques proposed are the classical 'stretch and spray' and injections with a small amount of local anesthetic or simply with dry needles. According to Melzack et al,[11] acupuncture points and MTPs show a high degree of correspondence between both the spatial distribution and the associated pain patterns. In my opinion ear acupuncture can show an analogous correspondence,

and the best way to prove this was to identify the auricular points which best could modify the clinical features of MTPs with needle contact.

A series of 52 consecutive patients with chronic pain syndromes involving the neck, the shoulder girdle and the arm was examined. The exclusion criteria for my evaluation were: psychiatric disorders, cognitive impairment, intake of analgesics, psychoactive drugs and corticosteroids administered less than 12 hours previously.

All patients were examined sitting or lying down and each painful area was palpated in order to individuate the tender points and the MTPs. Every tender spot was marked with ink and the following four characteristics were recorded for each one: (i) tenderness within a palpable band; (ii) irradiation of pain at distance from the pressed point; (iii) local twitch response; (iv) pain in response to movement and/or limited range of motion.

The 52 patients totalled 142 tender spots (average 2.7); 81 (57%) spots had at least two clinical features which could be considered typical of an MTP.

After the search for MTPs, the tenderness of the auricle on the same side as the pain was tested with PPT and every sensitive point was marked with ink. NCT was then performed on every point and the result of this stimulation was checked after 1 minute on each tender spot of the body. No more than three attempts were made to test a singular MTP, to avoid the therapeutic effect of the palpation itself.

Of the 81 MTPs, 53.1% completely lost any tenderness during the minute following NCT, the local twitch response was no longer obtainable, and range of motion improved. Only a reduction of tenderness was seen in 30.9% of the total, but in the majority of cases the typical features of an MTP could no longer be evoked. In 16%, however, the tenderness of the trigger area was unchanged despite the three attempts made.

Thanks to this study I could represent the MTPs of some muscles on the ear: some of them are represented on the lateral surface, as for example the sternocleidomastoid, the pectoralis major and the biceps brachii (Fig. 8.6A). The majority of muscles, however, are represented on the medial surface, such as the splenius capitis, the upper trapezius, the levator scapulae, the triceps brachii and the latissimus dorsi (Fig. 8.6B). Furthermore, some muscles have a double representation on

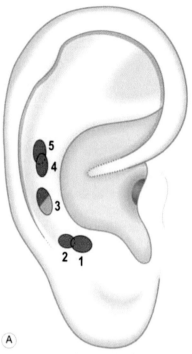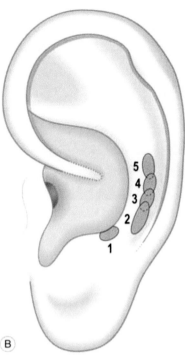

Fig. 8.6   Representation of the myofascial trigger points (MTPs) of some muscles of the neck, shoulder girdle and arm on the lateral surface (A) and on the medial surface (B). (A) 1 = masseter; 2 = sternocleidomastoid; 3 = supraspinatus (represented both on lateral and medial surface); 4 = biceps brachii; 5 = pectoralis (dark pink). (B) 1 = splenius capitis; 2 = trapezius; 3 = levator scapulae; 4 = triceps brachii; 5 = latissimus dorsi (pale pink).

both surfaces, such as the supraspinatus and the deltoid. The representation of other muscles not belonging directly to the neck and shoulder girdle may, however, be overlapping, such as the masseter and the sternocleidomastoid. The following case studies describe how best to correlate an auricular point with the corresponding MTP.

CASE STUDY 1

A 70-year-old male patient had a fall when on a bus and strained his right biceps brachii muscle. Soon he began to suffer with anterior shoulder pain, weakness, restricted elevation of the arm and also some autonomic phenomena such as numbness of the forearm. After several sessions of physiotherapy had brought no benefit he asked to be treated with acupuncture.

When asked to raise his arm he could not do so beyond 90°. An MTP was found in a taut band of the distal portion of the muscle, palpation was painful and the referred pain typically extended upward to the shoulder. With PPT I found a point on the anthelix between the Chinese location of the shoulder (SF4–SF5 *jian*) and thoracic vertebrae (AH11 *xiongzhui*). On Nogier's map the point corresponds to the area located between the shoulder and chest. NCT was performed for about 10 seconds and the patient was astonished to be able to raise his arm to an angle of 120° (Fig. 8.7). A semi-permanent needle was inserted on the day of consultation and another close by 3 days later because the pain was not completely under control. Two weeks later he was free from pain.

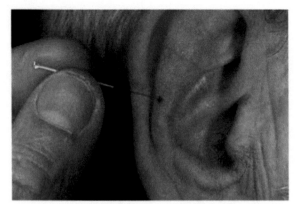

Fig. 8.7   NCT for neutralizing a myofascial trigger point in the right biceps brachii muscle and improving range of motion in elevation in a 70-year-old male.

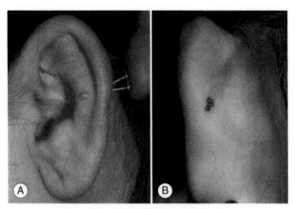

Fig. 8.8   (A) Double NCT and insertion of needles for neutralizing myofascial trigger points in the long head of triceps brachii and in the latissimus dorsi in a 42-year-old female. (B) In the same patient single-use steel implants (ASP, Sedatelec) for reducing pain and improving range of motion.

CASE STUDY 2

A 42-year-old female had been suffering with left posterior shoulder pain, worsening at night, for 20 days, due to overload from repeatedly lifting her 2-year-old child. Two tender spots were found on the posterior arm and on the posterior axillary fold: both had clinical features of MTPs and were attributed respectively to the triceps brachii and to latissimus dorsi. PPT performed on the whole auricle identified two tender points close together on the medial surface. Both were tested with NCT: the first point gave a very good result on the MTP of the triceps, whereas the second neutralized the local twitch response and the irradiation of pain to the arm of the MTP of the latissimus dorsi.

Both needles were inserted immediately after NCT and left for 30 minutes (Fig. 8.8A). The extension of the left elbow and internal rotation of the arm improved instantly: the needles were then removed and replaced by three ASP (Fig. 8.8B).

The case above illustrates how the medial surface of the ear should be considered together with the corresponding lateral surface: especially in musculoskeletal disorders involving the totality of a joint such as the shoulder or the knee, both sides of the auricle should be thoroughly examined.

FOR MUSCULAR HYPERTONUS: OUR EXPERIENCE WITH CRANIOMANDIBULAR DISORDERS

While it is easy enough to apply NCT for challenging a painful condition, it is more difficult to demonstrate that needle contact can reduce muscular hypertonus.

I have always been interested in finding an ideal research model in which the stimulation of one auricular point could change the hypertonus of a given muscle. One day, by chance, while examining a patient with bruxism with Dr Renzo Ridi, we found the right key: the patient, sitting in the dentist's chair, presented neck stiffness he had had since awakening. I tried to relax his muscles with ear acupuncture but surprisingly I did not find any sensitive point on the commonly accepted representation of the neck and the cervical vertebrae.

Moving the tip of the algometer downward to the ear lobe, however, I found a very sensitive point which I later realized to be located within the Chinese occiput area (AT3 *zhen*). On that morning the patient was scheduled for an EMG investigation according to the technique proposed by Jankelson.[12] In this procedure some electrodes are attached bilaterally on fixed areas corresponding to masticatory muscles such as temporalis anterior, masseter, digastric and temporalis posterior. However, in this case and in the trial which followed, using Myotronics EM2, we replaced the recording on the latter with the sternocleidomastoid.

After a base recording I pressed the sensitive point with the tip of the algometer as usual in the PPT, and we were excited to notice that the first two muscles in particular lost their tension, measured in mV, during the following minutes. This fortunate case was the first of a series which led us finally to devise a randomized controlled trial (RCT) for demonstrating the value of ear acupuncture in reducing muscular hypertonus.

In a pilot study made on 10 consecutive patients with bruxism, we tried first to find an answer to the question: to what extent do diagnostic maneuvers act as a confounding factor and provoke a variation of muscular tension?

Actually, whatever auricular diagnostic technique is chosen, it may act per se as a therapeutic stimulation; this fact does not usually receive sufficient consideration.

We first evaluated ESRT, which we thought was the least invasive procedure. Indeed, the pressure exerted on the skin by the spring-loaded electrode can be considered negligible (see Ch. 6); however, we did not know if the electrical current flow through the ear could also be considered negligible. We decided to test the point with the lowest electrical resistance within the occiput area. One hour before starting EMG, comparing the right and left auricles only one point was chosen. The point was marked with ink and 1 hour later, after a base recording of 5 minutes, it was again identified with Agiscop. A further period of 14 minutes continuous recording was then performed (Fig. 8.9A). Taking this opportunity we decided to evaluate also the stimulation effect of NCT, and after needle contact for 10 seconds we carried out a second EMG recording for the same period of 14 minutes (Fig. 8.9B).

Comparing the EMG variations in the two periods, we can see that the electrical current flow through the occiput point during the ESRT procedure temporarily reduces muscular tension. In the last 5 minutes compared to the first 5 minutes, however, the muscular tension worsens significantly in a possible rebound effect (Table 8.1). The response to NCT is different and the reduction of muscular tension is progressive during the whole period of recording, and the last 5 minutes show a significant improvement compared to the first.

Apart from the opposite influence of ESRT and NCT on muscular tension, this pilot study gave us essential information regarding the physiology of auricular acupuncture. NCT performed on one side could induce a significant EMG variation not only on the ipsilateral but also on the contralateral temporalis anterior muscle (Table 8.1).

Our findings led us to organize an RCT[13] on three homogeneous groups of patients with malocclusion rated with Helkimo's index of the clinical and dysfunctional state (CDI) of the masticatory system.[14]

The patients belonged to a selected group that I had treated previously with acupuncture for disorders such as chronic neck and back pain, vertigo, atypical facial neuralgia, migraine, etc. One common characteristic in these patients was that the result of the treatment had been rated by me in the follow-up as unsatisfactory and not durable. Given the possibility that craniomandibular disorders may be responsible for postural changes in the case of chronic myofascial pain, Dr Ridi made a complete evaluation of the stomatognathic system of these patients, including EMG.

The patients were included on the day of experimentation if their values of muscular tension in mV, in at least one muscle, were higher than the normal range established by Myotronics-EM2. The normal range was 1.5–2.5 mV for temporalis anterior, 1.0–2.0 mV for the masseter and 1.5–2.5 mV for the digastric muscle. Out of a total of 61 subjects examined, only 43 were included and randomized in three groups. In the first group NCT was performed for 10 seconds and in the second a 0.20×15 mm needle was placed on the same point; the third group acted as the control group and received no intervention for the whole period of observation. The EMG recording time was brought up to 30 minutes for a total of 120 consecutive recordings.

The EMG variations on the total number of eight muscles were compared with t-test for independent samples (Table 8.2). Both stimulations were superior to the control group in reducing the electrical activity of all muscles except the sternocleidomastoid. As regards the comparison between the insertion of the needle and the simple contact, acupuncture results were superior to NCT only for the right temporalis and left digastric. The reaction to the stimulation of the sternocleidomastoid was different than in the other muscles but it has to be pointed out that the sternocleidomastoid does not participate directly in mastication. This is a further reason for possibly considering the occiput area as specific for bruxism and malocclusion.

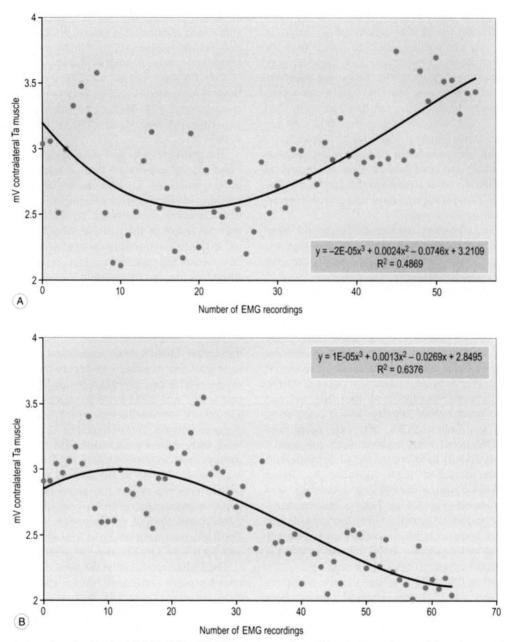

Fig. 8.9 Cubic regression line for muscular tension (mV) and consecutive EMG recordings of contralateral temporalis anterior (Ta) muscle according to the modified Myotronics EM2 procedure in 10 patients with bruxism; after electrical detection of the identified point (A); after NCT for 10 seconds of the identified point (B). Twenty recordings correspond approximately to 5 minutes.

Table 8.1 Comparison between the mean values of muscular tension in the ipsilateral and contralateral temporalis anterior (Ta) muscle, after ESRT and subsequently after NCT

| | Method | Mean value | | Mean difference | 95% C.I. | | P |
		First 20 EMG recordings (mV)	Last 20 EMG recordings (mV)		Lower	Upper	
Ipsilateral Ta	ESRT	2.93	3.57	−0.64	−0.89	−0.39	<0.001
	NCT	3.25	2.50	0.75	0.57	0.93	<0.001
Contralateral Ta	ESRT	2.78	3.21	−0.42	−0.68	−0.17	<0.005
	NCT	2.88	2.24	0.64	0.51	0.76	<0.001

Ta = temporalis anterior

Table 8.2 Comparison, with t-test for independent samples, of the EMG variations in the eight muscles of three groups (acupuncture, needle contact, control)

| Muscle | Acupuncture vs. control | | NCT vs. control | | Acupuncture vs. NCT | |
	t-test	P value	t-test	P value	t-test	P value
Right Ta	8.429	<0.005	6.346	<0.005	3.308	<0.005
Left Ta	7.012	<0.005	5.884	<0.005	0.681	NS
Right Mm	4.425	<0.005	6.750	<0.005	1.590	NS
Left Mm	6.542	<0.005	3.580	<0.005	0.888	NS
Right Da	5.101	<0.005	3.948	<0.005	1.936	NS
Left Da	6.360	<0.005	3.481	<0.005	4.647	<0.005
Right SCM	0.246	NS	1.855	NS	−2.077	<0.05
Left SCM	−4.167	<0.005	0.157	NS	−4.987	<0.005

Ta = temporalis anterior; Mm = masseter; Da = digastric; SCM = sternocleidomastoid

The conclusions of our RCT were that:

we had the rare opportunity to study the stimulation effect of a single point, how it has been possible with the acupuncture point PC6 on nausea. The result in our group of patients indicates the possibility that EMG could be a sensitive tool for measuring the effects of auricular stimulation also in other medical conditions. As regards NCT, this modality most probably should be considered an intermediate method of stimulation between true acupuncture and non stimulation.[13]

CASE STUDY

A 25-year-old female employee working several hours a day at a computer had been suffering for 2–3 years with bilateral neck stiffness and pain. She also had tension headache with occasional dizziness. Four months previously she had suffered for the first time with sciatic pain on her right side. Recently she had complained again of back pain, especially before getting up in the morning. Dr Ridi examined her and on opening the patient's mouth found that she had a lateral deviation of the mandible to the left and a left temporomandibular joint (TMJ) painful on palpation. The left temporal and external pterygoids were also tender on palpation. Dentition was complete with extensive reconstruction of the occlusal surfaces of the premolar and molar teeth. A point with low electrical skin resistance (ESR) within the left occiput area was identified with Agiscop (−) (Fig. 8.10). EMG recording with faithful application of the technique, according to the original instructions, showed an electrical activity which was higher than normal on both digastric and masseter muscles, on the right temporalis anterior and especially on both temporalis posterior muscles (Fig. 8.11A). Five minutes after NCT was performed on the left occiput point, a significant reduction of activity could be recorded on all

muscles except the right digastric muscle (Fig. 8.11B). These variations remained unchanged throughout 30 minutes of EMG recording. Dr Ridi suggested making the patient a neuromuscular bite to wear regularly every night. This device steadily reduced her neck stiffness and no more back pain was observed in the follow-up (time of observation 8 years).

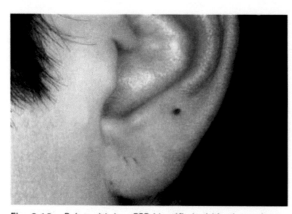

Fig. 8.10   Point with low ESR identified within the occiput area in a 25-year-old patient with neck pain and malocclusion.

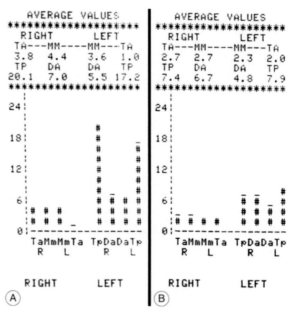

Fig. 8.11   EMG (Myotronics-EM2) average values in mV, before NCT (A); 5 minutes after NCT on the marked point of Figure 8.10 (B). Ta = temporalis anterior muscle; Mm = masseter muscle; Tp = temporalis posterior muscle; Da = digastric muscle

References

[1] Marcelli S. Il test dei punti attivi. Torino: Edizioni Libreria Cortina; 1995.

[2] Facco E, Liguori A, Petti F et al. Traditional acupuncture in migraine: a controlled randomized study. Headache 2008;3:398–407.

[3] Streng A, Linde K, Hoppe A et al. Effectiveness and tolerability of acupuncture compared with metoprolol in migraine prophylaxis. Headache 2006;10:1492–502.

[4] Diener HC, Kronfeld K, Boewing G et al. Efficacy of acupuncture for the prophylaxis of migraine: a multicentre randomised controlled clinical trial. Lancet Neurol 2006;4:310–6.

[5] Vickers AJ, Rees RW, Zollman CE et al. Acupuncture of chronic headache disorders in primary care: randomised controlled trial and economic analysis. Health Technol Assess 2004;8:1–35.

[6] Melchart D, Thormaehlen J, Hager S et al. Acupuncture versus placebo versus sumatriptan for early treatment of migraine attacks: a randomized controlled trial. Intern Med 2003;2:181–8.

[7] Allais G, De Lorenzo C, Quirico PE et al. Acupuncture in the prophylactic treatment of migraine without aura: a comparison with flunarizine. Headache 2002;9:855–61.

[8] Hesse J, Møgelvang B, Simonsen H. Acupuncture versus metoprolol in migraine prophylaxis: a randomized trial of trigger point inactivation. J Intern Med 1994;5:451–6.

[9] Romoli M, Allais G, Airola G et al. Ear acupuncture in the control of migraine pain: selecting the right acupoints by the 'needle-contact test'. Neurol Sci 2005;26(Suppl. 2):158–61.

[10] Travell JG, Simons DG. Myofascial pain and dysfunction – the trigger point manual. Vol. 1. Baltimore: Williams and Wilkins; 1983.

[11] Melzack R, Stillwell DM, Fox EJ. Trigger points and acupuncture points for pain: correlations and implications. Pain 1977;3:3–23.

[12] Jankelson RR. Neuromuscular dental diagnosis and treatment. St Louis: Ishiyaku EuroAmerica Inc Pub; 1990.

[13] Romoli M, Ridi R, Giommi A. Electromyographical changes in bruxism after auricular stimulation. A randomized controlled clinical study. Minerva Med 2003;1(Suppl. 4):9–15.

[14] Helkimo M. Studies on function and dysfunction of the masticatory system. II. Index for anamnestic and clinical dysfunction and occlusal state. Swed Dent J 1974;2:101–21.

Chapter 9

How to interface auricular diagnosis with clinical status

THE VALIDATION OF AURICULAR DIAGNOSIS

The term auricular diagnosis was first proposed officially by Terry Oleson in 1980.[1] His study, conducted at the department of anesthesiology at the UCLA School of Medicine in Los Angeles, belongs to the history of ear acupuncture. Its aim was to evaluate the claims by French and Chinese acupuncturists that a somatotopic mapping of the body is represented upon the external ear. Forty patients were examined by a physician to determine which of 12 reported areas of their body suffered musculoskeletal pain (Fig. 9.1). Each patient was then covered with a sheet to conceal any visible physical problems. A second physician afterwards carried out a blind examination of the patient's auricles for areas of higher tenderness or reduced electrical skin resistance. The ear points corresponding to body areas where the subject reported musculoskeletal pain were designated as 'reactive points', while 'non-reactive points' corresponded to areas of the body where the patient experienced no discomfort.

The results of Oleson's study were as follows:

1. The correct identifications summed to 75.2%. In 12.9% of the total the points were false-positive and in 11.9% the points were false-negative; the association was highly significant with χ^2 ($P<0.001$). In 37 of the 40 subjects there were more correct identifications than incorrect, which was rated as significant by the sign test ($P<0.01$).
2. Both mean electrical conductivity and dermal tenderness at ear points related to specific areas

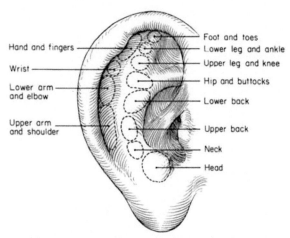

Hand and fingers

Wrist

Lower arm
and elbow

Upper arm
and shoulder

Foot and toes
Lower leg and ankle
Upper leg and knee
Hip and buttocks
Lower back
Upper back
Neck
Head

Fig. 9.1 The somatotopic mapping of musculoskeletal pain on the auricle according to Oleson *(with permission of the author)*.

of the body where pain problems were present were significantly higher with *t*-test ($P<0.01$).

3. As regards the laterality for ear points relative to the side of a body problem, the mean electrical conductance was significantly higher if the problem was ipsilateral ($P<0.01$); the mean tenderness of ear points, in the case of unilateral problems, did not differ between the right and left ear.

4. There were no significant differences in either auricular conductance or auricular tenderness between recent and old pain problems. Recent pain problems were defined as having occurred within the 6 months prior to the study, old problems as having occurred more than 6 months previously.

5. It was observed in 15% of the subjects that there was a localized region of white, flaky scaling of the dermis on the auricular areas corresponding to the part of the body where musculoskeletal pain was present. Oleson wrote on this subject: 'although infrequently observed, abnormal morphological characteristics on the auricular surface were highly predictive of the presence of pathology in the corresponding area of the body'.

The interesting conclusions of the article by Oleson and colleagues were that:

this study also indicated that the auricular diagnosis technique is often sensitive to pathological problems of which the patient is only minimally

aware. When some patients were told of their auricular diagnosis results, they suddenly remembered having a minor or old pain problem in that bodily area, a problem which they had neglected to mention during the medical evaluation. Since these post-hoc results were derived after the ear diagnosis had been made, these instances were not included in any statistical analyses. Nonetheless, such observations do suggest that auricular diagnosis may be effectively employed as part of a general medical evaluation designed to reveal all organic aspects of a patient's pain complaint. Since there are also ear points for abdominal and thoracic bodily organs, auricular diagnosis could also be utilized with standard diagnostic procedures for analyzing pathological conditions related to internal pain or referred pain.[1]

Since then Oleson's research has become the major reference study and has been cited in several articles on ear acupuncture. A recent paper, however, re-examined the question of whether auricular maps were reliable for chronic musculoskeletal pain disorders.[2] Fortunately the authors had no intention of replicating Oleson's study but only of proposing a different method for validating auricular diagnosis by using a 250 g algometer. The main shortcomings of this study were the limited number of patients examined (only 25), the lack of importance given to the posterior surface of the ear, which was not examined at all, and the adoption of an arbitrary somatotopic arrangement of the auricular zones which does not faithfully correspond either to the French or to the Chinese map. For example the knee was reproduced twice on two different areas roughly representing it, according to the schools just mentioned. It is not reported in the article which of the two the blind assessor had to consider as corresponding to a painful knee, or whether both corresponded. In contrast, in Oleson's study the 12 different auricular regions chosen for the research were the faithful somatotopic representation of the body according to the Chinese map.

In my opinion the concept of parallelism between a topographical area of the body and the corresponding somatotopic auricular area expressed by Oleson has to be considered innovative. Actually, in the diagnostic process we need to speak about areas, especially if we are learning, or teaching beginners to select the most effective points for treatment within each area.

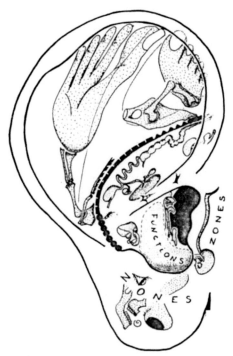

Fig. 9.2 The representation of the homunculus according to Bossy *(with permission of the author).*

Bourdiol in particular introduced the concept of somatotopic area early, but the most interesting interpretation of the body's representation on the auricle is probably that of Jean Bossy,[3] former director at the Montpellier Institute of Anatomy and author of several books and articles on the neurophysiological basis of acupuncture. His representation of the homunculus on the auricle[4] is probably more realistic and useful for the practitioner than the well proportioned fetus which we see on the common drawings of the ear. As in the *homunculus sensitivus* and *motorius* of Penfield, the hand and the thumb have a large representation as well as the lips, the nose and the jaws (Fig. 9.2).

A NEW PROJECT FOR VALIDATING AURICULAR DIAGNOSIS

Starting from Oleson's historical paper I tried to create a project for validating auricular diagnosis which could be acceptable and reproducible.

METHODOLOGY

Each new patient was invited to fill in a form with his past and recent symptoms and diseases in decreasing order of importance; the most relevant were listed at the top, the less important at the bottom. The patient was also asked to write down the type and number of surgical interventions experienced as well as any hospital admissions and injuries, and to list medication taken regularly, especially analgesic and psychoactive drugs, and their time of intake. My assistant had the task of removing any diagnostic material such as X-rays or laboratory tests which could influence my diagnosis.

The patient, seated, was invited to remain silent for a while and not give any information about his health. Inspection was the first diagnosis I performed, followed in random order by the pressure pain test (PPT) or the electrical skin resistance test (ESRT). For each method I used different sheets of the Sectogram, transcribing all possible symptoms and diseases I thought to be related with the topography of skin alterations or the location of the points identified with PPT and ESRT.

My assistant afterwards appeared on the scene and compared my diagnosis with the complaints listed by the patient. He had the delicate task of working out the number of consistent symptoms, but was free to interpret them as best he could, also speaking to the patient. For example, a 'pain in the arm' could be reinterpreted as a 'painful shoulder' or 'cervical–brachial pain'; when the clinical condition was uncertain both terms could be retained. With mental disorders the different terms reported by the patient had to be harmonized. For example, 'tension' or 'irritation' were evaluated as anxiety, and 'sadness' or 'melancholy' were evaluated as depression.

PATIENT CHARACTERISTICS

Between 2002 and 2007 I examined a total of 506 patients: 371 females (average age 48.1 years, SD 14.6, range 17–84) and 135 males (average age 46.5 years, SD 14.9, range 13–80). The total number of symptoms reported/identified in my population of patients was 5641 (females averaged 11.9 symptoms, males averaged 9.2 symptoms).

The higher number of female patients attending my clinic is not unusual for therapists practicing complementary techniques. Several factors could explain this phenomenon: in my opinion it could be related to what today seems to be a stronger desire

Table 9.1   Classification and percentage of 5641 symptoms declared/identified in 506 patients

Symptom	%
Musculoskeletal	32.7%
Psychological/psychiatric	22.5%
Gastrointestinal	14.7%
Cardiovascular	6.8%
Nervous system (central/peripheral)	4.6%
Dermatological	4.6%
Genitourinary	3.7%
Ear, nose and throat	2.9%
Endocrine and metabolic	2.7%
Teeth and temporomandibular joint	2.3%
Other	2.5%
Total	100%

in females compared to males to preserve their health at its best, or perhaps to the search for alternative treatments to drugs with pronounced side-effects or which are feared to be potentially harmful.

Another characteristic in the patient population I examined was the relatively high percentage aged >60 years (22.3%). This factor is possibly due to the greater presence of musculoskeletal disorders in this phase of life. Indeed, if we consider the 5641 symptoms reported the most numerous are those related to the musculoskeletal system (32.7%), followed by psychological/psychiatric symptoms (22.5%). Table 9.1 lists further symptoms related to other organs and systems in decreasing order of frequency.

It is possible that every practitioner may find or treat varying types of symptoms in his patients, according to his experience and interest in specific fields of medicine. Nevertheless my impression is that acupuncture for musculoskeletal pain is the most common application for the majority of therapists.

RESULTS

The aim of my validation was to find answers to the following questions:

1. Were the different diagnostic methods quantitatively equivalent in unveiling the patient's problems?

2. Were the different methods equivalent in diagnosing recent and past problems?
3. In the case of musculoskeletal disorders, were the different methods equally effective in detecting the prevalent side of pain?

Were the different diagnostic methods quantitatively equivalent in unveiling the patient's problems?

The three diagnostic methods used had different success rates for the identification of patients' symptoms. First came inspection with 52.2%, followed by PPT with 33.7% and ESRT(−) with 33.2%. Interestingly, if a symptom had been identified by at least one method there was a success rate of 78.6% (Table 9.2a). The significance of this is evident: the experienced practitioner, who generally applies all the proposed methods, acquires a better understanding of patients' conditions. This result is confirmed by the significantly higher diagnostic potentiality of the three methods together compared to the inspection alone (Table 9.2b).

As expounded in Appendix 2, the Agiscop device used in the diagnostic procedures reported in this book allows a double electrical test, choosing either the minus (−) or the plus (+) modality. In 202 patients out of the total group of 506 we added the + modality, even though the average number of identified points is usually lower than with the − modality and consequently appears to identify a lower number of disorders in the patient. The success rates according to the four methods employed were as follows: (i) inspection 52%; (ii) PPT 34%; (iii) ESRT(−) 33.3%; (iv) ESRT(+) 20.4%. Thus, as expected, the + modality showed a lower success rate than the − modality; nevertheless its application as a fourth diagnostic modality increased the total success rate to 80.9% (Table 9.3).

Were the different methods equivalent in diagnosing recent and past problems?

If the three methods adopted had different success rates in identifying recent and past problems, we applied the categorization used by Oleson in his study. Recent problems (defined as occurring in the previous 6 months) had an average of 62 days; old problems (occurred more than 6 months previously) had an average of 11.8 years.

The success rates in identifying these two categories of symptoms were very similar for all three diagnostic methods. It has to be stressed that the

Table 9.2 Diagnostic success rates (%) obtained in the identification of 5641 symptoms in 506 patients with three methods: inspection, PPT and ESRT(−) (a); comparison of the different methods with paired samples t-test (b)

a)

	Inspection	PPT	ESRT(−)	Three methods together
Diagnostic success rate	52.2%	33.7%	33.2%	78.6%

b)

		95% CI of the difference		P
Comparison	Mean	Lower	Upper	
Inspection – PPT	18.5%	16.8%	20.3%	<0.001
Inspection – ESRT(−)	19.0%	17.2%	20.9%	<0.001
PPT – ESRT(−)	0.5%	−1.1%	2.1%	NS
Inspection – three methods together	−26.4%	−27.6%	−25.3%	<0.001

Table 9.3 Diagnostic success rates (%) obtained in the identification of 2495 symptoms in 202 patients with four methods: inspection, PPT, ESRT(−) and ESRT(+) (a); comparison of the different methods with paired samples t-test (b)

a)

	Inspection	PPT	ESRT(−)	ESRT(+)	Four methods together
Diagnostic success rate	52.0%	34.0%	33.3%	20.4%	80.9%

b)

		95% CI of the difference		P
	Mean	Lower	Upper	
Inspection – PPT	18.0%	15.4%	20.6%	<0.001
Inspection – ESRT(−)	18.7%	16.0%	21.4%	<0.001
Inspection – ESRT(+)	31.6%	29.1%	34.2%	<0.001
PPT – ESRT(−)	0.7%	−1.7%	3.1%	NS
PPT – ESRT(+)	13.6%	11.3%	16.0%	<0.001
ESRT(−)– ESRT(+)	12.9%	10.9%	15.0%	<0.001
Inspection – four methods together	−28.9%	−30.7%	−27.2%	<0.001

group of recent disorders scored only 11.2% of the total; this is a further sign that my population of patients asking for help from acupuncture was composed of people suffering especially with chronic recurrent ailments. I was somewhat surprised by the results for inspection, which I expected would have a much higher importance in diagnosing older problems. Nevertheless, inspection showed a better diagnostic success rate in both cases compared to PPT and ESRT. The latter, however, showed no significant difference either for recent or old problems (Tables 9.4 and 9.5).

Table 9.4   Diagnostic success rates (%) obtained in the identification of 570 symptoms, occurring in the prior 6 months, with three methods: inspection, PPT and ESRT(−) (a); comparison of the different methods with paired samples t-test (b)

a)

	Inspection	PPT	ESRT(−)	Three methods together
Diagnostic success rate	48.2%	33.7%	30.7%	74.7%

b)

		95% CI of the difference		P
Comparison	Mean	Lower	Upper	
Inspection – PPT	14.6%	9.1%	20.0%	<0.001
Inspection – ESRT(−)	17.5%	11.8%	23.3%	<0.001
PPT – ESRT(−)	3.0%	−2.0%	7.9%	NS
Inspection – three methods together	−26.5%	−30.1%	−22.9%	<0.001

Table 9.5   Diagnostic success rates (%) obtained in the identification of 5071 symptoms, having occurred at ≥6 months, with three methods: inspection, PPT and ESRT(−) (a); comparison of the different methods with paired samples t-test (b)

a)

	Inspection	PPT	ESRT(−)	Three methods together
Diagnostic success rate	52.6%	33.7%	33.4%	79.1%

b)

		95% CI of the difference		P
Comparison	Mean	Lower	Upper	
Inspection – PPT	19.0%	17.1%	20.8%	<0.001
Inspection – ESRT(−)	19.2%	17.3%	21.1%	<0.001
PPT – ESRT(−)	0.3%	−1.4%	2.0%	NS
Inspection – three methods together	−26.4%	−27.6%	−25.2%	<0.001

In the case of musculoskeletal disorders, were the different methods equally effective in detecting the prevalent side of pain?

In my blind examination of the patient I had three options for determining the prevalent side of pain: right, left and bilateral. In diagnosing musculoskeletal pain disorders I obtained the following success rates for ipsilateral (right- or left-sided) pain: (i) inspection 51.7%; (ii) PPT 25.3%; (iii) ESRT (−) 14.6% (Table 9.6). If the pain was bilateral or without prevalence for one side, the success rates were, as expected, higher: (i) inspection 85.2%; (ii) PPT 56.2%; (iii) ESRT (−) 20.7% (Table 9.7). These results show that it is easier to identify a bilateral pain disorder on the auricle, especially with inspection and PPT.

Table 9.6   Diagnostic success rates (%) obtained in the identification of 633 unilateral (right or left) musculoskeletal pain disorders with three methods: inspection, PPT and ESRT(−) (a); comparison of the different methods with paired samples t-test (b)

a)

	Inspection	PPT	ESRT(−)	Three methods together
Diagnostic success rate	51.7%	25.3%	14.6%	66.5%

b)

Comparison	Mean	95% CI of the difference		P
		Lower	Upper	
Inspection − PPT	26.4%	21.5%	31.4%	<0.001
Inspection − ESRT(−)	37.2%	32.5%	41.9%	<0.001
PPT − ESRT(−)	10.8%	6.7%	14.8%	NS
Inspection − three methods together	−14.7%	−17.5%	−11.9%	<0.001

Table 9.7   Diagnostic success rates (%) obtained in the identification of 755 bilateral musculoskeletal pain disorders with three methods: inspection, PPT and ESRT(−) (a); comparison of the different methods with paired samples t-test (b)

a)

	Inspection	PPT	ESRT(−)	Three methods together
Diagnostic success rate	85.2%	56.2%	20.7%	92.1%

b)

Comparison	Mean	95% CI of the difference		P
		Lower	Upper	
Inspection − PPT	29.0%	25.0%	33.0%	<0.001
Inspection − ESRT(−)	64.5%	60.7%	68.3%	<0.001
PPT − ESRT(−)	35.5%	31.2%	39.8%	NS
Inspection − three methods together	−6.9%	−8.7%	−5.1%	<0.001

CONCLUSIONS

The conclusions of my validation can be summarized as follows:

1. Inspection is an essential part of auricular diagnosis, alone or in combination with one or more detection techniques. Its superiority over the other methods confirms the importance given by Chinese authors to this procedure apparently neglected in Western countries. The combination of as many diagnostic methods as possible permits the experienced physician to achieve a relevant diagnostic versatility in suspecting health disorders of various origin in his patients.

2. Inspection is furthermore superior to PPT and ESRT in diagnosing either recent or past problems; these methods, however, do not show any significant difference between themselves.

These findings coincide with the results of Oleson's study, where the mean auricular conductivity and the mean auricular tenderness of the areas identified in the two groups with recent or past problems were not statistically different.

3. In the case of musculoskeletal pain of any origin, auricular examination seems to be more important in diagnosing a bilateral disorder than an ipsilateral one. Inspection, however, once again seems to be superior to PPT and ESRT in evidencing both an ipsilateral or bilateral pain disorder. The reasons for the low success rate (especially with PPT and ESRT) in determining the side of pain may be correlated with the peculiar auricular physiology which probably does not strictly separate the somatotopic representations of structures and functions of the human body. Nogier himself stated that:

a large number of various and repeated observations could not permit me to state a priori that a certain auricular zone could be active on the ipsilateral or contralateral side of the body. A series of thorough investigations indeed allowed me to ascertain that the same region could act either on one side or the other. By means of all researches I have done, I am now convinced that the confounding factor was due to an interaction between the symmetrical points of the two auricles. When we are going to stimulate point A on the right ear we stimulate at the same time point A' on the left ear. This explains the crossed action of the auricular points: even if the stimulated point originally corresponds to the ipsilateral side of the body, the active point is in this case located symmetrically on the opposite ear.[5]

AURICULAR POINTS/AREAS INTERFACING WITH A PATIENT'S CLINICAL CONDITION

Once the consistency of auricular diagnosis in revealing the health problems of the subject has been demonstrated, we must learn more about how to correctly interface an auricular point/area with the clinical condition of the patient. Since every subject, especially among the elderly, has multiple disorders, we need to adopt a strategy concerning different aspects of the process, for example:

1. the topography of the identified auricular point/area
2. the interpretation of a false-positive or false-negative auricular diagnosis
3. the symmetrical/asymmetrical distribution of the points on the auricles
4. the variation in the distribution of the auricular points over time, particularly when other treatments have been given or are in progress (surgery, drugs, rehabilitation, etc.).

THE TOPOGRAPHY OF THE IDENTIFIED AURICULAR POINT/AREA

In the formulation of a diagnostic hypothesis the concept of auricular topography is essential. It is possible that at the start we may be unable to match the identified zones with the patient's symptoms. We need therefore to single out some key areas: in this deductive work medical knowledge is important and the therapist should be free to obtain more information from laboratory tests and imaging techniques.

In my opinion one or more of the following criteria are necessary for an area to be considered essential for diagnosis and selectable for treatment:

a. The area should contain at least two skin alterations or two points close to each other with marked tenderness or reduced electrical resistance.
b. At least two skin alterations or two points with greater tenderness or reduced electrical resistance may be located on the same line according to Nogier's principle of alignment (see Ch. 3) or may be found in the same sector.
c. The identified skin alterations may be sensitive to pressure.

As regards criterion a, the diagnostic importance of the identified area is proportional to the number of points on it.

As regards criterion b, strictly applying Nogier's principle of alignment (as described in Ch. 3) could in my opinion reduce the information to be obtained from the patient. Therefore for diagnostic purposes I proposed in Chapter 4 ('Does inspection have the same value in all sectors of the outer ear?') to consider also the skin alterations pertaining to the same sector. The importance of inspection should be stressed here once more because it identified in my patients a higher rate of skin alterations on the same sector compared to points identified with PPT and ESRT: respectively 46.4%, 16.1% and 14.4% of the total.

As reported in the section of Chapter 4 mentioned above, only 23.6% of the aligned skin alterations were found on the same part of the ear: the practitioner should be prepared therefore to pay attention to any other parts of the auricle carrying pairs of aligned skin alterations (see Plates IIA, VID, IXD).

Regarding the last of the above criteria, criterion c, Chinese acupuncturists have stressed the importance of palpating skin alterations for distinguishing a 'false appearance' from a 'positive reaction point' (Ch. 4). About 50% of skin alterations are indeed tender to palpation and this phenomenon adds a higher value to the identified somatotopic area.

Figure 9.3 shows the right ear of a 64-year-old male patient who asked to be treated with acupuncture because he suffered with recurrent backache, especially on the right side. The inspection of the right auricle did indeed show a little hyperemia of the anthelix corresponding to the thoracolumbar junction and some telangiectasia on the representation of the Chinese knee. My attention was attracted, however, by a linear telangiectasia crossing the liver area. PPT identified two tender points on it which were furthermore aligned with point

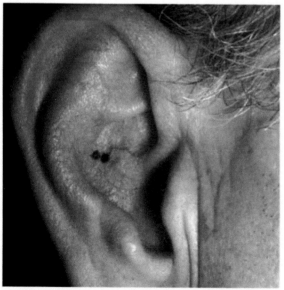

Fig. 9.3 Tender points on a telangiectasia of the upper concha in a 64-year-old male patient carrying a hepatic steatosis due to excessive drinking.

zero. My question to the patient about possible liver problems was affirmative: he had hepatic steatosis with abnormal concentration of serum glutamic pyruvic transaminase due to excessive drinking. Both points, however, were included in the treatment of his lumbar pain and he was warmly recommended to treat his liver with greater respect.

The systematic palpation of skin alterations as proposed by the Chinese is an interesting diagnostic procedure and may be helpful for the selection of points to treat (see Ch. 10). Nevi can also be checked for their tenderness but it is preferable not to include them in treatment. Another method is to limit the palpation of the skin alterations to the area representing the affected part of the body. For example, in the case of chronic shoulder pain it may be best to select directly the tender skin alterations of the shoulder area and the clavicle area. Since shoulder pain is often associated with neck problems it is useful also to check the skin alterations possibly located on the neck area and on the cervical vertebrae.

The last, less frequent aspect related to the topography of the identified area is the activation of an area bearing a scar, for example caused by piercing. It is rather difficult to demonstrate that piercing can primarily induce some specific symptoms in time. In some cases simple advice could be offered to patients with this kind of scar.

A 52-year-old female patient suffered with migraine and was treated successfully with ear acupuncture. Occasionally she suffered also with Ménière's disease. During a vertigo attack a sensitive area was found overlapping the representation of the internal ear according to the Chinese. Of the four tender points one coincided with the scar of a second piercing of the ear lobe. Beyond the treatment of the tender points I advised the patient to take off the earring with the aim of reducing possible mechanical stimulation of a reactive area of the ear (Fig. 9.4).

FALSE-POSITIVE AND FALSE-NEGATIVE AURICULAR DIAGNOSIS

This is probably the most complex problem that the therapist has to overcome to get the correct information about a patient's health problems.

A *false-positive* diagnosis in an asymptomatic subject is probably less confounding for the practitioner than a *false-negative* diagnosis in a patient with various known ailments. In the former the

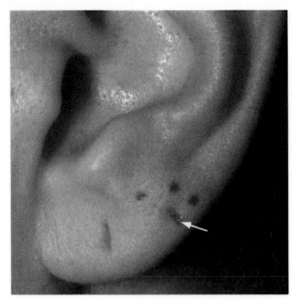

Fig. 9.4 Tender points of the ear lobe of a 52-year-old female patient with current vertigo attack. One tender point coincides with the scar of piercing.

identified auricular areas may be the representation of parts of the body which have been injured in the past, leaving almost no after-effects. A second possibility is the detection of a tendency to allergy or food intolerance, or a predisposition to diabetes and hypertension, when these disorders are shared by other members of the patient's family. A third possibility is that of indicating hitherto unexpressed stress-related symptoms or somatization disorders in apparently healthy subjects.

A *false-negative* diagnosis is much more limiting and frustrating for the practitioner when the patient is affected by a series of different diseases. The suspicion arises especially when PPT and ESRT identify points which do not fit at all with the patient's current or past problems. Another possibility is that PPT and ESRT may show a particularly low number of points (average ≤2) which keep the practitioner from making a sufficient diagnosis. Different reasons can explain this, for example a particularly high pain threshold at PPT or the particularly high electrical skin resistance of the subject.

However, I have long been aware of the possibility that some specific drugs may interfere with auricular diagnosis. Ceccherelli et al[6] examined

two groups of patients affected by disorders of the upper digestive system, scheduled to undergo endoscopy of the esophagus, stomach and duodenum the following day. The first group was under regular treatment with benzodiazepines; the second was not taking any medication of this type. The author found a fivefold higher number of tender points in the second group. Ceccherelli's conclusions were that in clinical practice we must investigate if a patient is taking benzodiazepines for any reason; in that case auricular diagnosis is not reliable.

The drop of points with PPT was explained by the author by the decrease of reactivity to nociceptive afferents shown by this class of drugs on the central nervous system. Despite the great difference in the half-life of drugs such as diazepam, lorazepam, triazolam, etc., administered with both a sedative and a hypnotic objective, the disappearance of tender points still took place.

In several further studies we (Romoli and Van der Windt) tried to control this interference by excluding from the clinical trial patients who had taken antidepressants or benzodiazepines less than 12 hours previously or NSAIDs less than 6–8 hours previously.[7] The aim was to avoid a false-negative detection of auricular points in the group to be treated with ear acupuncture, but the temporal range proposed was based only on clinical impressions. It is indeed rather difficult, outside an experimental setting, to calculate the real half-life of a drug in every patient.

For instance, it is interesting to notice how unpredictable the interference of nimesulide is on PPT and ESRT in patients with musculoskeletal pain disorders. Some subjects still show a reduced number of tender points 48 or 72 hours after the intake of 100 mg of nimesulide. The auricular findings in these patients are, however, consistent with their statement that they are able to control pain only with two or three doses a week. Some other drugs can have further unpredictable effects, for example antihypertensive drugs or aspirin, even in low doses (100 mg). In general, every drug may interfere specifically with the auricular diagnosis of areas related to the symptom which the drug is supposed to cure. This aspect has, however, to be checked if we are planning, for example, to combine ear acupuncture with drugs with the intention of reducing the amount of drug needed to maintain the same therapeutic effect, as in the following case.

CASE STUDY

A 46-year-old female patient wanted to reduce the amount of the antidepressant she was taking, because of its side-effects. When I examined her for the first time I found only a few points related to backache, which she had been suffering from recurrently; I was not able to find any further point or area related to the depressive disorders of the patient (Fig. 9.5, red dots). She was also taking antihypertensive drugs and I informed her that it would be impossible for me to identify the points relevant to her case. With her consent and with the approval of her psychiatrist we planned the following strategy of exclusion. At first we excluded hypertensive drugs for 12 and 24 hours. This brought no change or appearance of new points. We then reduced the antidepressant (sertraline hydrochloride 100 mg) which the patient took twice a day, in the morning and in the evening. The exclusion of one pill did not

change the auricular reactivity after 7 hours; the exclusion also of a second pill, about 30 hours after the last intake, was finally able to reveal a series of points which were definitively associated to her depressive disorders and treated consequently with ear acupuncture (Fig. 9.5 gray dots).

There are further factors interfering with correct auricular diagnosis. An important factor seems to be the presence of foci, as has been asserted by practitioners of neural therapy. The reader will allow me to make a short digression on this method which is possibly one of the less recognized non-conventional techniques in the English speaking population. According to the World Health Organization's 2001 review *The Legal Status of Traditional Medicine and Complementary/Alternative Medicine: A Worldwide Review*, neural therapy (German *Neuraltherapie*) or procaine injection therapy is officially

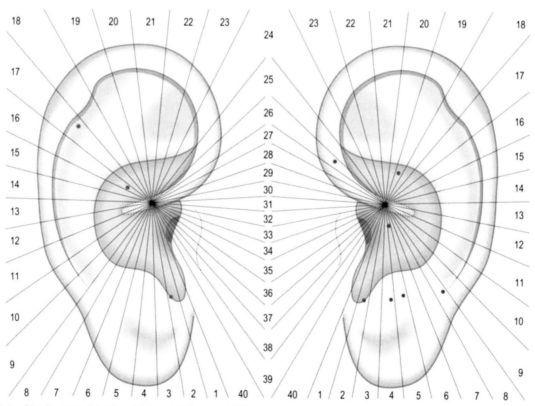

Fig. 9.5 Distribution of tender points in a 46-year-old female patient with depressive disorder taking 200 mg a day of sertraline hydrochloride (Zoloft®) (red points); the same patient about 30 hours after the last intake (gray points).

recognized in only a few countries, for example Germany, Austria and Hungary. The founders of the method were the German physicians Walter and Ferdinand Hüneke who in the 1920s and 1930s discovered the effects of injecting procaine into tissues of the human body carrying foci or 'fields of disturbance'. It is interesting to note the differences in the definition of 'focus' across the different languages. In Dorland's Medical Dictionary focus is defined as the chief center of a morbid process; Roche's Medical Dictionary for German practitioners defines it more extensively as a circumscribed damaged area of tissue due to infection, inflammation, degeneration, etc. which may induce a pathological reaction or loss of function in further associated districts or in the whole body. Typical examples of foci are post-traumatic or postoperative scars which may cause local or regional pain, weakening of muscle groups of the same neurological segment, but also remote vegetative nervous phenomena. Injecting procaine or other local anesthetics such as lidocaine appears to have a membrane potential stabilizing effect on the tissues in which fields of interference are located. Restoring the electrophysiological stability of the cells involved corrects the abnormal emission of afferent signals to the spinal cord, regulating the responses of the autonomic nervous system.

In the case of scars, in my opinion another interesting hypothesis is related to the entrapment of neural endings during the process of cicatrization and their chronic stimulation due to the mechanical effect of traction. This hypothesis seems to be supported by the fact that scars which need to be treated respond to the injection of a simple physiological saline solution as well as they do to procaine. In my opinion the possible effect of this procedure could be attributed to the 'ungluing' of the minute adhesions within the different layers of the scar. Even the advice given to the patient to massage the tender parts of the scar is of value and probably reduces the above-mentioned effect of traction.

I want for a moment to return to the issue of scars confounding auricular diagnosis. It is sometimes possible for the practitioner to identify a point on the auricle, in a fixed location, which remains tender to pressure despite multiple treatments with acupuncture or other methods of stimulation. In this case the notion that a scar of any origin may be located on the corresponding area of the body should not be dismissed. It may be an old or forgotten scar, responsible through chronic irritation for unclear painful syndromes in distant parts of the body. Should such a suspicion arise, the whole of the patient's skin needs to be checked for both major and minor scars, especially on the side of the body corresponding to the tender auricular point. Every scar should then be palpated along its entire length and all painful spots should be marked with ink. On completion of the examination the therapist has two options: he can apply the needle contact test on the auricular point to confirm the interrelationship, or he may treat the scar and observe its effect on the tender point. Although neural therapy recommends treating the whole length of the scar, in my opinion it is sufficient to infiltrate only the sensitive portion. If treatment is successful the therapist will witness the prompt disappearance of any tenderness in the corresponding auricular point.

CASE STUDY

A 68-year-old female patient underwent surgery on her right lateral malleolus for a fracture she suffered 4 months previously. As well as ankle pain the patient also suffered from recurrent backache which had worsened in the previous weeks. This symptom was explained by her compensatory asymmetrical gait shifting her weight onto her left leg. The ankle was furthermore swollen and movements of eversion were limited. A first session for treatment of the most tender points of the right auricle resulted in relief from pain for some days; however, a second session brought no further relief. A tender point was still present in a fixed position from one session to the other (Fig. 9.6). Suspecting the scar to be responsible for this tenderness I examined it thoroughly along its entire length. On palpation I found a very tender spot of about 10 mm (see arrows in Fig. 9.7). A 30 second massage of the scar evoked referred pain in the whole area, overlapping with the bothersome sensation the patient had become used to feeling. I obtained a reduction in tenderness of the auricular point but not its total relief. Therefore I proposed to the patient the infiltration of the scar with a few drops of mepivacaine hydrochloride 1%. Immediately after the injection the auricular point completely lost its tenderness and the patient felt some relief. After a second infiltration 2 weeks later the patient was finally free of her symptoms and able to benefit fully from her rehabilitation program.

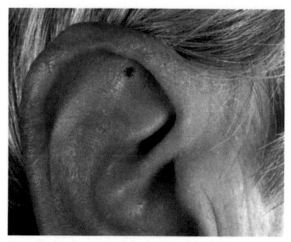

Fig. 9.6 Tender point of the ipsilateral anthelix in a 68-year-old female patient who 4 months previously had experienced a fracture of the lateral malleolus and who still suffered after-effects of surgery.

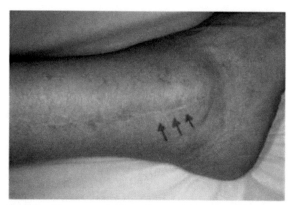

Fig. 9.7 The arrows indicate the sensitive part of the scar at palpation; the infiltration of the scar with mepivacaine made the tenderness of the point shown in Figure 9.6 disappear.

THE SYMMETRICAL/ASYMMETRICAL DISTRIBUTION OF THE POINTS ON THE AURICLES

As we saw in Chapter 4, there is no significant difference in the number of skin alterations identified on the right and left ears. Nevertheless, another confounding aspect for the practitioner can be the asymmetrical distribution of points on the auricles. The asymmetry may involve the different extension of the same somatotopic area, the total number of points scored on both ears, the variable and uneven distribution of points on the sectors of the Sectogram.

As reported in Chapter 4, we know that the human body presents several irregularities in its anatomy which are obvious, as in the case of liver and spleen; other parts located on the midline of the body show a less apparent asymmetry and only careful examination reveals that the cardia and the pylorus are basically located to the right of the midline and the greater curvature of the stomach to the left (see p. 82). This asymmetry is reflected on the auricle and should always be considered in the diagnostic process.

Another issue regarding the irregularity of distribution of auricular points is that skin alterations, but also points with greater tenderness and lower electrical resistance, tend, for reasons still to be understood, to be concentrated on particular sectors (see Figs 4.7, 5.5, 7.1). It is possible that these clusters of high value are the representation of recurrent diseases with a higher rate of symptoms in specific areas of the body, as for example backache and neck pain reported respectively by 82.6% and 74.3% of my patients. Another hypothesis which has already been discussed is that this asymmetry, respecting Bossy's homunculus principle, may also be correlated with the functions of the body regulated by the autonomic nervous system. Therefore the representation of ganglion and plexus related to the cervical sympathetic and cranial parasympathetic systems could be represented on sectors 5–11 of the Sectogram and the abdominal sympathetic system could be represented on sectors 15–19.

Asymmetrical distribution of auricular points and musculoskeletal pain

The easiest way to understand asymmetrical distribution is of course to study musculoskeletal pain, for which we may observe different pattern combinations:

1. The most frequent is a consistent ipsilaterality as regards post-traumatic and postoperative pain, or arthritic pain disorders in single joints.
2. Secondly there is the possibility that a bilateral pain of the same area of the spine is represented asymmetrically on the auricles as in Figure 9.8. In these cases vertebral manipulation often reduces the number of tender points at PPT.
3. A third option is that bilateral pain can be recognized only on one side. Besides the possibility of a crossed action of the auricular points, as assumed by Nogier himself, there may be other reasons for explaining this phenomenon. For example, in

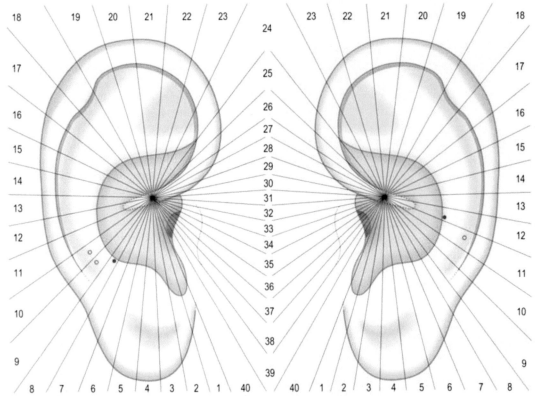

Fig. 9.8 Asymmetrical distribution of the tender points in a 55-year-old female patient affected by bilateral neck pain for several years. Dots = lateral surface; circles = medial surface.

some cases a stress reaction or a somatization disorder could contribute to a prevalent unilateral activation of the auricle (see next section).

4. Last but not least, a symptom could be represented on the contralateral side in specific disorders such as trigeminal neuralgia or other forms of neuropathic pain.

Asymmetrical distribution of auricular points in case of postural disorders

The most simple case of uneven distribution is perhaps that resulting from hip replacement in serious coxarthrosis. Orthopedist Dr Gianluigi Da Campo examined nine patients before surgery and found, as expected, a higher concentration of points on the ipsilateral ear representing the hip which had to be replaced (Fig. 9.9). After 2 weeks, the pain decreased in intensity and this decrease was paralleled by a reduction in the number of tender points. After 3 months, the concentration of auricular points was higher on the non-operated side (Fig. 9.10). This may be due to the change of posture shifting the body's weight to the contralateral side in the recovery phase and/or to the sensitization of the contralateral hip area corresponding to degenerative changes of the same type. What is noticeable in Da Campo's research is the sensitization of the cervical and shoulder area also. This phenomenon might be interpreted as the expression of either general postural imbalance involving also the neck muscles or muscular strain caused by the daily use of crutches.

The most complex asymmetries of auricular points, however, concern postural disorders associated with the onset of myofascial trigger points.

The reader will allow me to make a digression concerning the practice of posturology, which relies on interdisciplinary collaboration aimed at resolving the problems of a patient frequently affected by recurrent pain disorders of the cervical and lumbar areas. This interdisciplinary approach to the patient with postural problems was introduced by chiropractors and osteopaths and was subsequently

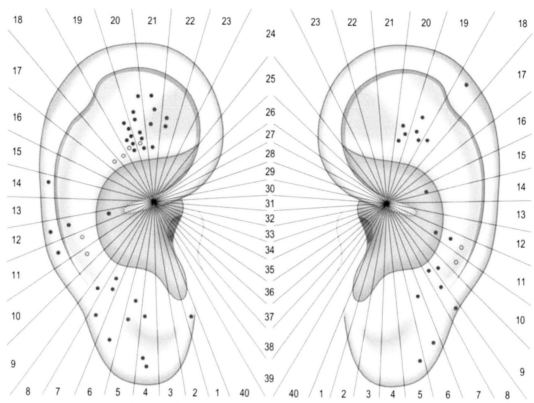

Fig. 9.9 Asymmetrical distribution of tender points in nine patients scheduled for arthroplastic surgery of the right hip *(unpublished data, with permission of Da Campo).* Dots = lateral surface; circles = medial surface.

further developed by dentists, ophthalmologists and podiatrists. Acupuncturists too play a role in the investigation of postural disorders in patients with recurrent back problems; for example they can individuate and test any scars for a negative influence on the patient's harmonious postural balance.

Returning to auricular diagnosis, it is possible that an uneven distribution of points may lead the practitioner to suspect postural disturbance. The best way to demonstrate this is to examine the patient twice, once lying and once in the standing position. First the patient is invited to lie down for 5 minutes, holding cotton splints between his jaws. This procedure allows him to relax those muscles of the neck, shoulder girdle and hip girdle related to posture. After 5 minutes, investigation of the auricles is carried out using PPT. Any tender points are marked with ink and their location transcribed on the Sectogram. The patient is then invited to take out the cotton splints and stand on firm flooring, remaining still for at least

5–10 minutes: carpets and any soft materials under the feet that could minimize structural asymmetries must be avoided. A second investigation with PPT is then performed and the new points appearing on the auricles are transcribed on a new sheet of the Sectogram.

After 5–10 minutes in the standing position several areas became sensitive, among them the right hip and the left shoulder area, either on the lateral or the posterior surface where the postural muscles of the hip and shoulder girdle are represented. I examined 25 patients with postural disorders of various origins with this procedure. Figure 9.11 shows the new points I found between the lying and the standing position. The right hip and left shoulder areas often correspond to the common pattern of postural disturbance noticeable also in the absence of a shorter leg. In this pattern the right iliac crest often appears raised and rotated forwards as does the left shoulder.

Since postural disorders, especially in patients with chronic disorders, are often caused by multiple

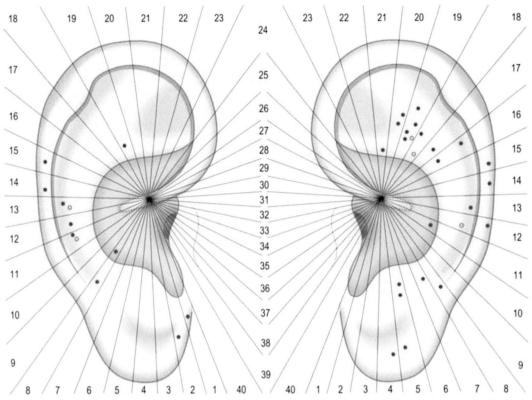

Fig. 9.10 Distribution of tender points in the same patients as in Figure 9.9 3 months after surgery *(unpublished data, with permission of Da Campo)*. Dots = lateral surface; circles = medial surface.

disturbing factors, it is highly advisable for auricular diagnosis to be accompanied by a thorough clinical examination covering dental occlusion, foot contact with the ground, ocular convergence, etc. An interdisciplinary approach to these kinds of disorders, in collaboration with the specialists in these areas, is therefore recommended.

Possible associations between a subject's dominant side and the asymmetrical distribution of auricular points

An uneven distribution of points in the absence of any other disorder such as musculoskeletal pain or postural disturbance is a puzzle that has intrigued me for many years. Only when I started to study the stress response on the ear did I become aware that the stress reaction itself, or stress-prone patients, could show an asymmetrical activation of areas as reported in Chapter 5. One question which remains open is understanding why, following a life event, biological mechanisms

and behavioral changes in humans should be accompanied by a prevalent sensitization of one ear. Basically, in the whole group of 506 patients, no significant difference was found between the right and left auricle as regards the total number of points with higher/greater tenderness or lower electrical resistance. But if we consider a single patient we may often observe an asymmetrical distribution of points which does not exactly match the patient's symptoms. Also, healthy or asymptomatic people may show an uneven location of points, which are not easily interpretable.

In all these cases the problem of cerebral asymmetry and the subject's dominant side has been frequently advanced by practitioners regularly applying ear acupuncture. The first were Nogier[5] and Bourdiol,[8] who introduced the concepts of 'dominant auricle' and 'auricular laterality'. They supposed that in right-handers the dominant ear (also called the 'active ear') was the right ear and that it had a more pronounced sympathetic activity. The left was therefore the non-dominant ear (also

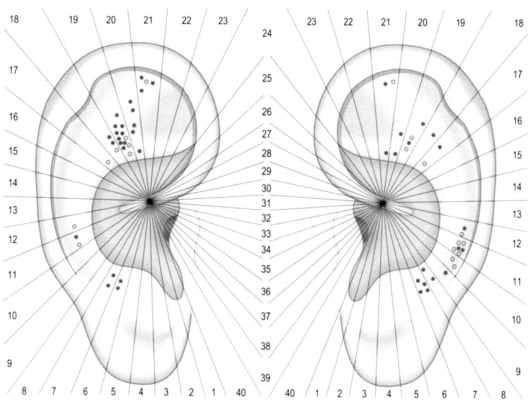

Fig. 9.11 Sensitization of the auricles in 25 patients with postural disturbances (without lower leg inequality) passing from the lying to the erect position. Dots = lateral surface; circles = medial surface.

called the 'passive ear'), which showed a prevalent parasympathetic activity. The reverse situation obviously held for left-handers. This dichotomous or split consideration of the brain in the 1960s probably derived from the limited knowledge of the cerebral functions existing at that time. The still popular simplification attributes to the left hemisphere, besides the function of speech, other functions such as the logical, sequential and analytical patterns of thought. The functions of the right hemisphere are supposed to be the simultaneous, holistic, intuitive and creative patterns of thought.

Nogier and Bourdiol proposed different methods such as auricular massage, magnetic and electrical stimulation with different polarities to correct laterality disturbances, as for example dyslexia, learning disabilities and attention deficit disorders. Nogier proposed the 'tragus master point' too, also called the 'master oscillation point', which he located on the tragus (see Fig. A1.17 on the right) where Bourdiol represented the corpus callosum (Fig. 9.12). It is not clear to what extent

the proposed treatments, supposed to regulate hemispheric integration, could correct these disturbances permanently, as the authors themselves declared. However, they recommended using dominance tests such as clapping hands, clasping hands, folding arms, eye gaze, etc. to identify subjects with mixed dominance who needed to be treated with particular care, as they might not respond at all to auricular treatment or have hypersensitive reactions to the prescribed medication.

The topic of cerebral asymmetries is of great interest and many scientific articles have been written on their association with dominance and human behavior. Since the majority of studies have been performed on neurological patients, one of the issues was to confirm and quantify the association between hand and language dominance in healthy people. Deppe, Knecht and colleagues tackled this issue and examined healthy volunteers with functional transcranial Doppler ultrasonography (fTCD).[9] They assessed the perfusion changes in the vascular territories of the language areas with fTCD

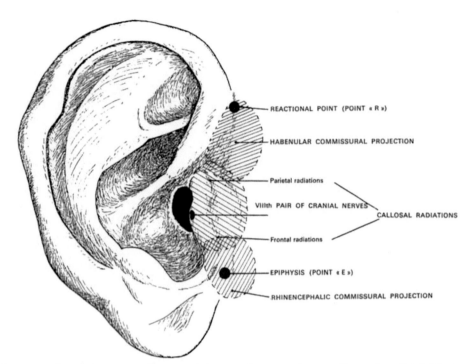

REACTIONAL POINT (POINT « R »)

HABENULAR COMMISSURAL PROJECTION

Parietal radiations

VIIIth PAIR OF CRANIAL NERVES

CALLOSAL RADIATIONS

Frontal radiations

EPIPHYSIS (POINT « E »)

RHINENCEPHALIC COMMISSURAL PROJECTION

Fig. 9.12   Representation of the corpus callosum and the commisura anterior according to Bourdiol *(with permission).*

during a word generation task. The distribution of hemispheric language dominance in 326 healthy volunteers varied significantly with the degree of handedness assessed by the Edinburgh Handedness Inventory (EHI), which ranges from −100 for strong left-handedness to +100 for strong right-handedness. The authors found that the more right-handed the subjects, the lower the relative incidence of right hemisphere language dominance. For example, in extreme right-handers its incidence was 4% compared to 27% in extreme left-handers.[10]

My experience regarding lateral preference and asymmetrical distribution of auricular points

When I discovered the importance of the auricular *Sanjiao* area as a major representation of a patient's reaction to life events,[11] I could not imagine that this experience would induce me to study the issue of dominance.

The reader will allow me to make a short digression on Oldfield's Edinburgh Handedness Inventory (EHI),[12] which is a 10-item questionnaire asking which hand one prefers for writing, drawing, throwing, using scissors, using a toothbrush,

using a knife (without fork), using a spoon, using a broom (upper hand), striking a match and opening a box (lid). Two supplementary items regard which foot one uses for kicking a ball and which eye one uses alone (for example looking at a spot through a hole or shooting a target with a rifle).

Applying Oldfield's inventory I found a significantly higher concentration of tender points on areas 5 and 6 of the left auricle in strong right-handers[13] (see Ch. 5). Since then I have considered the increased sensitization of the left auricle as a marker of stress response in a right-hander; the left auricle shows a higher number of points in left-handers also, but the ratio is significantly lower than in a right-hander.

The auricles therefore appear to show a linear relationship to handedness which is definitely not of binary right–left type but also includes ambidextrous subjects and those with mixed-handedness. As is well known, ambidextrous people perform certain types of tasks either with their right or left hand, while mixed-handed or cross-dominant people favor one hand for some tasks and the opposite for others. For example, a cross-dominant person might write with their left hand but throw a ball more skillfully with their right hand.

Table 9.8 Distribution (%) of preferences in 124 subjects applying Oldfield's Edinburgh Handedness Inventory

Dominance	Type	n	%
Handedness (10 items)	Strong right-handers	76	61.3%
	Mixed-handed	33	26.6%
	Ambidextrous	12	9.7%
	Strong left-handers	3	2.4%
Footedness (1 item)	Right-footedness	108	87.1%
	Left-footedness	11	8.9%
	Ambidextrous	5	4.0%
Eyedness (1 item)	Right-eyedness	84	67.8%
	Left-eyedness	36	29.0%
	Ambidextrous	4	3.2%

For this book I tried to make a further contribution to this issue by examining a group of 124 unselected subjects using PPT: the tender points on their right and left auricles were transcribed on the Sectogram. The assessment of lateral preferences was made independently by my assistant. The percentages shown in Table 9.8 show that there is a significantly lower percentage of left-handers compared to left-footers and left-eyed people; moreover there is a non-negligible rate of cross-dominant or mixed-handed people (26.6%). In connection to the first observation, my data are possibly consistent with those expressed in the literature regarding the more pronounced environmental influence for right-handedness as for right-footedness or eyedness.

As regards the second observation, my percentages are consistent with those found by Annett:[14] about 30% of the right-handed population preferentially carry out a variable number of tasks with the left hand.

The literature tells us that true ambidexterity is a rare condition; nevertheless Oldfield's questionnaire allows for the possibility of answering 'either right or left' if the task in question can be performed by either hand.

We carried out a linear regression analysis between the EHI scoring and the number of tender points respectively of the left and right auricle (Figs 9.13, 9.14). The significance tests of the regression coefficients are reported in Tables 9.9 and 9.10.

The regression lines show the possibility of an association between the side of preference for the hand and the opposite auricle. We are at a loss to understand the physiology of this association and whether it has to be considered a regular feature of all subjects or a sign of dysfunction manifesting itself in a particular subgroup of patients. In my opinion, however, all reported observations on auricular laterality are not only theoretical but allow the practitioner to have a holistic approach to the patient and to obtain better results in practice.

VARIATION IN THE DISTRIBUTION OF THE AURICULAR POINTS OVER TIME

The practitioner might be surprised at how often the distribution of auricular points changes over time. These variations may occur between one session and another as the result of the treatment itself, or may be the expression of a patient's spontaneous recovery. For example, Figure 9.15A shows the tender points detected at the first examination in 31 patients with sore throat,[15] when a culture was obtained by swabbing the pharynx and both tonsils or tonsillar fossae for identifying β-hemolytic streptococci. Symptoms such as temperature, oropharyngeal color, oropharyngeal enanthems, cervical adenopathy and cervical adenitis were scored using the tonsillopharyngitis score of Schachtel (TSS),[16] ranging from 0 to 10. As the culture plates were incubated and

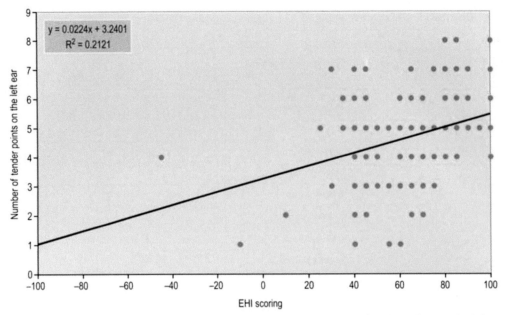

Fig. 9.13 Regression line in 124 subjects between the EHI scoring and the number of tender points on the left ear (−100 = strong left-handedness; +100 = strong right-handedness).

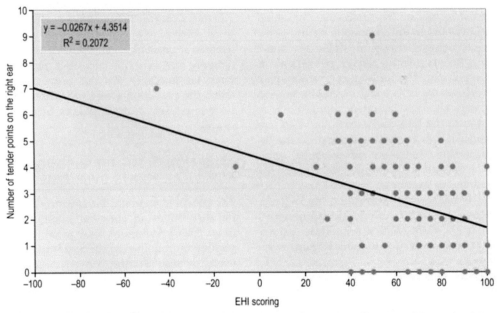

Fig. 9.14 Regression line in 124 subjects between the EHI scoring and the number of tender points on the right ear (−100 = strong left-handedness; +100 = strong right-handedness).

interpreted only within 18–24 hours, amoxicillin and clavulanic acid (675 + 325 mg twice a day) were administered to all patients from the first day for 6 days. One week later they were again scored with the TSS and their auricles re-tested

with PPT (Fig. 9.15B). The TTS score and the number of points dropped respectively by 65% and 70%, but no significant difference was found between 10 patients with a positive culture for group A β-hemolytic streptococci and the rest of

Table 9.9 Significance test of the regression coefficients related to Figure 9.13

	Coefficient	SE	t	P
Intercept.	4.35	0.33	13.20	<0.001
EHI scoring	−0.03	0.00	−5.65	<0.001

Table 9.10 Significance test of the regression coefficients related to Figure 9.14

	Coefficient	SE	t	P
Intercept.	3.24	0.27	11.9	<0.001
EHI scoring	0.02	0.00	5.73	<0.001

the group. The conclusion drawn in this article was that also the presumed viral infection in 21 patients with negative culture test could be responsible for the drop in auricular tender points following spontaneous recovery.[15]

However, the original aim of my study had been to solve the puzzle of the representation of the Chinese helix areas 1–4 (HX9 *lunyi*, HX10 *luner*, HX11 *lunsan*, HX12 *lunsi*), with their common indication for tonsillitis. I was rather surprised to find that pharyngotonsillitis activates not only the occiput area and the aligned trigeminal area but also the whole helix including sectors 19 and 20.

Questions on this subject remaining open are: should the helix actually be considered representative of tonsils, or should its great sensitization be regarded as the result of the activation of an important focal area such as the tonsillar fossa, as assumed by neural therapy. It may be surprising

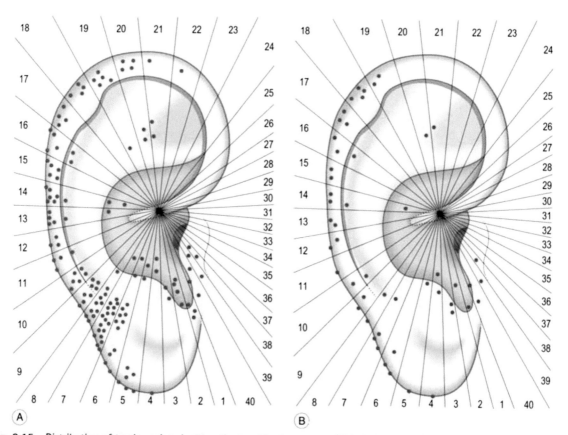

Fig. 9.15 Distribution of tender points in 31 patients with pharyngotonsillitis before antibiotic treatment (A); distribution of tender points in the same group 1 week later (B).

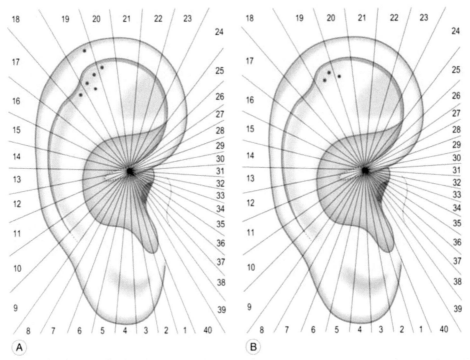

Fig. 9.16 Injury of the right hand with a fracture of the thumb in a worker aged 50; tender points on the ipsilateral auricle on the same day of the accident (A); distribution of tender points 20 days later (B).

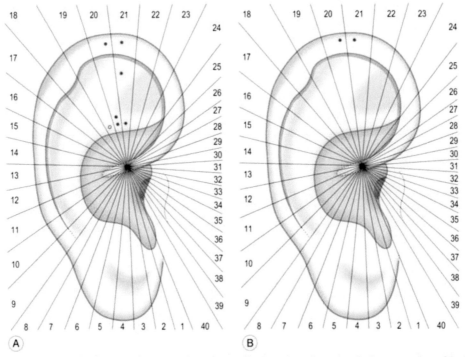

Fig. 9.17 Lumbar–sciatic pain in protrusion of L5–S1 disk: distribution of tender points before a session of body acupuncture (A); distribution of tender points after the session (B). Dots = lateral surface; circles = medial surface.

to notice that this area lies on the boundaries of different neural territories belonging to the fifth, seventh, ninth and tenth cranial nerves. This various and complex innervation in many ways recalls that of the auricular area and possibly explains why the tonsillar fossa and the retromolar area may reflect symptoms in distant parts of the body when they become 'fields of disturbance'.

Among the possible variations of distribution are surgery and traumatic injuries.

Figure 9.16 shows the case of a patient who crushed his right hand at work. He had a large wound on the back of his hand and a fracture of the last phalanx of the thumb. The day of the accident he had at least six tender points covering an area consistent with the representation of the hand and the wrist (Fig. 9.16A). After 20 days the number of points had dropped to three (Fig. 9.16B).

Further variations can be seen in patients after vertebral manipulation, injection in a joint or during a course of physiotherapy. A session of acupuncture on meridian points can also change the number and the location of auricular points. Figure 9.17 shows the case of a patient who was affected by lumbar–sciatic pain in protrusion of the L5–S1 disk; the search for tender points was made before a session of body acupuncture; a series of aligned points was found mainly on sectors 20 and 21 (Fig. 9.17A). Immediately after the session, the number of points dropped and only two tender points remained on the helix (Fig. 9.17B). This is in my opinion a procedure for indirectly controlling the effect of body acupuncture: good treatment should reduce the number of tender auricular points as much as possible. At the same time it is possible to increase the therapeutic response subsequently including the left points into treatment, as in the former case, inserting one or more semi-permanent needles.

References

[1] Oleson TD, Kroening RJ, Bresler DE. An experimental evaluation of auricular diagnosis: the somatotopic mapping of musculoskeletal pain at ear acupuncture points. Pain 1980;8:217–29.

[2] Andersson E, Persson AL, Carlsson CP. Are auricular maps reliable for chronic musculoskeletal pain disorders? A double-blind evaluation. Acupunct Med 2007;3:72–9.

[3] Bossy J. Bases neurobiologiques des réflexothérapies. 3rd ed. Paris: Masson; 1983.

[4] Bossy J. Actes VII journées d'Acupuncture, d'Auriculothérapie et de Médecine. Besançon: September; 1971.

[5] Nogier PFM. Traité d'auriculothérapie. Moulins-les-Metz: Maisonneuve; 1969.

[6] Ceccherelli F, Altafini L, Varotto E et al. The effect of benzodiazepines administration on auricular symptomatological evidence. Acupunct Electrother Res 1990;2:95–106.

[7] Romoli M, van der Windt D, Giovanzana P et al. International research project to devise a protocol to test the effectiveness of acupuncture on painful shoulder. J Altern Complement Med 2000;3:281–7.

[8] Bourdiol RJ. Elements of auriculotherapy. Moulins-les-Metz: Maisonneuve; 1982.

[9] Deppe M, Knecht S, Papke K et al. Assessment of hemispheric language lateralization: a comparison between fMRI and fTCD. J Cereb Blood Flow Metab 2000;20:263–8.

[10] Knecht S, Dräger B, Deppe M et al. Handedness and hemispheric language dominance in healthy humans. Brain 2000;12:2512–8.

[11] Romoli M, Giommi A. Ear acupuncture in psychosomatic medicine: the importance of the *sanjiao* (Triple Heater) area. Acupunct Electrother Res 1993; 3–4:185–94.

[12] Oldfield RC. The assessment and analysis of handedness: the Edinburgh Inventory. Neuropsychol 1971;9:97–113.

[13] Romoli M, Giommi A. Ear acupuncture and psychosomatic medicine: right–left asymmetry of acupoints and lateral preferences (Part II). Acupunct Electrother Res 1994;1:11–7.

[14] Annett M. Handedness and cerebral dominance: the right shift theory. Neuropsychiatry 1998;10:459–69.

[15] Romoli M, Giommi A. The puzzle of the Chinese map's auricular points 'tonsil' and 'helix'. Giorn Ital Riflessoter Agopunt 1997;1:3–9.

[16] Schachtel BP, Fillingim JM. Subjective and objective features of sore throat. Arch Intern Med 1984;144: 497–500.

Chapter 10

From diagnosis to therapy: how to select points for treatment

INTRODUCTION

Once auricular diagnosis has been completed in all its aspects, it is time to start to treat. The therapist will need to make a selection of points which will be more or less complicated, according to his objective and the specific health problems presented by each patient. For example, to treat knee pain he will need to select one or more points in the area in which the knee is represented, be it French or Chinese. If instead he has identified a larger number of points and the syndrome is more complex, he will need to select those which are more effective and at the same time most suitable for a specific patient. Whatever the procedure he decides to adopt, there is an unwritten golden rule which says one should obtain the best result with the lowest number of points. This rule derives from body acupuncture which holds that a higher number of points does not produce better results but rather increases the risk of 'hyperstimulation syndrome' as defined by Pontinen,[1] which can manifest by exacerbating pain in the 24–48 hours following an acupuncture session. This phenomenon is surely much less frequently observed in ear acupuncture which probably depends on the fact that ear stimulation is based on different reflexes than body acupuncture, or that auricular diagnosis correctly performed identifies the points which are strictly necessary to the patient. This selection therefore reduces the risk of stimulating a wrong or inappropriate auricular area.

Every physician will adopt his own strategy but in any case he will need to be fully acquainted with the patient's condition and should be prepared, especially if symptoms are still insufficiently clear, to seek professional advice from other colleagues.

Another important factor in planning treatment is the evaluation of the patient's compliance. Abbate[2] wrote on this subject:

to enhance compliance, inform your patients of the treatment plan and prognosis and provide them with written instructions of all directives. However, recognize that some variables are beyond our control as practitioners. The patient may not keep appointments or change certain lifestyle factors. Personal resources (i.e., money, transportation, social support for treatment) are oftentimes limited, as is the ability to follow self-treatment instructions.

THE COMBINATION OF DIAGNOSTIC METHODS FOR SELECTING POINTS TO TREAT: A REVIEW OF THE LITERATURE

It is possible to produce a detailed review of the long sequence of books published on ear acupuncture since the publication of Paul Nogier's historic treatise in French (1969) and in English (1972).[3] A probably incomplete list of texts in English, French, German, Italian and Chinese is reported in Table 10.1.[2-53] These different authors have detailed a variety of diagnostic methods, according to their skill, experience and will to describe a particular method. If we exclude the books featuring only one specific method we get an average of 2.2 methods per author. There are some major differences to note when comparing authors oriented more toward either the French or the Chinese schools of ear acupuncture. The former do not give primary importance to inspection and include the vascular autonomic signal (VAS) phenomenon among their diagnostic procedures. Physicians following the Chinese school, on the other hand, attribute major importance to inspection and do not follow any method related to the specific pulse diagnosis proposed by Nogier himself. However, all authors consider the contribution of the pressure pain test (PPT) and the electrical skin resistance test (ESRT) equally important in the detection and selection of auricular points to treat.

Some new methods possibly deserve attention, such as the 'very point' technique (VPT) proposed mainly by German authors, and the needle contact test (NCT) proposed by myself as a modification of Marcelli's 'active point test' (see Ch. 8).

The reader will allow me a short digression on VPT, a diagnostic–therapeutic procedure which has some similarities to NCT. The technique was first proposed by Gleditsch[54] for identifying body acupuncture points and other specific points such as those of mouth acupuncture. He used a short, fine injection needle for gently tapping out the skin area presumed to contain the acupuncture point to treat. The *verum punctum* or 'very point' corresponds to the center of the acupuncture point and when it is correctly identified it shows the following characteristics:

1. The patient indicates its particular tenderness through facial and verbal expression.
2. The needle penetrates the *verum punctum* more easily than its surroundings.
3. The superficial penetration quite regularly provokes a *de qi* effect not dissimilar to the same effect evoked by deep needling as commonly practiced in body acupuncture.

According to Gleditsch, VPT can safely be proposed to the beginner but is not intended to replace the classical methods of needle manipulation.

Angermaier[18] and Rubach[17] applied VPT to the auricle, tapping repeatedly or scraping the skin lightly with a very fine needle measuring 0.3 μm in diameter. This method does not traumatize the skin and any micro-bleeding of a point is part of the treatment itself and denotes local stagnation.

VPT should not be confused with Nogier's treatment of larger auricular areas by 'multiple puncture'. The discoverer of auriculotherapy employed this method empirically, according to the traditional rules for handling energy in acupuncture:

- gold needles to correct disorders resulting from insufficiency
- silver needles to correct disorders resulting from excess
- steel needles to obtain a balanced, moderating action.[3]

RESULTS OF A SURVEY CARRIED OUT ON 109 MEDICAL DOCTORS

A total of 136 colleagues, practicing members of the Federazione Italiana Società di Agopuntura (FISA), participated in a survey which I organized in 2002 for identifying the most important factors in the evaluation of adequate acupuncture treatment.[55]

Table 10.1   Review of the diagnostic methods proposed by 52 textbooks on ear acupuncture/auriculotherapy

Ear acupuncture textbook	Year of publication	Language	Number of diagnoses	Type of diagnosis
Nogier R[4]	2008	English	3	PPT, ESRT, VAS
Rouxeville Y, Meas Y, Bossy J[5]	2007	French	4	INSP, PPT, ESRT, VAS
Scoppa F[6]	2006	Italian	4	INSP, PPT, ESRT, VAS
Ouyang B, Gao J, Yang X[7]	2006	Chinese/French	1	INSP
Cheng J[8]	2005	Chinese	2	INSP, PPT
Frank BL, Soliman NE[9]	2005	English	4	INSP, PPT, ESRT, VAS
Strittmatter B[10]	2004	English	3	PPT, ESRT, VAS
Chen P[11]	2004	English	3	INSP, PPT, ESRT
Abbate S[2]	2004	English	1	INSP
Oleson T[12]	2003	English	4	INSP, PPT, ESRT, VAS
Romoli M[13]	2003	Italian	5	INSP, PPT, ESRT, VAS, NCT
Carmignola C, Speronello MR, Zampieri F[14]	2003	Italian	3	INSP, PPT, ESRT
Ogal HP, Kolster BC[15]	2003	German	4	INSP, PPT, ESRT, VPT
Sponzilli O[16]	2001	Italian	3	INSP, PPT, ESRT
Rubach A[17]	2001	German/English	5	INSP, PPT, ESRT, VAS, VPT
Angermaier M[18]	2000	German	4	PPT, ESRT, VAS, VPT
Nogier R[19]	2000	French	2	PPT, ESRT
Rouxeville Y[20]	2000	French	1	VAS
Noack M[21]	2000	German	3	INSP, PPT, ESRT
Linde N[22]	2000	German	4	INSP, PPT, ESRT, VAS
Huang L[23]	1999	English	1	INSP
Helling R, Feldmeier M[24]	1999	German	1	VAS
Nogier P[25]	1998	French/German/English	3	PPT, ESRT, VAS
Greenlee DL[26]	1997	English	3	INSP, PPT, ESRT
Chen K, Cui Y[27]	1997	English	3	INSP, PPT, ESRT
Huang L[28]	1996	English	3	INSP, PPT, ESRT
Hecker U[29]	1996	German	2	PPT, VAS
Liu S[30]	1996	English	1	INSP
Xiao Fei, Wei Lishuang[31]	1996	English	3	INSP, PPT, ESRT
Postneek F[32]	1995	German	2	ESRT, VAS

Continued

Table 10.1   Review of the diagnostic methods proposed by 52 textbooks on ear acupuncture/auriculotherapy—cont'd

Ear acupuncture textbook	Year of publication	Language	Number of diagnoses	Type of diagnosis
Xinghua B[33]	1994	English	3	INSP, PPT, ESRT
Bucek R[34]	1994	German	3	INSP, PPT, ESRT
Nogier R[35]	1993	French	1	VAS
Bahr FR[36]	1993	German	3	VAS, PPT, ESRT
Elias J[37]	1990	German	1	VAS
Kiener E, Roths A[38]	1989	French	3	PPT, ESRT, VAS
Lange G[39]	1987	German	4	INSP, PPT, ESRT, VAS
Rosenstiel-Heller P, Amar M[40]	1987	French	3	PPT, ESRT, VAS
Yu M[41]	1987	English	3	INSP, PPT, ESRT
Nogier PFM, Nogier R[42]	1987	French/English	4	INSP, PPT, ERT, VAS
Caspani F[43]	1985	Italian	3	INSP, PPT, ESRT
Kropej H[44]	1984	German/English	3	INSP, PPT, ESRT
Nogier PFM[45]	1983	French/English	3	PPT, ESRT, VAS
Mastalier O[46]	1983	German	2	ESRT, VAS
Bourdiol RJ[47]	1982	French/English	2	PPT, ESRT
Bourdiol RJ[48]	1981	French	1	VAS
Lu HC[49]	1975	English	3	INSP, PPT, ESRT
Grobglas A, Levy J[50]	1975	French	3	INSP, PPT, ESRT
Academy of TCM[51]	1975	English	3	INSP, PPT, ESRT
Ear Acupuncture Compiling Group of Nanjing Military Headquarters[52]	1973	Chinese/English/Italian	3	INSP, PPT, ESRT
König G, Wancura I[53]	1973	German	3	INSP, PPT, ESRT
Nogier PFM[3]	1972	French/English/German	3	PPT, ESRT, VAS

INSP = inspection; PPT = pain pressure test; ESRT = electrical skin resistance test; VAS = vascular autonomic signal; VPT = very point technique; NCT = needle contact test

The aim was to develop a possible scale to be used for systematic reviews on acupuncture.

A second questionnaire regarded the modalities of auricular diagnosis and therapy. A total of 109 medical practitioners answered the following questions:

1. Do you use auricular diagnosis before inserting needles?
2. Which methods do you use for diagnosis and selection of points?
3. Which combination of diagnostic methods do you consider best for the selection of points?
4. Do you apply the principles of traditional Chinese medicine (TCM) when selecting points for therapy?
5. Do you apply the principle of Nogier's phases when selecting points/areas for therapy?
6. Do you apply formula acupuncture recommended by the textbooks for treating specific disorders?

Table 10.2 Diagnostic methods and selection of auricular points according to 109 physicians practicing ear acupuncture

Auricular diagnosis	Yes	67.0%
	No	17.4%
	Sometimes	15.6%
	Total	100%
Diagnostic methods used (%)	Pain pressure test (PPT)	35.3%
	Inspection	33.6%
	Needle contact test (NCT)	16.4%
	Electrical skin resistance test (ESRT)	11.8%
	Vascular autonomic signal (VAS)	2.9%
	Total	100%
Combination of diagnostic methods (%) (in 81 physicians; 74.3% of the total)	Inspection + PPT	30.9%
	Inspection + PPT + NCT	25.9%
	Inspection + PPT + ESRT	9.9%
	Inspection + PPT + ESRT + NCT	8.6%
	Inspection + ESRT	3.7%
	PPT + NCT	3.7%
	Other combinations	17.3%
	Total	100%
Points selection according to TCM	Yes	36.7%
	No	37.6%
	Sometimes	25.7%
	Total	100%
Phases of Nogier	Yes	8.2%
	No	78.0%
	Sometimes	13.8%
	Total	100%
Formula acupuncture	Yes	14.7%
	No	52.3%
	Sometimes	33.0%
	Total	100%

The answers to the questionnaire are reported in Table 10.2.

It is evident that the majority of doctors (67%) questioned prefer to make an auricular diagnosis before starting treatment. The most popular diagnosis is PPT (35.3%) followed by inspection (33.6%), NCT and ESRT; VAS has a very low rate of application and only 2.9% of the doctors questioned seem to make use of it regularly.

A total of 28 practitioners use only one method; the other 81 (74.3% of the total) combine different methods to obtain the best information on a patient's condition. Inspection and PPT together are most popular with 30.9%, whereas inspection + ESRT totals only 3.7%. The combination of inspection + PPT + NCT is second most popular (25.9%).

It is interesting to note that more than 50% of the practitioners participating in the survey more or less regularly select points according to the principles of TCM. This may indicate that this group has been trained in recognizing symptoms and syndromes according to Chinese medicine.

Nogier's phases which are fundamental in auriculomedicine are recognized and used regularly in practice by only a minority of doctors (8.2%).

Finally, the majority of the practitioners (52.3%) do not like formula acupuncture, but at least one-third sometimes choose the set of points recommended in the various textbooks for treating specific disorders.

WHICH STRATEGY SHOULD BE USED IN SELECTING POINTS?

In time every therapist will develop his own style of treatment and may follow the steps proposed here more or less systematically.

1. Select first the areas which have been identified by more than one procedure

As reported in Chapter 9 ('The topography of the identified auricular point/area'), the auricular somatotopic arrangement is essential for formulating a diagnostic hypothesis.

The practitioner who combines different methods may adopt his personal strategy in selecting the points to treat. For example, in the patient shown in Figure 10.1, who was affected by recurrent panic attacks, two areas were taken into consideration for treatment. The first, below the root of the helix, corresponding consistently to the Chinese esophagus area (CO2 *shidao*), was identified by inspection, PPT and ESRT. The second area, corresponding to Nogier's fear area and the Chinese anterior ear lobe (LO4 *chuiqian*), was identified with PPT and ESRT. In this session the points detected on the antitragus with ESRT (possibly

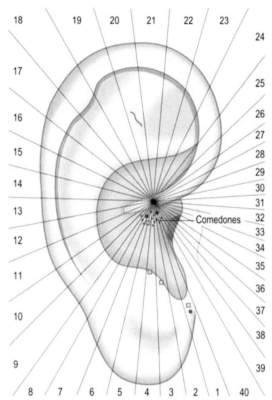

Fig. 10.1 Selection of points in a female patient aged 45 years suffering with panic disorder. Dots = points detected with PPT; squares = points detected with ESRT.

related to a past migraine) were not selected for treatment; neither was the Shen men area detected only by inspection (telangiectasia).

2. In the identified areas select the most important points in order of importance

This procedure is particularly evident if we are going to examine the patient's auricle with PPT. The principle of 'relativity of tenderness', described in Chapter 5, is based on the progressively upward shift of the pain threshold of the points, after repeated examinations.

It is therefore possible to reduce the number of points to treat by minimizing the discomfort of therapy to the patient and preventing any side-effects due to inappropriate stimulation. The patient in Figure 10.2 asked for help because he was suffering with chronic back and neck pain; further symptoms were depressive mood, fatigue, bruxism and constipation. PPT identified 15

tender points spread over the whole ear (Fig. 10.2A). Detection was repeated immediately with the purpose of shifting the pain threshold to a higher level. The number of tender points actually dropped to six; three of them on the back were mainly related to pain and stiffness along the lumbar and cervical spine. The point on the posterior part of the antitragus was related to bruxism and malocclusion; the point on the middle part of the antitragus to depression; and finally the point on the tragus was related to fatigue and chronic stress (Fig. 10.2B). All points were included in treatment; the patient was also advised to attend back care classes and to check his jaw occlusion with a dentist in order to correct any possible negative effects on his cervical and lumbar muscles.

A hierarchical order can be established also with ESRT, when too many points have been detected, shifting the sensitivity knob from lower to higher values of electrical resistance discontinuity. In Figure 10.3 ESRT was applied to a patient affected by fibromyalgia and insomnia. Eight points were identified with the knob on level 4 (corresponding to a discontinuity of ~1 MΩ – see Fig. A2.3) (Fig. 10.3A). Shifting the knob from level 4 to 2, three points were still identifiable: two on the scapha corresponding to the representation of the intermediolateral nuclei of the lateral horn according to Nogier (see Fig. A1.3), the third on the antitragus associated with the patient's sleep disorders. All these points were selected for treatment (Fig. 10.3B).

3. Select the most effective points in case of pain and limited range of motion

When the area which is more or less topographically related to the pain syndrome has been identified with auricular diagnosis, use the NCT. The patient in Figure 10.4 suffered with a painful shoulder and reduced range of motion during flexion and elevation. Using PPT I identified nine tender points covering at least the Chinese areas of representation of the shoulder (SF5 *jian*), neck (AH12 *jing*) and cervical vertebrae (AH13 *jingzhui*) (Fig. 10.4A). When PPT was repeated, the number of tender points had dropped to four, but the shoulder was still painful during flexion and elevation. NCT was performed on point 1 without results; only the contact on point 2 improved the range of motion (Fig. 10.4B).

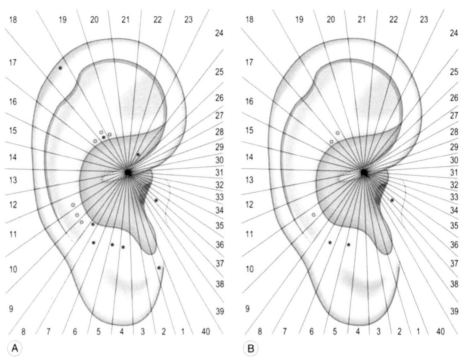

Fig. 10.2 Selection of the most tender points in hierarchical order after two consecutive detections (A and B) in a 36-year-old male patient suffering with recurrent back and neck pain. Dots = lateral surface; closed circles = medial surface.

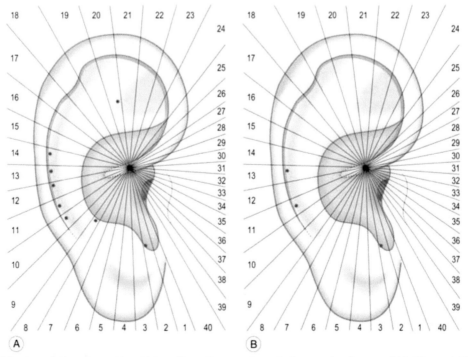

Fig. 10.3 Selection of the points with a higher skin resistance discontinuity, passing from ∼1 MΩ (A) to ∼5 MΩ (B) in a 48-year-old female patient suffering with fibromyalgia and sleep disorders.

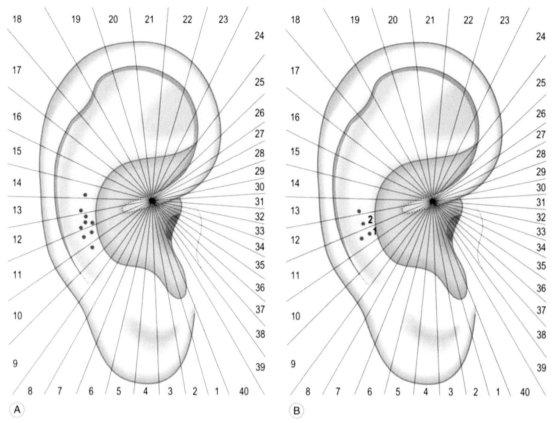

Fig. 10.4   Tender points in a 57-year-old male patient suffering with painful shoulder with a limited range of motion in flexion and elevation of the shoulder (A); selection of points combining PPT and NCT (points 1 and 2) (B).

4. Select the points according to a given medical diagnosis and consider them as having a pseudo-pharmacological activity

In the patient in Figure 10.5 the main symptom prompting consultation with the acupuncturist was tiresome hot flushes in menopause. Secondary symptoms were neck stiffness, constipation and hemorrhoids. Seven tender points were identified with PPT (Fig. 10.5A). The selection of points in the first session was directed particularly on the areas commonly related to a climacteric syndrome: the antitragus and the fossa ovalis. Two points were selected on the antitragus: one within the genital or gonadotropinic area of Nogier, corresponding to the Chinese forehead area (AT1 *e*), the second on the lower part of the antitragus within the area of dysthymia and depression, corresponding to the French hypothalamus and Chinese temple (AT2 *nie*). One tender point was selected on the fossa triangularis, within the area

which was recently considered to be related to the ovary (see Fig. 5.48). The rationale for treating hot flushes with these three points (Fig. 10.5B) was to try, from a pseudo-pharmacological point of view, respectively to reset the endocrine activity of the gonadotropinic system, to obtain an antidepressant effect and to enhance the residual production of estrogen by the ovary.

In the patient in Figure 10.6 the main symptom to treat was a relapse of chronic backache. The patient had no irradiating pain to the legs but showed a marked stiffness of the spine on flexion. The majority of points was concentrated on the right ear, even if the patient did not show a clear prevalence of pain on this side (Fig. 10.6A). Most of the points were located in correspondence with the dorsolumbar tract; secondary points were also found on the back of the ear, corresponding to the representation of the neck muscles. Two further points were found on the representation of the right Chinese knee (AH4 *xi*) and toe (AH2 *zhi*)

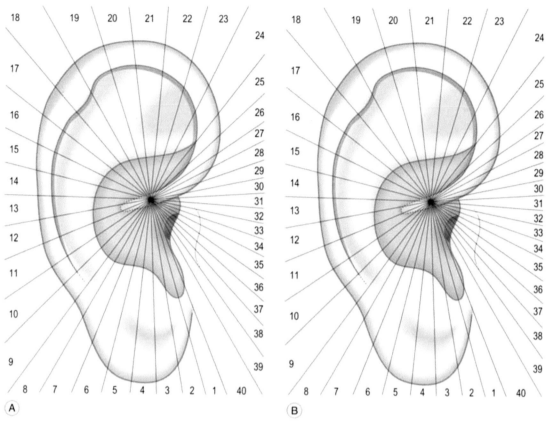

Fig. 10.5 Tender points in a 52-year-old female patient with hot flushes and depression (A); selection of points with a possible pseudo-pharmacological effect on these symptoms (B). Dots = lateral surface; circles = medial surface.

as the possible expression of a postural disorder connected with foot asymmetry. The point located on the root of the helix, on the left auricle, was instead considered to belong to the stomach, as an expression of possible gastritis due to the recurrent intake of NSAIDs. In the first session, however, only the two points of the lower root of the anthelix were selected with the aim of obtaining an analgesic (diclofenac-like) effect, and the three points of the medial surface to get a reasonable muscle-relaxing (baclofen-like) effect (Fig. 10.6B).

5. Select the points corresponding to one or more syndromes described by TCM

This selection may be of particular interest to therapists who treat mental disorders and visceral dysfunctions according to TCM. As ESRT seems to have a higher rate than PPT in identifying this kind of problem, the practitioner may rely more often on this diagnosis in combination with auricular inspection.

The patient in Figure 10.7A, for example, suffered from chronic migraine; the secondary symptoms were eczema, which worsened especially in spring and autumn, blepharitis and constipation. From the point of view of TCM, migraine was defined as the expression of excessive *yang* and heat in the Liver. Among the points identified with ESRT, four points were selected: first were the temple area (former location of *taiyang* EX2 point) and the liver point. It is noteworthy that the antitragus presented a tiny dyschromia very close to the identified point. The other two points were selected for their internal–external relation with each other (Lung–Large Intestine). In particular, constipation was considered as 'heat in the large intestine' and eczema was considered as heat in the blood. Lung is well known to relate with the external surface of the body and allergy.

The patient in Figure 10.7B suffered from anxiety and sleep disorders; secondary symptoms were neck stiffness and dyspepsia. Among the points

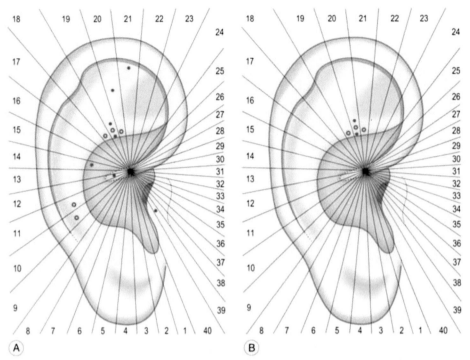

Fig. 10.6 Tender points in a 60-year-old male patient with back pain associated with foot asymmetry (A); selection of points, on the medial surface, with a possible pseudo-pharmacological effect on back pain and stiffness (B). Dots = lateral surface; circles = medial surface.

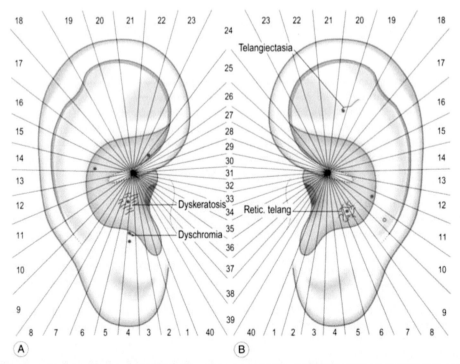

Fig. 10.7 Selection of points of reduced electrical skin resistance, according to TCM, in a 35-year-old female patient suffering with migraine and eczema (A); selection of points of reduced electrical resistance, according to TCM, in a 25-year-old female patient suffering with anxiety, insomnia and dyspepsia (B). Dots = lateral surface; circles = medial surface.

identified with ESRT, four points were selected: the Shen men point and heart area to calm the spirit and to 'regulate the deficit of *qi* and blood of the Heart'. The spleen point and the neck muscles point of the medial surface were selected to 'strengthen the spleen and the stomach' for dyspepsia and to reduce muscular tension. It is noteworthy that the heart area was identifiable at inspection and was covered by a reticular telangiectasia; the Shen men area moreover was identifiable by a telangiectasia nearby the point identified with ESRT.

6. Select the 'reference points' for each disease

This is an interesting strategy in selecting points for treatment, even if it requires long and systematic work collecting cases with the same symptoms. Despite the great variability of response in different human beings to the same etiological factor, there are nevertheless some common recurrent symptoms which characterize a given disease. The same phenomenon occurs on the auricles with regard to the prevalent sensitization of particular areas. The term 'reference points' was introduced by the doctors of the Nanjing garrison and applied to 52 patients with 'accurately diagnosed' glomerulonephritis. The text does not specify whether the diagnosis referred to acute, subacute or chronic forms and whether nephritis was perhaps secondary to hemolytic streptococcal infection. What is interesting, however, in the list of 21 different tender points identified in the above-mentioned patients, is the variable rate of sensitization. The identified points were converted to areas according to the standardized Chinese map (Fig. 10.8) and the sensitization rates are reported in Table 10.3. As we can see, a 100% sensitization was found for only three points/areas (nephritis, kidney, endocrine), whereas a decreasing per cent was found for other areas such as Shen men, bladder, esophagus, lumbosacral vertebrae, etc. Nephritis point, represented on helix area HX12, is of course the most puzzling point since there are no indications of kidney-related symptoms, but rather indications such as tonsillitis, upper respiratory tract infections and fever which could be associated to the possible streptococcal infection in these patients. Another puzzling area, with a high sensitization rate (90.4%), is the representation of the esophagus. All other areas can be interpreted in decreasing

order, as preferred, either with medical or with TCM diagnosis (Fig. 10.8).

7. Select personal points as soon as possible

The more each practitioner examines the auricles of his patients systematically, the more he will find new points and combinations of areas not yet described by the leading schools. He will develop specific experience in using these new points and will be able to foresee and measure their therapeutic effect, especially in the case of unique symptoms. He needs, however, to report both the points identified by auricular diagnosis and those selected for treatment systematically on the Sectogram. Examining the patient from one session to the next in this way, the therapist will be able to understand which points are more effective and in which combination they may be treated to obtain the best results. In my opinion this approach should be open-minded and not limited by the existing ear maps.

One less recognized effect in Western countries is, for example, the antihistaminic effect of some points. There is a point on the tip of the auricle used by Nogier to counteract allergy (Fig. A1.17); the point has been reported as the ear apex point *erjian* and is indicated for conjunctivitis, hypertension and insomnia (Fig. A1.16). My impression, after several observations of patients with urticaria, was that this point was not isolated; indeed I discovered that the whole upper and posterior part of the helix, HX7 and HX8 for the Chinese, was often sensitized by an allergic reaction. I was rather surprised furthermore to note how this area was effective in reducing the itching of some allergic conditions such as urticaria. Why the helix points of an area belonging to the lower thoracic segments should show antihistaminic properties is hard to say. It has to be remembered that in the same area there are other points and areas which the Chinese associate with an allergic reaction, as for example Wind stream *fengxi* (see Table 4.12).

In the case shown in Figure 10.9A, the 30-year-old female patient came to my practice with an urticaria spreading over the thighs and abdomen, which was presumed to be caused by her intake of amoxicillin. The rash had been present for a few hours and itching was scored verbally by the patient as between 7 and 8 on a scale of 10. With PPT I identified seven tender points, two on the scapha and five scattered on the helix of sectors 17–21. Acupuncture

Fig. 10.8 The standardized Chinese areas corresponding to the 'reference points' for nephritis in 52 patients (see Table 10.3 for key).

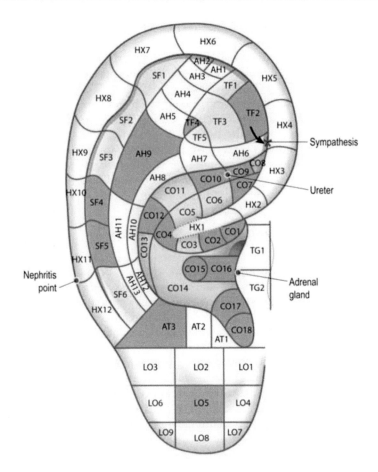

Table 10.3 Percentage of tender 'reference points' in 52 patients with nephritis according to the Ear Acupuncture compiling group of Nanjing Military Headquarters[52] (see Fig. 10.8).

100%	Kidney (CO10), nephritis point, endocrine (CO18)
98.1%	Bladder (CO9), Shen men (TF4)
90.4%	Esophagus (CO2)
82.7%	Lumbosacral vertebrae (AH9)
59.6%	Shoulder joint (SF4,5), stomach (CO4)
51.9%	Triple energy (CO17)
48.8%	Ureter
46.1%	Occiput (AT3)
40.4%	Large intestine (CO7), heart (CO15), mouth (CO1)
36.5%	Trachea (CO16), internal genitals (TF2), adrenal gland
32.7%	Sympathesis
21.1%	Liver (CO12), eye (LO5)

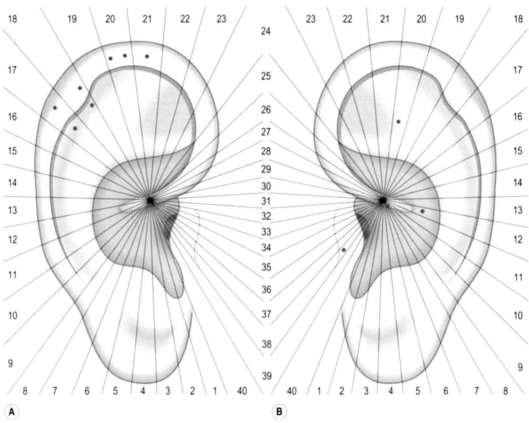

Fig. 10.9 Tender points in acute urticaria in a 30-year-old female patient (A); tender points tested with NCT for relieving pregnancy-related nausea in a 33-year-old female patient (B).

stimulation on these points reduced itching to 50% in the following 10 minutes.

Another example of a personal point is that for treating nausea during pregnancy. For this symptom Chinese acupuncturists use mainly the cardias area (CO3 *benmen*). German physicians instead use a so-called nausea point on the posterior auricular incisure.

My goal was to find out an auricular point with the same efficacy as PC6 (*neiguan*). As reported by a recent systematic review,[56] PC6 stimulation may be beneficial for various conditions involving nausea and vomiting, even if the added value to modern antiemetics remains unclear. However, few acupuncturists expressed their opinion on the fact that the application of only one needle (two, considering the symmetrical stimulation on both sides) is really unusual in acupuncture. Experts in TCM and practitioners of westernized acupuncture both know that the same acupuncture point often treats different symptoms, or a combination of different

points may treat the same syndrome. Nevertheless, starting from this evidence I tried to identify a specific point which alone could modify the intensity of nausea. I tested several areas without great results. When pregnant women ask to be treated they have often been suffering for several days or weeks and expect a full and rapid effect from treatment. Unfortunately, despite their expectations and frequent anxiety, it can take time for the patients to feel relief from nausea. Given the difficulty in modifying intense nausea after 10 seconds of needle contact, I adopted the following personal solution: having noted previously that PC6 is sensitive to pressure during nausea, on one or both sides, I tried to modify its tenderness with NCT on selected auricular points. When the most effective point in reducing the tenderness of PC6 had been identified, I inserted a needle for at least 30 minutes and measured the effect on nausea. Subsequently I took out the needle and replaced it with a semi-permanent one for the following days, inviting the patient to press the needle as many times as necessary to keep the nausea under control.

In the 33-year-old pregnant lady in Figure 10.9B I adopted this procedure and after some attempts I found a point on the root of the helix immediately below point zero which reduced her nausea after 30 minutes by 30–50%.

I am sure the effectiveness of the treatment could be increased by adding further points or personalizing the treatment on the patient. It would also be worthwhile, in a larger group, to identify predictors of response so that pregnant women could optimize ear acupuncture therapy.

References

[1] Pontinen PJ. Hyperstimulation syndrome. Am J Acup 1979;7:161–5.

[2] Abbate S. Chinese auricular acupuncture. Boca Raton: CRC Press; 2004.

[3] Nogier PFM. Treatise of auriculotherapy. Moulins-les-Metz: Maisonneuve; 1972.

[4] Nogier R. Auriculotherapy. Stuttgart: Thieme; 2008.

[5] Rouxeville Y, Meas Y, Bossy J. Auriculothérapie – Acupuncture auriculaire. Paris: Springer; 2007.

[6] Scoppa F. Lineamenti di auricoloterapia. Bologna: Martina; 2006.

[7] Ouyang B, Gao J, Yang X. The ear reflexology zone massage. Jiangsu Science and Technology Press; 2006.

[8] Cheng J. Ear acupuncture therapy for many diseases. Beijing: People's Military Medical Press; 2005.

[9] Frank BL, Soliman NE. Auricular therapy. Bloomington: AuthorHouse; 2005.

[10] Strittmatter B. Identifying and treating blockages to healing. Stuttgart: Thieme; 2004.

[11] Chen P. Modern Chinese ear acupuncture. Brookline: Paradigm; 2004.

[12] Oleson T. Auriculotherapy manual. 3rd ed. Edinburgh: Churchill Livingstone; 2003.

[13] Romoli M. Agopuntura auricolare. Turin: UTET; 2003.

[14] Carmignola C, Speronello MR, Zampieri F. Auricoloterapia cinese. Spinea: Prosa Edizioni; 2003.

[15] Ogal HP, Kolster BC. Ohrakupunktur für Praktiker. Stuttgart: Hippokrates; 2003.

[16] Sponzilli O. Reflessologia auricolare e cranica. 2nd ed. Rome: Marrapese; 2001.

[17] Rubach A. Principles of ear acupuncture. Stuttgart: Thieme; 2001.

[18] Angermaier M. Leitfaden der Ohrakupunktur. Munich: Urban and Fischer; 2000.

[19] Nogier R. Auriculothérapie personnalisée–1er degré. Montpellier: Sauramps; 2000.

[20] Rouxeville Y. Acupuncture auriculaire personnalisée. Montpellier: Sauramps; 2000.

[21] Noack M. Arbeitsbuch Ohrakupunktur. Berlin: Akapit; 2000.

[22] Linde N. Ohrakupunktur: ein Leitfaden für Theorie und Praxis. 3rd ed. Stuttgart: Sonntag; 2000.

[23] Huang L. Auricular diagnosis. Bellaire: Longevity Press; 1999.

[24] Helling R, Feldmeier M. Aurikulomedizin nach Nogier. Stuttgart: Hippokrates; 1999.

[25] Nogier P. Introduction pratique à l'auriculothérapie. 2nd ed. Brussels: SATAS; 1998.

[26] Greenlee DL. The healing ear. Kelseyville: Earthen Vessel; 1997.

[27] Chen K, Cui Y. Handbook to Chinese auricular therapy. Beijing: Foreign Languages Press; 1997.

[28] Huang L. Auriculotherapy diagnosis and treatment. Bellaire: Longevity Press; 1996.

[29] Hecker U. Ohr-Schädel-Mund-Handakupunktur. Stuttgart: Hippokrates; 1996.

[30] Liu S. Auricular diagnosis, treatment, health preservation. Beijing: Science Press; 1996.

[31] Xiao Fei, Wei Lishuang. Auricular acupuncture therapy. Jinan: Shandong Science and Technology Press; 1996.

[32] Postneek F. Ohrakupunktur bei weiblichen Fertilitätsstörungen. Stuttgart: Hippokrates; 1995.

[33] Xinghua B. Chinese auricular therapy. Beijing: Scientific Technical Documents Publishing House; 1994.

[34] Bucek R. Lehrbuch der Ohrakupunktur. Heidelberg: Haug; 1994.

[35] Nogier R. Introduction pratique à l'Auriculomédecine–la photoperception cutanée. Brussels: Haug International; 1993.

[36] Bahr FR. Systematik und Praktikum der wissenschaftlichen Ohrakupunktur für Fortgeschrittene. Braunschweig: Skriptum; 1993.

[37] Elias J. Lehr- und Praxisbuch der Ohrakupunktur. Teningen: Sommer-Verlag; 1990.

[38] Kiener E, Roths A. Acupuncture dentaire, auriculothérapie, réflexothérapie facio-buccale. Paris: Guy Trédaniel; 1989.

[39] Lange G. Akupunktur der Ohrmuschel. Schorndorf: WBV; 1987.

[40] Rosenstiel-Heller P, Amar M. L'auriculothérapie sans aiguille. Paris: Robert Laffont; 1987.

[41] Yu M. Auricular acupuncture. Academy of Chinese Acupuncture, 1987.

[42] Nogier PFM, Nogier R. The man in the ear. Saint-Ruffine: Maisoneuve; 1987.

[43] Caspani F. Auricoloterapia. Como: Edizioni red; 1985.

[44] Kropej H. The fundamentals of ear acupuncture. 2nd ed. Heidelberg: Haug; 1984.

[45] Nogier PFM. From auriculotherapy to auriculomedecine. Moulins-les-Metz: Maisonneuve; 1983.

[46] Mastalier O. Herd- und Störfeldtestmethoden der Ohrakupunktur fur Zahnärzte und Ärzte. Braunschweig: Friedrich Vieweg; 1983.

[47] Bourdiol RJ. Elements of auriculotherapy. Moulins-les-Metz: Maisonneuve; 1982.

[48] Bourdiol RJ. L'auriculo-somatologie. Moulins-les-Metz: Maisonneuve; 1981.

[49] Lu HC. A complete textbook of auricular acupuncture. 2nd ed. Vancouver: Academy of Oriental Heritage; 1975.

[50] Grobglas A, Levy J. Traité d'acupuncture auriculaire. Paris: Publi Réal; 1975.

[51] Academy of TCM. Beijing: Foreign Language Press; 1975.

[52] Ear Acupuncture Compiling Group of Nanjing Military Headquarters. Shanghai: People's Publishing House; 1973.

[53] König G, Wancura I. Einführung in die chinesische Ohrakupunktur. 2nd ed. Heidelberg: Karl Haug; 1973.

[54] Gleditsch JM. Mundakupunktur. Schorndorf: WBV; 1979.

[55] Romoli M, Allais G, Giovanardi CM et al. What are the most important factors in the evaluation of adequate acupuncture treatment: developing a possible scale to be used for systematic reviews on acupuncture. Clin Acup Orient Med 2004;4:109–13.

[56] Ezzo J, Streitberger K, Schneider A. Cochrane systematic reviews examine P6 acupuncture-point stimulation for nausea and vomiting. J Altern Complement Med 2006;5:489–95.

Conclusions

Paul Nogier (1908–1996) would today be very proud to see how many 'adoptive children' he has around the world. In my opinion, ear acupuncture is one of the most intriguing discoveries of the last 50 years.

Two lessons have ensued from Nogier's experience: the first is that even a single physician, without expensive and sophisticated instruments, can perform good research, following his clinical instinct and rigorously analyzing his observations. The second is that every revolutionary approach in the field of medicine has to struggle before being accepted by the scientific community. Over the last 20 years the great increase in complementary/alternative methods has brought an equally increasing request among therapists and patients for evidence-based information on their efficacy. Ear acupuncture is no exception, and a full knowledge of the range of its possibilities needs to be brought to light.

It can be freely stated that there is still much work to do with both auricular diagnosis and auricular therapy. As regards diagnosis there are still portions of the auricle which have to be thoroughly explored, for example the ear lobe, the helix and the medial surface of the auricle. To imagine that the central nervous system is represented on the ear lobe does not mean that we have the key consistently to identify the areas corresponding to specific parts of the brain. The simplification expressed commonly by Western researchers that one auricular zone is the representation of one anatomical structure is probably wrong, and we should convince ourselves that the same organ can have multiple representations

on the ear as has been expressed by both Chinese practitioners and Western physicians practicing auriculomedicine.

Therefore we need specific methodology to discover these associations with direct and indirect methods. The direct methods, through modern imaging techniques such as fMRI, PET, etc., could evaluate which structures of the brain are activated by auricular stimulation, either in healthy subjects or in patients with pain or other neurological disorders.

The indirect methods, however, using the diagnostic procedures proposed in this book, may help the clinician to identify recurrent auricular areas associated with different symptoms or syndromes. This is furthermore necessary because there is often no complete consensus between the different schools concerning the somatotopic representations of the body.

The interpretation of these multiple clusters of points brings to mind someone doing a jigsaw puzzle with no knowledge of the final picture.

One of the aims of this patient and perhaps endless work is to attribute finally much more importance to the autonomic nervous system which thus far seems so insufficiently investigated. Contemporary anatomists do not study the morphology of this system and it is unlikely that they are given adequate grants or funding for such research. Consequently medical students still receive the same information on a few pages of their anatomy books as they did 20–30 years ago. The autonomic nervous system, however, is essential for all functions of our body and auricular diagnosis gives us the opportunity to examine the concha which it should be remembered is the only zone of the body where the tenth cranial nerve comes to the surface.

As regards auricular therapy, there is a lot of work to do on the following aspects:

First, despite great interest in ear acupuncture throughout the world, there is still a lack of evidence-based information about the fields in which auricular treatment could be applied more advantageously. Some evidence has been found for the treatment of pain disorders such as lumbago, cervical pain and migraine. Further evidence has been found for the treatment of drug addiction and obesity as well as for anxiety and insomnia. Auricular therapy for the treatment of psychosomatic disorders seems to be promising and should in my opinion be proposed as a complementary therapy in association with psychoactive drugs.

Another interesting therapeutic combination could be the inclusion of ear acupuncture in rehabilitation programs, to reduce the number of sessions and the total cost of rehabilitation.

The second important aspect of auricular therapy, which has not yet been taken into consideration adequately, is the measurement of the therapeutic effect of non-invasive stimulation of the auricle such as massage, magnetic pearls, *Vaccaria* seeds, electrical and laser stimulation, etc. This is an important issue because many therapists are not medical doctors and in several countries are not allowed to insert needles. The peculiarity of the auricle from the neurophysiological point of view seems to support the hypothesis that light, non-invasive stimulation may have a significant therapeutic effect. There is an urgent need to face these issues in order to place ear acupuncture definitively among the evidenced-based complementary therapeutic methods.

Appendix 1

The auricular charts

The auricular charts in this appendix should be consulted *cum grano salis* (literally with a grain of salt; i.e. with discernment). They should not be considered as having absolute value but rather be interpreted freely, adapted and updated with regard to location, dimension and the intrinsic clinical value of each somatotopic area. This will depend on the personal experience of each practitioner and the diagnostic method adopted. To offer readers an easy and advantageous comparison of the auricular representation of the body according to different medical traditions and schools of thought, the maps have been arranged in pairs, allowing face to face consultation of the French map on the left page with the corresponding Chinese map on the right-hand page.

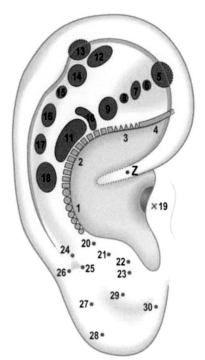

No.	Representation	No.	Representation
1	Cervical spine C1-C7	16	Elbow
2	Thoracic spine Th1-Th12	17	Arm
3	Lumbar spine L1-L5	18	Shoulder
4	Sacrum-coccyx	19	Internal ear (internal surface)
5	Foot	20	Occipital bone
6	Tibia-fibula	21	Parietal bone
7	Knee	22	Frontal bone
8	Thigh	23	Frontal sinus
9	Hip	24	TMJ
10	Diaphragm	25	Upper jaw
11	Chest	26	Lower jaw
12	Thumb	27	Tongue
13	Fingers	28	Lips
14	Wrist	29	Eye
15	Forearm	30	External nose

Fig. A1.1 The somatotopic representations of the body and of the cephalic extremity according to Nogier[1,2,3,4] (z = point zero).

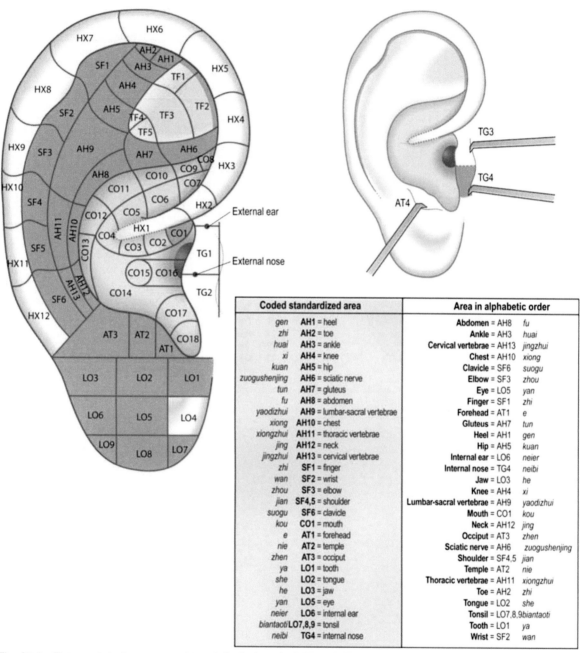

External ear

External nose

Coded standardized area		Area in alphabetic order	
gen	**AH1** = heel	**Abdomen** = AH8	fu
zhi	**AH2** = toe	**Ankle** = AH3	huai
huai	**AH3** = ankle	**Cervical vertebrae** = AH13	jingzhui
xi	**AH4** = knee	**Chest** = AH10	xiong
kuan	**AH5** = hip	**Clavicle** = SF6	suogu
zuogushenjing	**AH6** = sciatic nerve	**Elbow** = SF3	zhou
tun	**AH7** = gluteus	**Eye** = LO5	yan
fu	**AH8** = abdomen	**Finger** = SF1	zhi
yaodizhui	**AH9** = lumbar-sacral vertebrae	**Forehead** = AT1	e
xiong	**AH10** = chest	**Gluteus** = AH7	tun
xiongzhui	**AH11** = thoracic vertebrae	**Heel** = AH1	gen
jing	**AH12** = neck	**Hip** = AH5	kuan
jingzhui	**AH13** = cervical vertebrae	**Internal ear** = LO6	neier
zhi	**SF1** = finger	**Internal nose** = TG4	neibi
wan	**SF2** = wrist	**Jaw** = LO3	he
zhou	**SF3** = elbow	**Knee** = AH4	xi
jian	**SF4,5** = shoulder	**Lumbar-sacral vertebrae** = AH9	yaodizhui
suogu	**SF6** = clavicle	**Mouth** = CO1	kou
kou	**CO1** = mouth	**Neck** = AH12	jing
e	**AT1** = forehead	**Occiput** = AT3	zhen
nie	**AT2** = temple	**Sciatic nerve** = AH6	zuogushenjing
zhen	**AT3** = occiput	**Shoulder** = SF4,5	jian
ya	**LO1** = tooth	**Temple** = AT2	nie
she	**LO2** = tongue	**Thoracic vertebrae** = AH11	xiongzhui
he	**LO3** = jaw	**Toe** = AH2	zhi
yan	**LO5** = eye	**Tongue** = LO2	she
neier	**LO6** = internal ear	**Tonsil** = LO7,8,9	biantaoti
biantaoti	**LO7,8,9** = tonsil	**Tooth** = LO1	ya
neibi	**TG4** = internal nose	**Wrist** = SF2	wan

Fig. A1.2 The somatotopic representations of the body and of the cephalic extremity according to the Chinese standardization.[5,6]

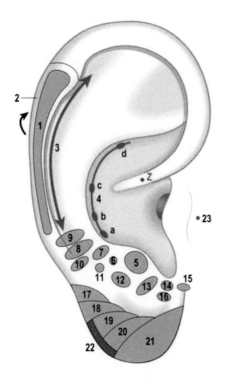

No.	Representation
1	Spinal cord (sensitive roots on the lateral surface)
2	Spinal cord (motor roots on the medial surface)
3	Intermediolateral nuclei of the lateral horn (till Th11)
4	Sympathetic lateral-vertebral ganglia
	a) cervical superior ganglion
	b) cervical middle ganglion (marvellous point)
	c) cervical inferior ganglion
	d) thoracic ganglia (Th10–L1)
5	Thalamus
6	Red nucleus
7	Cerebellum
8	Reticular formation
9	Medulla oblongata
10	Pons
11	Locus niger
12	Hypothalamus
13	Striatum
14	Amigdala
15	Cingular circonvolution
16	Hippocampus
17	Occipital cortex
18	Parietal cortex
19	Temporal cortex
20	Frontal cortex
21	Prefrontal cortex
22	Trigeminal nerve
23	Corpus callosum (so called Tragus Master-Point)

Fig. A1.3   The somatotopic representations of the nervous system according to Nogier[1,2,3,4] (z = point zero).

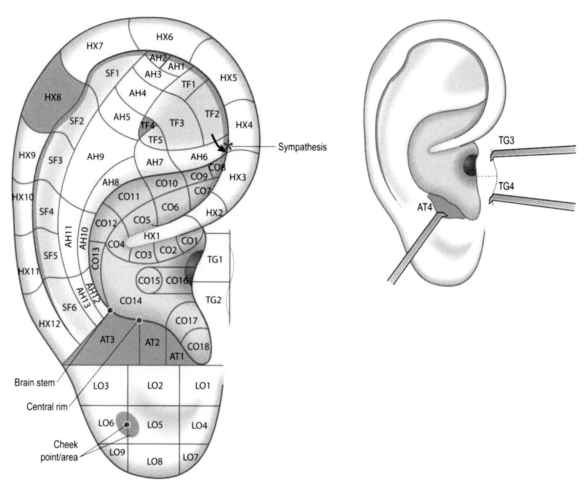

Fig. A1.4 The representation of some areas related to symptoms/disorders of the nervous system according to the Chinese standardization.[5,6]

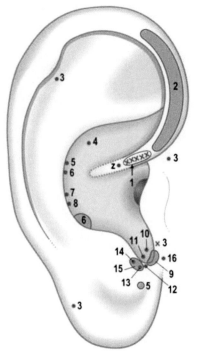

No.	Representation
1	Ovary/testicle (internal surface)
2	Adrenal gland
3	Adrenocorticotropic hormone (ACTH) multiple points
4	Pancreas
5	Mammary gland, twice represented
6	Thymus, twice represented
7	Parathyroid
8	Thyroid
9	Hypophysis
10	Prolactin
11	Somatotropic hormone (STH)
12	Thyroid-stimulating hormone (TSH)
13	Luteotropic hormone (LTH)
14	Follicle-stimulating hormone (FSH)
15	Gonadotropic or genital area
16	Epiphysis

Fig. A1.5 The somatotopic representations of the endocrine system according to Nogier[1,2,3,4] (z = point zero).

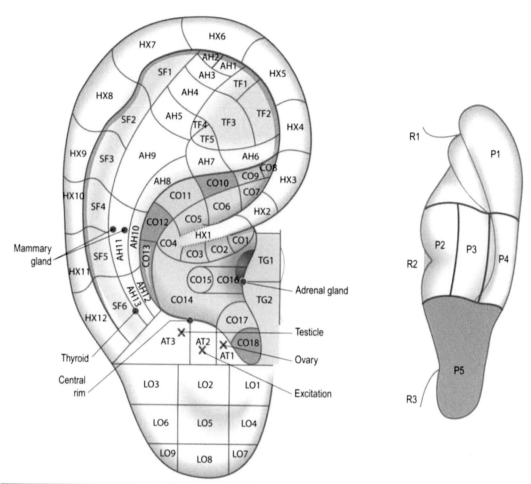

Coded area and name	Symptom
CO4 *wei* = stomach	Obesity
CO10 *shen* = kidney	Menstrual disorders
CO11 *yidan* = pancreas-gallbladder	Diabetes
CO12 *gan* = liver	Menstrual disorders, premenstrual syndrome, climacteric syndrome
CO13 *pi* = spleen	Obesity, menstrual disorders
CO17 *sanjao* = triple energizer	Obesity
CO18 *neifenmi* = endocrine	Hypopituitarism, menstrual disorders, hyperthyroidism
TG1 *shangping* = upper tragus	Diabetes
TG2 *xiaping* = lower tragus	Obesity, hyperthyroidism
Adrenal gland *shenshangxian*	Asthenia, hypotension, inflammatory diseases, allergic diseases
Central rim *yuanzhong*	Acromegaly
P5 *erbeishen* = kidney of the medial surface of the auricle	Menstrual disorders
The following points of the auricle belong historically to the auricular chart preceding the standardisation:	
Mammary gland (double representation) *ruxian*	Premenstrual syndrome
Thyroid gland *jiazhuangxian*	Thyroid gland disorders
Testicle *gaowan* (on the internal surface of the antitragus)	Hypogonadism
Excitation *xingfen* (on the internal surface of the antitragus)	Hypogonadism
Ovary *luanchao* (on the internal surface of the antitragus)	Menstrual disorders, hypogonadism

Fig. A1.6 The representation of some areas related to disorders of the endocrine system and the metabolism according to the Chinese standardization[5,6] (in pale pink the areas associated with diabetes and obesity).

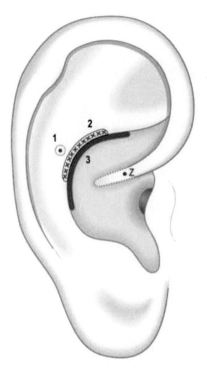

No.	Representation
1	Heart (medial and lateral surface)
2	Heart (internal surface)
3	Circulatory system

Fig. A1.7   The somatotopic representations of the cardiovascular system according to Nogier[1,2,3,4] (z = point zero).

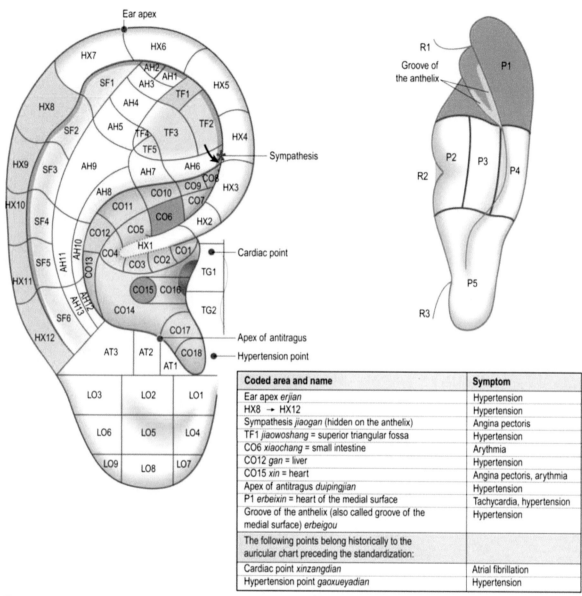

Coded area and name	Symptom
Ear apex *erjian*	Hypertension
HX8 → HX12	Hypertension
Sympathesis *jiaogan* (hidden on the anthelix)	Angina pectoris
TF1 *jiaowoshang* = superior triangular fossa	Hypertension
CO6 *xiaochang* = small intestine	Arythmia
CO12 *gan* = liver	Hypertension
CO15 *xin* = heart	Angina pectoris, arythmia
Apex of antitragus *duipingjian*	Hypertension
P1 *erbeixin* = heart of the medial surface	Tachycardia, hypertension
Groove of the anthelix (also called groove of the medial surface) *erbeigou*	Hypertension
The following points belong historically to the auricular chart preceding the standardization:	
Cardiac point *xinzangdian*	Atrial fibrillation
Hypertension point *gaoxueyadian*	Hypertension

Fig. A1.8 The representation of some areas related to symptoms/disorders of the cardiovascular system and hypertension according to the Chinese standardization[5,6] (in pale pink the areas associated with hypertension).

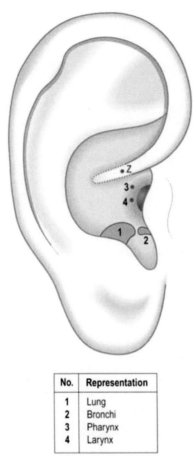

No.	Representation
1	Lung
2	Bronchi
3	Pharynx
4	Larynx

Fig. A1.9   The somatotopic representations of the respiratory system according to Nogier[1,2,3,4] (z = point zero).

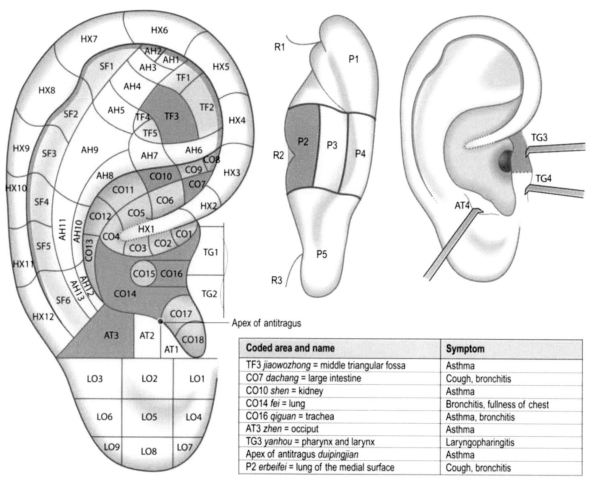

Coded area and name	Symptom
TF3 *jiaowozhong* = middle triangular fossa	Asthma
CO7 *dachang* = large intestine	Cough, bronchitis
CO10 *shen* = kidney	Asthma
CO14 *fei* = lung	Bronchitis, fullness of chest
CO16 *qiguan* = trachea	Asthma, bronchitis
AT3 *zhen* = occiput	Asthma
TG3 *yanhou* = pharynx and larynx	Laryngopharingitis
Apex of antitragus *duipingjian*	Asthma
P2 *erbeifei* = lung of the medial surface	Cough, bronchitis

Fig. A1.10   The representation of some areas related to symptoms/disorders of the respiratory system according to the Chinese standardization.[5,6]

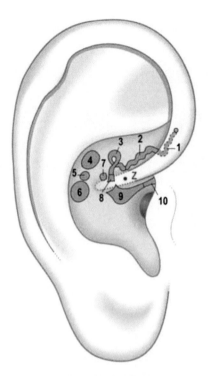

No.	Representation
1	Rectum
2	Large intestine
3	Small intestine
4	Pancreas
5	Spleen
6	Liver
7	Gallbladder
8	Duodenum
9	Stomach
10	Esophagus

Fig. A1.11   The somatotopic representations of the digestive system according to Nogier[1,2,3,4] (z = point zero).

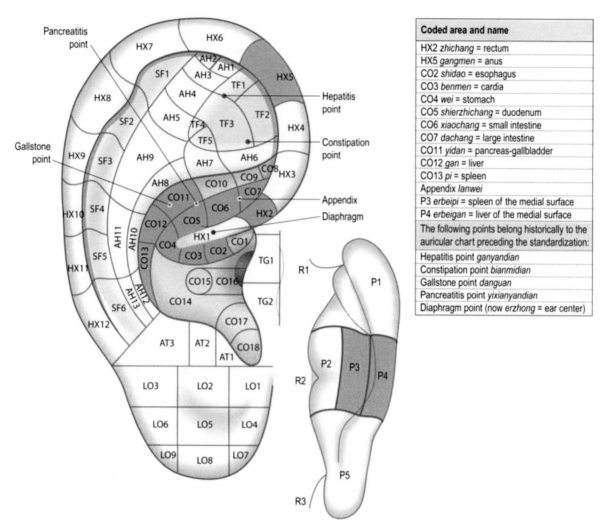

Fig. A1.12 The representation of the areas related to the digestive system according to the Chinese standardization.[5,6]

Coded area and name
HX2 *zhichang* = rectum
HX5 *gangmen* = anus
CO2 *shidao* = esophagus
CO3 *benmen* = cardia
CO4 *wei* = stomach
CO5 *shierzhichang* = duodenum
CO6 *xiaochang* = small intestine
CO7 *dachang* = large intestine
CO11 *yidan* = pancreas-gallbladder
CO12 *gan* = liver
CO13 *pi* = spleen
Appendix *lanwei*
P3 *erbeipi* = spleen of the medial surface
P4 *erbeigan* = liver of the medial surface
The following points belong historically to the auricular chart preceding the standardization:
Hepatitis point *ganyandian*
Constipation point *bianmidian*
Gallstone point *danguan*
Pancreatitis point *yixianyandian*
Diaphragm point (now *erzhong* = ear center)

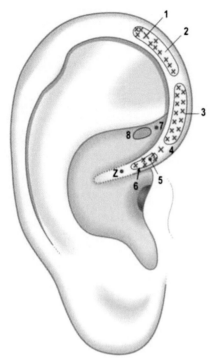

No.	Representation
1	Kidney (on the internal surface of the helix)
2	Ureter (on the internal surface of the helix)
3	Uterus/prostate (on the internal surface of the helix)
4	Vagina (on the internal surface of the helix)
5	External genitals
6	Ovary/testicle (on the internal surface of the helix)
7	Urethra
8	Bladder

Fig. A1.13   The somatotopic representation of the genitourinary system according to Nogier[1,2,3,4] (z = point zero).

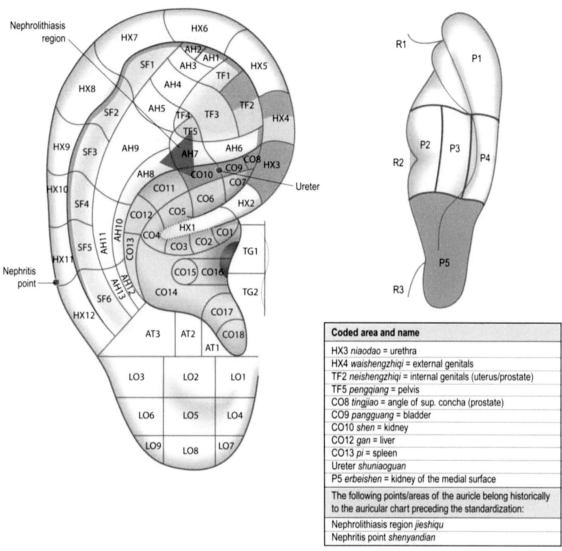

Coded area and name
HX3 *niaodao* = urethra
HX4 *waishengzhiqi* = external genitals
TF2 *neishengzhiqi* = internal genitals (uterus/prostate)
TF5 *pengqiang* = pelvis
CO8 *tingjiao* = angle of sup. concha (prostate)
CO9 *pangguang* = bladder
CO10 *shen* = kidney
CO12 *gan* = liver
CO13 *pi* = spleen
Ureter *shuniaoguan*
P5 *erbeishen* = kidney of the medial surface
The following points/areas of the auricle belong historically to the auricular chart preceding the standardization:
Nephrolithiasis region *jieshiqu*
Nephritis point *shenyandian*

Fig. A1.14 The representation of the areas related to the genitourinary system according to the Chinese standardization[5,6] (in pale pink the areas associated particularly with disorders of the female genital apparatus).

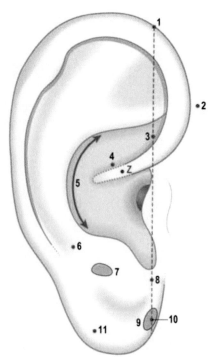

No.	Representation
1	Omega 2 (somatic stress)
2	Reactional Point (point R) of Bourdiol
3	Omega 1 (visceral stress)
4	Anxiety point
5	Sympathetic cervical ganglia
6	'Jérôme' point
7	Hypothalamus
8	Aggressiveness
9	Fear area
10	Omega (psychological stress)
11	Sadness point

Fig. A1.15 The somatotopic representations of some points/areas related to mental disorders according to Nogier and Bourdiol[1,2,3,7] (z = point zero).

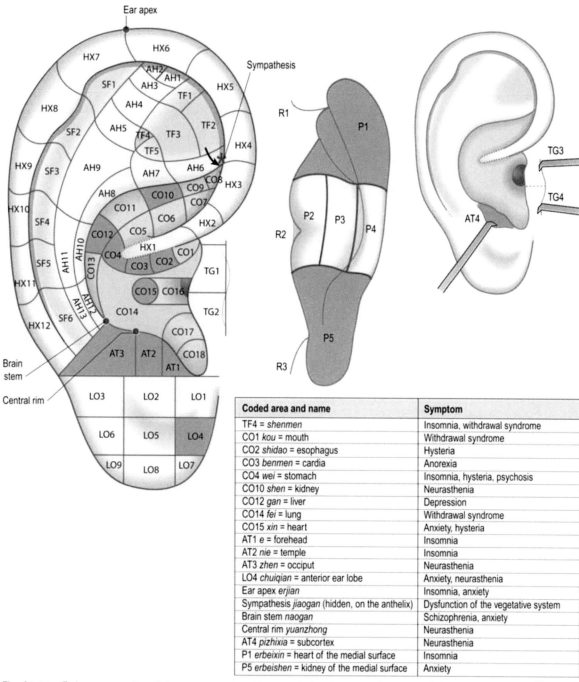

Coded area and name	Symptom
TF4 = *shenmen*	Insomnia, withdrawal syndrome
CO1 *kou* = mouth	Withdrawal syndrome
CO2 *shidao* = esophagus	Hysteria
CO3 *benmen* = cardia	Anorexia
CO4 *wei* = stomach	Insomnia, hysteria, psychosis
CO10 *shen* = kidney	Neurasthenia
CO12 *gan* = liver	Depression
CO14 *fei* = lung	Withdrawal syndrome
CO15 *xin* = heart	Anxiety, hysteria
AT1 *e* = forehead	Insomnia
AT2 *nie* = temple	Insomnia
AT3 *zhen* = occiput	Neurasthenia
LO4 *chuiqian* = anterior ear lobe	Anxiety, neurasthenia
Ear apex *erjian*	Insomnia, anxiety
Sympathesis *jiaogan* (hidden, on the anthelix)	Dysfunction of the vegetative system
Brain stem *naogan*	Schizophrenia, anxiety
Central rim *yuanzhong*	Neurasthenia
AT4 *pizhixia* = subcortex	Neurasthenia
P1 *erbeixin* = heart of the medial surface	Insomnia
P5 *erbeishen* = kidney of the medial surface	Anxiety

Fig. A1.16 The representation of the areas associated to mental disorders according to the Chinese standardization[5,6] (in pale pink the areas associated with the drug withdrawal syndrome).

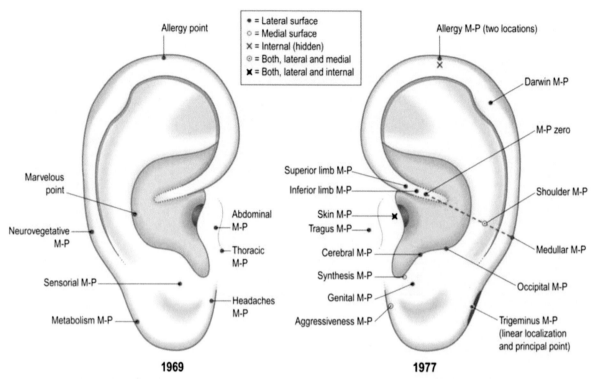

Fig. A1.17 Master Points (M-P) proposed by Nogier in two different periods of his clinical approach to the outer ear: in 1969 on the left;[8] in 1977 on the right.[9]

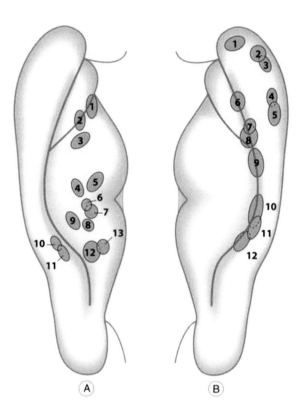

No.	Representation of some internal organs	No.	Representation of some parts of the musculoskeletal system
1	Prostate	1	Heel
2	Kidney	2	Thumb
3	Colon	3	Other fingers of the hand
4	Gallbladder	4	Wrist
5	Pancreas	5	Elbow
6	Duodenum	6	Knee
7	Stomach	7	Hip
8	Cardias	8	Muscles of the pelvic girdle
9	Esophagus	9	Muscles of the lumbar-thoracic tract
10	Thyroid gland	10	Muscles of the shoulder girdle
11	Larynx	11	Shoulder
12	Lung	12	Muscles of the neck
13	Heart		

Fig. A1.18 Representation of some internal organs on the medial surface (A); representation of some parts of the musculoskeletal system (B) according to Romoli.

References

[1] Nogier PFM. Treatise of auriculotherapy. Moulins-les-Metz: Maisonneuve; 1972.

[2] Nogier PFM, Petitjean F, Mallard A. Compléments des points réflexes auriculaires. Moulins-les-Metz: Maisonneuve; 1989.

[3] Nogier PFM. Handbook to auriculotherapy. 2nd ed. Brussels: SATAS; 1998.

[4] Nogier R. Auriculothérapie 1er degré. Montpellier: Sauramps; 2000.

[5] Auricular Points Chart. Institute of Acupuncture and Moxibustion – China Academy of TCM. Beijing: China Medico-Pharmaceutical Science and Technology; 1989.

[6] Technical Supervise Bureau of State. The nomenclature and location of ear acupuncture points. Beijing: Chinese Standard Publishing House; 1993.

[7] Bourdiol RJ. Elements of auriculotherapy. Moulins-les-Metz: Maisonneuve; 1982.

[8] Nogier PFM. Traité d'auriculothérapie. Moulins-les-Metz: Maisonneuve; 1969.

[9] Nogier PFM. Introduction pratique à l'auriculothérapie. Moulins-les-Metz: Maisonneuve; 1977.

Appendix 2

Observations on the Agiscop device

Filadelfio Puglisi

Since all of the clinical evaluations in this book were obtained using a commercial device, it is necessary to ascertain its consistency with the one specially built to take the measurements described in Chapter 6: Agiscop D, made by Sedatelec, France (see www.sedatelec.fr) does not use the single active electrode technique, but a double electrode.

The Agiscop is a small, portable, battery-operated apparatus, with a hand reference electrode held by the patient, while the operator holds a probe made of two concentric electrodes. The center one is a metal rod with a smoothed point 1 mm in diameter, surrounded by a coaxial electrode made from a metal tube with an external diameter of 3 mm (Fig. A2.1). Both electrodes are covered with an insulated coating except at their tip. The force to

be exerted when pressing the probe in Agiscop D varies from about 50 g (both electrodes securely in contact with the skin) to about 80 g (end of mechanical range for the springs loading the electrodes).

From what can be inferred from the documentation supplied and from direct examination, the apparatus first measures the skin resistance between one of the two electrodes and a reference metal hand piece held by the patient. In a second step, it measures the resistance between the other electrode and the reference. Then it subtracts the two values and indicates if they differ by more than a specified amount. The difference is set by the operator within a continuous range conventionally indicated by the numbers 0 to 6 and this amount diminishes when going from 0 to 6.

With a second knob the operator chooses whether to be informed of one of two possibilities:

1. The coaxial electrode has a lower resistance than the central electrode (knob set as −).
2. The coaxial electrode has a higher resistance than the central electrode (knob set as +).

In either case a beep is heard and an LED flashes if the difference is greater than the set amount. Nothing happens if the difference is smaller.

The amounts corresponding to the different knob positions were measured using resistors of known value and modeling the double contact with the circuit shown in Figure A2.2. When the sensitivity knob is set at '1', the amount of difference is about 20 MΩ, diminishing in an exponential fashion as shown in Figure A2.3. The values of resistance shown in this figure are only approximated, probably around 10% more or less, since

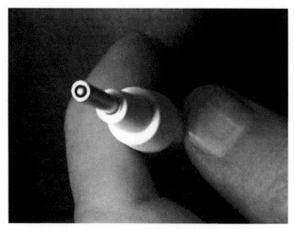

Fig. A2.1 Agiscop's central and coaxial electrodes.

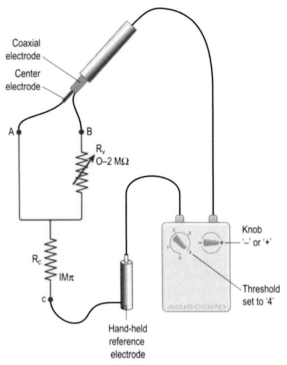

Fig. A2.2 Experimental setting for threshold measuring. The knob on the left regulates the threshold, the knob on the right decides the − or + modality.

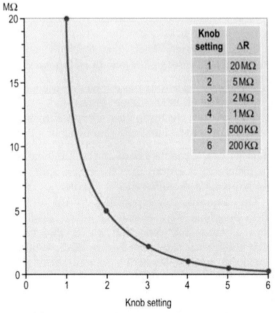

Knob setting	ΔR
1	20 MΩ
2	5 MΩ
3	2 MΩ
4	1 MΩ
5	500 KΩ
6	200 KΩ

Fig. A2.3 Approximated values of resistance difference for knob settings 1 to 6 when light and sound switch on.

the knob is small and there is a dead range at the beginning for switching the device 'on'.

Almost all the measurements in this book have been taken with Agiscop's sensitivity knob set at '4' since this seemed a good compromise between an almost absolute absence of signal points (sensitivity knob set to '1'), and practically all touches signaled by the device (knob to '6').

It is consistently observed that when Agiscop's probe explores ear skin, − points are always much more numerous than + points, usually in the ratio of about 2 to 1. According to the explanation given above, this would mean that the resistance under the coaxial electrode is more often below the resistance under the central electrode than the reverse. This is difficult to explain, because if at a given spot the center electrode has a higher resistance, by moving it by about 0.5 to 1 mm the situation should reverse, since now the center has moved onto the lower resistance region while the coaxial electrode is now on an area that includes the former high resistance spot. But this assumption is not often confirmed by practice.

Probably at least part of the behavior of Agiscop can be explained by observing Figure A2.4. It is possible that the indentation of the skin under the coaxial electrode is larger and more skin area is in contact with the coaxial rather than the central electrode. Therefore the resistance under the center one is constantly somewhat higher. This would explain why − findings with the Agiscop are so much more frequent than + findings. This problem is addressed to the maker, whereas for clinical purposes it is sufficient to know that spots signaled by Agiscop in position '4' indicate a difference in resistance of about 1 MΩ between two areas of skin, concentric with one another and falling within a circular surface about 3 mm in diameter.

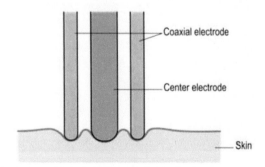

Fig. A2.4 Skin indentation at Agiscop's tip.

It is interesting to note that the value of position '4' (decided empirically by Dr Romoli) is not very far from the threshold (2 MΩ) adopted in Chapter 6 after examining the histogram in Figure 6.7. Part of the study presented in Chapter 6 was dedicated to evaluating whether such discontinuities revealed by Agiscop corresponded to the locations where the resistance between a single electrode on the skin surface and a large electrode hand-held by the patient was significantly lower.

As observed in Chapter 6, 118 of the 228 points tested were indicated by the Agiscop as 1 MΩ discontinuity points (with the Agiscop's sensitivity knob in position '4'), either of the − or of the + modality, the − points being about double the + points.

It appears therefore that if a spot on the ear skin has a local discontinuity of at least 1 MΩ, then it also has an absolute low skin resistance, as measured with a device such as the circuit in Figure A2.2. This is a remarkable finding, for which again there is no ready physiological explanation.

Summing up the results above, a minimum set of assumptions can be reasonably made on the Agiscop detected points:

- Agiscop measures discontinuities in electrical skin resistance (ESR).
- The discontinuity value that is signaled by the device depends on the position of the sensitivity knob, diminishing from 0 to 6.
- Most of the points detected by Agiscop, in the − or + setting, are also points with an absolute low ESR.
- It is more frequent to find − points than + points, probably in a ratio of 2 to 1.

Color Plates

FROM THE LABORATORY OF PROFESSOR PIERRE RABISCHONG

PLATE I SERIAL ANATOMY AND EXPERIMENTAL RESEARCH

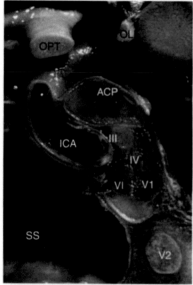

Plate IA Coronal section of the anterior part of the cavernous sinus showing the oculomotor nerves III, IV, VI and the ophthalmic branch (V1) of the trigeminal nerve.

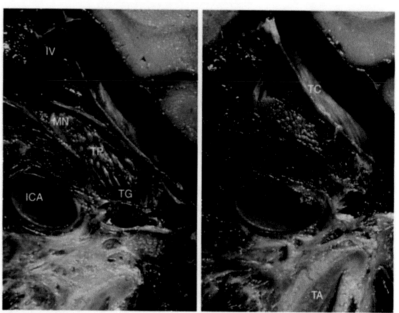

Plate IB Anterior view of a coronal section of the trigeminal motor and sensory roots: on the left, the trigeminal cavum; on the right, the entrance of the cavum.

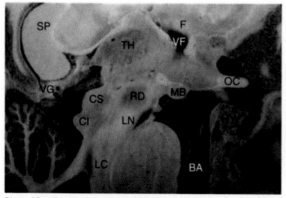

Plate IC Sagittal section of the mesencephalon and pons. Key for plates 1A, 1B, 1C

ACP	=	anterior clinoid process	OPT	=	optic tract
BA	=	basilar artery	RD	=	red nucleus
CI	=	colliculus inferior	SP	=	splenium
CS	=	colliculus superior	SS	=	sphenoid sinus
F	=	fornix	TA	=	tuba
HY	=	hypophysis	TC	=	tentorium cerebelli
ICA	=	internal carotid artery	TG	=	trigeminal ganglion
III	=	oculomotor nerve	TH	=	thalamus
IV	=	trochlear nerve	TP	=	triangular plexus
LC	=	locus coeruleus	VI	=	abducens nerve
LN	=	locus niger	V1, V2	=	first and second branch of trigeminal nerve
MB	=	mamillary body			
MN	=	masticatory nerve	VF	=	ventricular foramen
OC	=	optic chiasma	VG	=	vena Galeni
OLF	=	olfactory tract			

PLATE I SERIAL ANATOMY AND EXPERIMENTAL RESEARCH

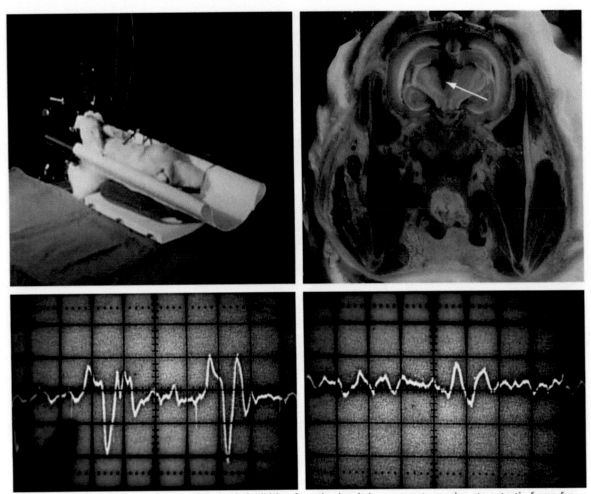

Plate ID Experimental demonstration of thalamic inhibition for pain signals by acupuncture using stereotactic frame for rabbit (upper left). Electrode implantation into the parafascicular thalamic nucleus (upper right, see arrow). Thalamic signal during painful stimulation of hind limb of rabbit before acupuncture (lower left) and after acupuncture (lower right). (Unit 103, INSERM, Montpellier, France.)

PLATE II SKIN ALTERATIONS RELATED TO VASCULARIZATION (PALENESS, HYPEREMIA, TELANGIECTASIA). (From the photographic archive of Dr Marco Romoli.)

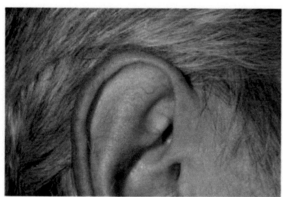

Plate IIA Paleness of the lower branch of the anthelix delimited by two telangiectasia in a 65-year-old male with herniation of the L4–L5 intervertebral disk. The telangiectasia lying behind and a third telangiectasia on the upper branch of the anthelix are aligned with Nogier's point zero.

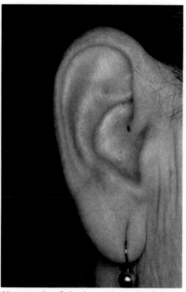

Plate IIB Hyperemia of the lower branch of the anthelix in a 63-year-old female suffering from chronic backache. Point zero has been marked with ink.

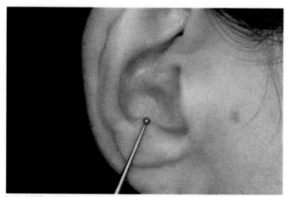

Plate IIC Hyperemia of the upper part of the inferior concha, below the helix root, in a 24-year-old female suffering with gastroesophageal reflux disease.

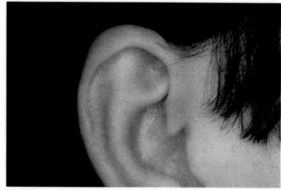

Plate IID Hyperemia of the triangular fossa in a 24-year-old female affected by polycystic ovaries and dysmenorrhea.

PLATE III SKIN ALTERATIONS RELATED TO VASCULARIZATION (PALENESS, HYPEREMIA, TELANGIECTASIA).

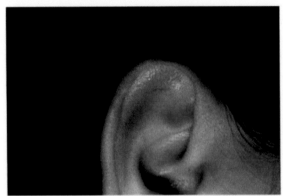

Plate IIIA Telangiectasia on the upper branch of the anthelix, caudally delimiting an area of paleness, in a 40-year-old female with a 12 month history of carpal tunnel syndrome on the right side. A reticular telangiectasia located on the representation of the elbow is possibly associated with the patient's respiratory allergy.

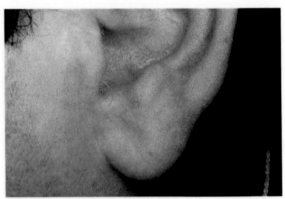

Plate IIIB Hyperemia and folliculitis of the anterior part of the antitragus in a 35-year-old male suffering with recurrent maxillary sinusitis.

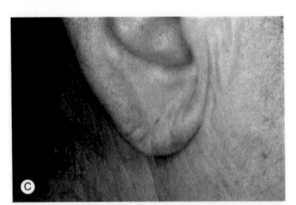

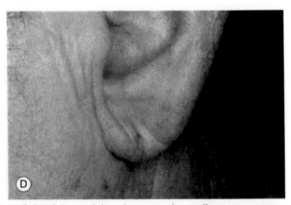

Plates IIIC and IIID Telangiectasia and spots on the lower border of the right ear lobe where two descending creases are going to meet together (C); paleness of the corresponding part of the left ear lobe (D) in a 66-year-old female affected by glaucoma and hypertensive retinopathy.

PLATE IV SKIN ALTERATIONS RELATED TO VASCULARIZATION (PALENESS, HYPEREMIA, TELANGIECTASIA).

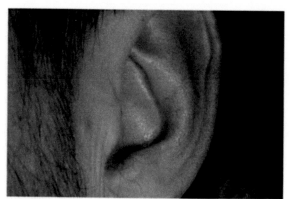

Plate IVA   Multiple telangiectasia on the anthelix in a 52-year-old male suffering from cervical-brachial pain syndrome at the C5–C6 level.

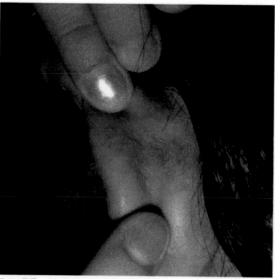

Plate IVB   Linear telangiectasia on the medial surface of the auricle, corresponding to Chinese *fengxi* (Wind Stream) area on the lateral surface in a 38-year-old female who had been suffering from hay fever for several years.

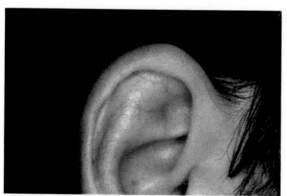

Plate IVC   Telangiectasia and spots on the upper branch of the anthelix in a 37-year-old male suffering with the after-effects of fracture of the right tibia that occurred 8 years previously. A further spot is visible on the concha.

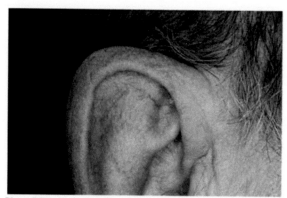

Plate IVD   Reticular telangiectasia on the scapha and a more pronounced telangiectasia on the upper branch of the anthelix in a 75-year-old male suffering with chronic degenerative gonarthritis.

PLATE V SKIN ALTERATIONS RELATED TO VASCULARIZATION (PALENESS, HYPEREMIA, TELANGIECTASIA).

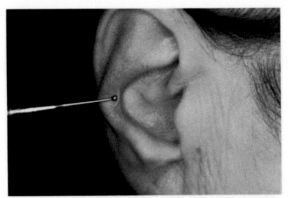

Plate VA   Linear telangiectasia on the right upper concha, delimiting a hypertrophic area of the root of the helix, in a 65-year-old female with chronic persisting hepatitis.

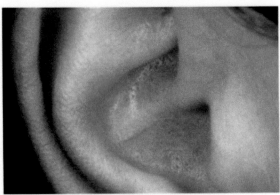

Plate VB   Linear telangiectasia on the concha in an 18-year-old female with dyspepsia caused prevalently by lactose intolerance.

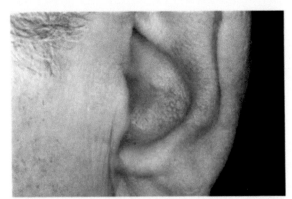

Plate VC   Reticular telangiectasia on the left lower concha in a 66-year-old male who had undergone coronary artery bypass surgery.

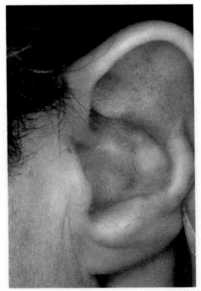

Plate VD   Reticular telangiectasia on the anthelix in chronic backache due to previous vertebral fracture of L1. Another reticular telangiectasia is appreciable on the upper and lower concha as an expression of anxiety with prevalent somatization on the digestive system.

PLATE VI SKIN ALTERATIONS RELATED TO VASCULARIZATION (PALENESS, HYPEREMIA, TELANGIECTASIA).

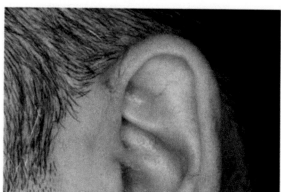

Plate VIA Thick telangiectasia on the ascending part of the helix and linear telangiectasia of the Shen men area in a 47-year-old male with ulcerative coloproctitis. A furfuraceous dyskeratosis is present on the digestive areas of the upper and lower concha.

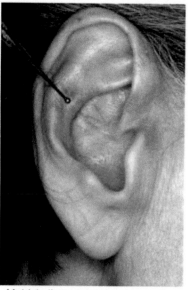

Plate VIB Multiple linear telangiectasia on the upper concha and hyperemia of the anthelix, both aligned on the same sectors, in a 70-year-old female affected by primary carcinoma of the liver. An angioma is furthermore visible on the upper part of the helix.

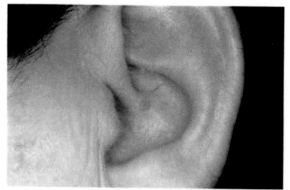

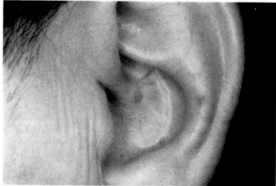

Plates VIC and VID Telangiectasia on the upper concha and pigmentation of the root of the helix in a 65-year-old female affected by diabetes mellitus treated with oral hypoglycemic drugs (C). The worsening of the patient's hyperglycemia 1 year later was accompanied by a darkening of the pigmented area, a higher evidentiation of telangiectasia on the upper concha and by the appearance of a new telangiectasia on the anthelix (D).

PLATE VII SKIN ALTERATIONS RELATED TO VASCULARIZATION (ANGIOMA).

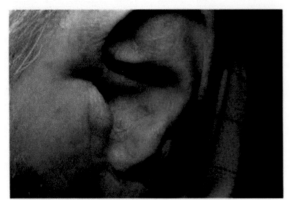

Plate VIIA   Angioma on the left lower concha in a
72-year-old patient with a squamous cell carcinoma of
the left lung.

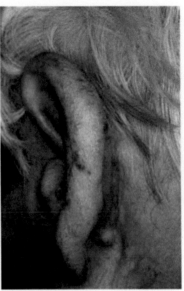

Plate VIIB   Multiple angioma on the helix in a 72-year-old
male affected by primary carcinoma of the liver.

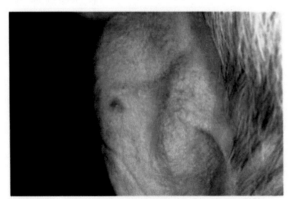

Plate VIIC   Angioma on the medial surface of the left
auricle in a 68-year-old male carrying an undifferentiated
adenocarcinoma of the posterior wall of the stomach.

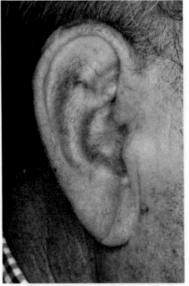

Plate VIID   Angioma allocated within a reticular
telangiectasia on the upper branch of the anthelix in a
73-year-old male; further punctiform angioma on the tail of
the helix and some incisures are visible on the upper part of
the helix. When the picture was taken, the first angioma was
related to the patient's prostate adenoma; 4 years later
unfortunately a further diagnosis of cancer of the rectum
was made.

PLATE VIII SKIN ALTERATIONS RELATED TO VASCULARIZATION (ANGIOMA).

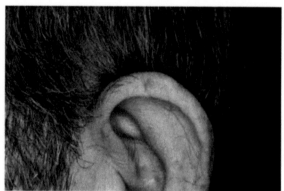

Plate VIIIA   Angioma on the upper part of the helix in a 69-year-old male with benign hypertrophy of the prostate.

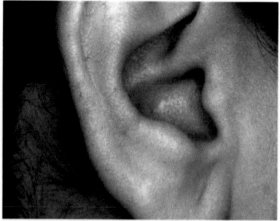

Plate VIIIB   Multiple punctiform angioma on the right anthelix and helix in a 46-year-old patient with fibroadenoma of the right breast.

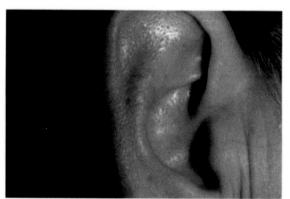

Plate VIIIC   A tiny angioma on the right anthelix in a 70-year-old female carrying an intracanalicular papilloma of the right breast.

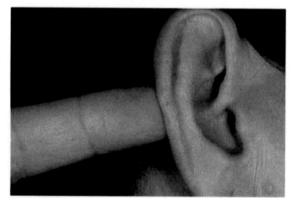

Plate VIIID   Angioma on the right helix in a 55-year-old female affected by adenocarcinoma of the left breast.

PLATE IX SKIN ALTERATIONS RELATED TO PIGMENTATION (DYSCHROMIA, MACULA, NEVUS).

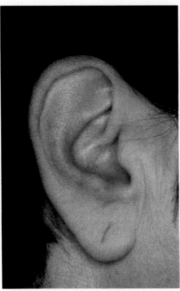

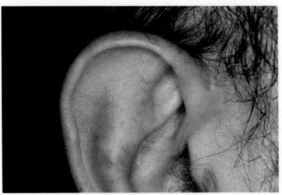

Plate IXB Multiple spots on the anthelix at the bifurcation into upper and lower branch in a 42-year-old male affected by congenital hip displacement. At least two telangiectasia are visible on the anthelix.

Plate IXA Two spots on the antitragus in a 45-year-old female who had been suffering with chronic migraine for 20 years.

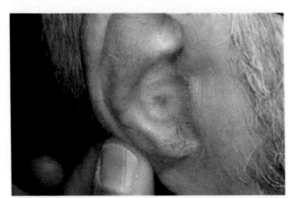

Plate IXC Pigmented area on the right lower concha in a 67-year-old male carrying lung cancer on the right side. The pigmentation was appreciated at least 2 years before any radiological sign of the tumor could be documented.

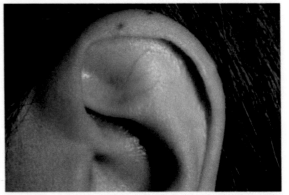

Plate IXD Spots and telangiectasia on the fossa triangularis and the upper branch of the anthelix on the left auricle. Aligned with these alterations and point zero are two nevi on the helix. The 41-year-old female had been operated on for a ovarian cyst on the left side and suffered with recurrent cystitis; her other symptoms were backache, migraine and asthma.

PLATE X SKIN ALTERATIONS RELATED TO PIGMENTATION (DYSCHROMIA, MACULA, NEVUS).

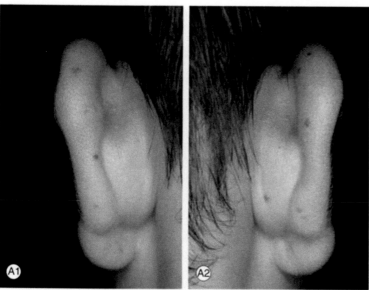

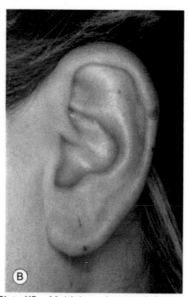

Plates XA1 and XA2 Multiple almost symmetrical nevi on the medial border of the left and right helix in a 28-year-old male suffering with chronic backache due to multiple intervertebral discs bulging in a congenital narrowing of the spinal canal.

Plate XB Multiple nevi on the left ear in a 43-year-old female with recurrent backache needing a lift block for a left short leg.

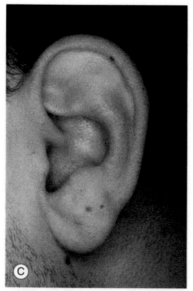

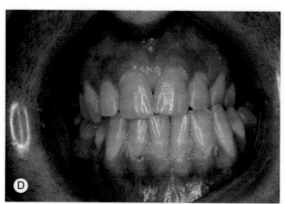

Plates XC and XD Multiple nevi on the left helix and ear lobe in a 25-year-old male suffering with recurrent neck and back pain (C); the same patient carrying a left crossbite with a drift of the lower median incisive line towards right. At inspection there was a reduced development of the hard palate on the left side (D).

PLATE XI SKIN ALTERATIONS RELATED TO PIGMENTATION (DYSCHROMIA, MACULA, NEVUS).

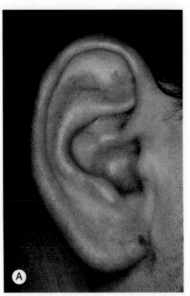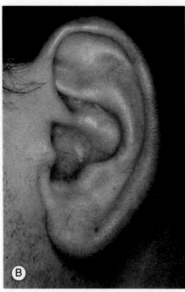

Plates XIA and XIB Multiple asymmetrical nevi on the right and left auricle in a 45-year-old male carrying a diagnosis of obsessive-compulsive disorder. Besides the particular concentration of nevi on the ear lobes, to be noted are linear telangiectasia on the right Shen men, liver and knee areas (A); on the left to be noted are a hypertrophy of the stomach area and linear telangiectasia on the anthelix and on the heart area of the left lower concha (B).

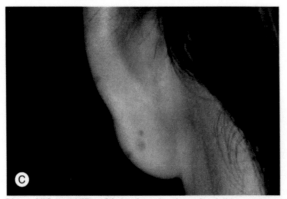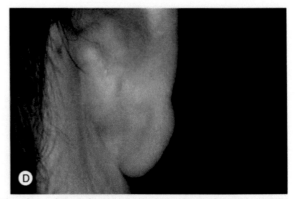

Plates XIC and XID Of the four dyschromia visible on the medial surface of the left ear only the three located on the ear lobe were sensitive to pressure (C). No explanation could be found for this phenomenon at the time when the pictures were taken because the 34-year-old male was symptom-free and the only drugs he took were benzodiazepines. In the following years the patient developed a severe depressive disorder which was treated with various drugs. This, however, did not prevent him from committing suicide 16 years later. The medial surface of the right ear seems to show a cutaneous depression (D) which is symmetrical to the area including the dyschromia on the left side.

PLATE XII SKIN ALTERATIONS RELATED TO CUTANEOUS STRUCTURE (DEPRESSED AREA, CREASE, INCISURE).

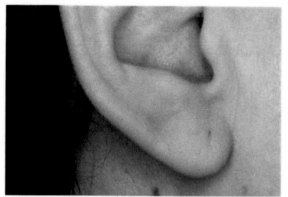

Plate XIIA Depressed area and hyperemia on the ear lobe in a 35-year-old female with otosclerosis (hearing loss and tinnitus).

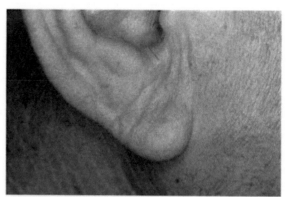

Plate XIIB Double crease on the ear lobe in a 70-year-old male affected by coronary heart disease and hypertension. Two further incisures on the border of the ear lobe are the possible expression of sensorineural hearing loss due to exposure to noise.

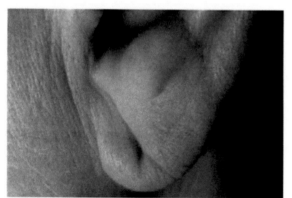

Plate XIIC Elongated depressed area between antitragus and ear lobe, sensitive on palpation, in a 63-year-old female affected by chronic depressive disorder.

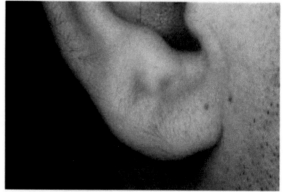

Plate XIID Bowl-shaped depressed areas and nevi on the ear lobe in a 27-year-old male with the double diagnosis of depression and addiction.

PLATE XIII SKIN ALTERATIONS RELATED TO CUTANEOUS STRUCTURE (DEPRESSED AREA, CREASE, INCISURE).

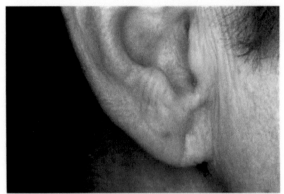

Plate XIIIA Multiple creases on the posterior part of the antitragus; a diagonal crease and a pigmented area on the ear lobe in a 67-year-old female affected by Parkinson's disease.

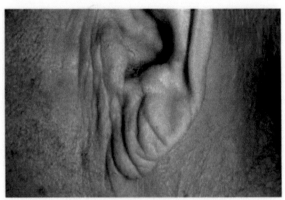

Plate XIIIB Multiple creases on the ear lobe and the tragus in an 87-year-old male with Alzheimer's disease.

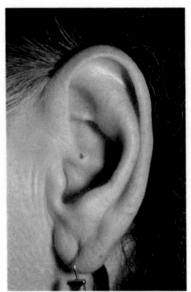

Plate XIIIC Cauterization for sciatica on the lower branch of the antitragus in a 57-year-old female.

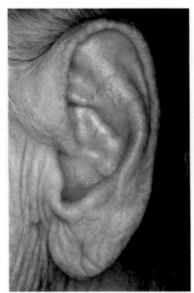

Plate XIIID The same patient as Plate XIIIC, 18 years later, with Alzheimer's disease. Multiple creases are visible on the ear lobe and the tragus.

PLATE XIV SKIN ALTERATIONS RELATED TO CARTILAGINOUS STRUCTURE (HYPERTROPHY i.e. THICKENING; HYPOTROPHY i.e. DEPRESSION).

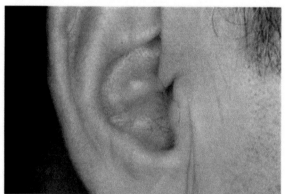

Plate XIVA Hypertrophy and telangiectasia on the root of the helix in a 62-year-old male suffering with gastroduodenitis associated with *Helicobacter pylori* infection.

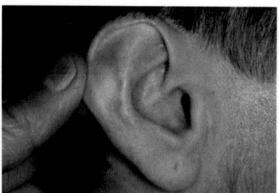

Plate XIVB Serpiginous hypertrophy of the anthelix in a 60-year-old female with widespread degenerative changes in the cervical spine.

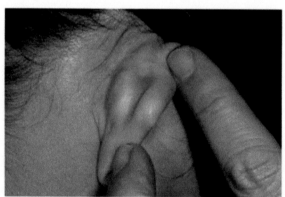

Plate XIVC Deepening of the groove of the anthelix in recurrent back and neck pain in a 36-year-old female.

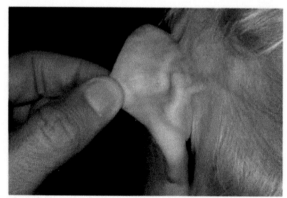

Plate XIVD Bowl-shaped depression on the groove of the anthelix in a 75-year-old female with chronic lumbago.

PLATE XV SKIN ALTERATIONS RELATED TO SEBACEOUS GLAND STRUCTURE (COMEDONES, SEBACEOUS CYSTS).

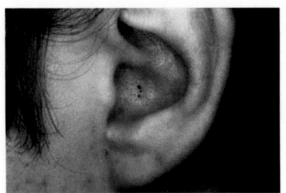

Plate XVA Comedones on the inferior concha in a 20-year-old female suffering with panic attacks.

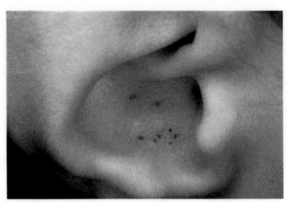

Plate XVB Comedones on the inferior concha in a 16-year-old male affected by allergic dermatitis.

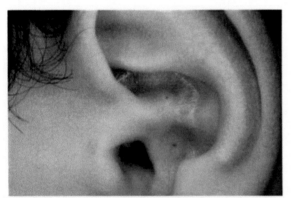

Plate XVC Comedones on the upper and lower concha in a 42-year-old female affected by irritable bowel syndrome in food hypersensitivity.

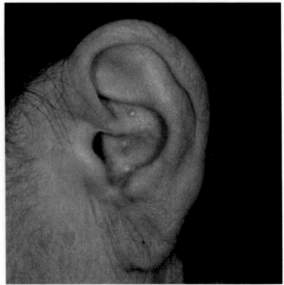

Plate XVD Multiple sebaceous cysts in a 65-year-old female with hypercholesterolemia and gallstones.

PLATE XVI SKIN ALTERATIONS RELATED TO KERATINIZATION (DYSKERATOSIS, DYSTROPHY).

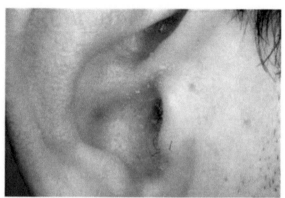

Plate XVIA   Furfuraceous microscales in a 28-year-old male bearing hypertriglycidemia.

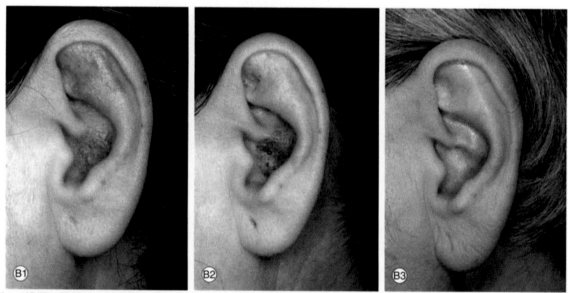

Plates XVIB1, XVIB2 and XVIB3   Dystrophy of the triangular fossa and the anthelix on the left auricle in a 48-year-old female with migraine, gastroesophageal reflux disease, asthenia and depression. Comedonic plaques were noticeable on the inferior concha (B). The same patient 2 years later after a careful and prolonged managing of her food intolerance; significant improvement of her medical condition and disappearance of the dystrophy on the auricle (C). The same patient 20 years later, still managing her food intolerance correctly; the medical condition is stable and only some residual telangiectasia are visible on the cardia area (D).

Case records sectogram

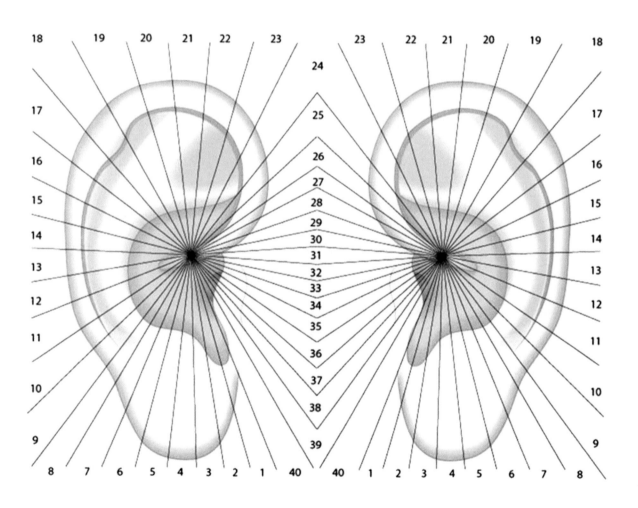

Index

nuclei
    brainstem, 29–30
        reticular formation, 32
    localization/identification, 31
    thalamus, 33
nucleus ambiguus, 29
nucleus of solitary tract, 29
nystagmus, 143, 144

O

obesity, 190
obsessive–compulsive disorder, 284
oculomotor nerves, 20, 273
Oleson, T.
    auricular diagnosis of
        musculoskeletal pain,
        207–8
    auricular zone system, 13
    graphic system, 47–8, 49
    representation of musculoskeletal
        pain, 208
opposed thumbs technique, 118–19
otosclerosis, 285
outer ear see auricle
ovarian cyst, 282
ovaries, 158–60

P

pain, 33
    electrical skin resistance test, 182–4
    gate control theory, 31
    needle contact test, 194–5, 196–7,
        199–200
    neurophysiology, 27–33
    the pain signal, 27
    pathways, 27–31
        brainstem level, 28–31
        spinal cord level, 27–8
pain control
    control centers
        brainstem reticular formation,
            32–3
        posterior horn selective gate,
            31–2
        thalamic selective filter, 33
    enkephaline in, 31
pain threshold in PPT, 114–15
palpation see auricular palpation
pancreas, 97
panic attacks, 288
    auricular inspection, 94, 95, 96
    PPT for, 128, 129, 134
        case study, 133
    selection of ponts for treatment,
        235–6

parasympathetic nervous system, 17,
    18
Parkinson's disease, 286
pars caudalis, 28
Percy, P.-F., 2
    cautery instruments, 2, 3
phobias, 95, 96
physiognomic classification of ear, 56
piercings, 215, 216
pinna
    evolution, 37–40
    measurements, 41
    shape classification, 42–4
pitted ear see fistula auris congenita
pituitary–hypothalamic system,
        representation of, 127
point of joy, 95
Pointoselect, 177
polycystic ovaries, 275
polysynaptic reflexes, 17
posterior horn selective gate, 31–2
postural disorders
    and auricular point distribution,
        220–2
    auricular sensitization, 223–4
posturology, 220–1
PPT see pressure pain test
pregnancy
    headache in, 113
    nausea during, 243–4
pressure pain test (PPT), 109–61
    allergic conditions, 138–40
    auricular palpation, 112–13
    background, 110–12
    cardiovascular system, 149–55
        hypertension-related points,
            152–5
    Chinese vs French systems, 149–60
    confounding factors, 114
    diagnostic success rates
        recent vs past disorders, 210,
            211–12
        'side of pain' detection, 212–13
        symptom identification, 210, 211
    dizziness/vertigo, 143–5
    ear, representation of, 141–3
    eye, representation of, 146–8
    false-positives/-negatives, 216
    with functional MRI, 110–12
    genital system, 156–60
        ovaries, 158–60
        uterus, 158
    headaches/neuralgia, 134–8
        case study, 113
        migraine/tension-type
            headache, 134–6
        trigeminal neuralgia, 136–8
    hierarchy of points, 236
    left/right ears, 115–16

    lesions causing interference, 142
    Nogier–Bourdiol experiment, 110
        with functional MRI, 111–12
    nose, representation of, 145–6
    pain threshold for auricular points,
        114–15
    physical areas
        fibromyalgia, 122–4
        lower limb, 117
        musculoskeletal system, 116–17
        spine
            cervical, 120–2
            thoracolumbar, 117–20
    popularity with practitioners, 235
    psychological/psychiatric areas,
        124–34
        anxiety
            with depression, 130–3
            phobic, 128–30
        sleep disorder, 128
        stress response, 125–8
    'relativity of tenderness', 115, 236
    scoring, 115
    teeth/temporomandibular joint,
        representation of, 148–9
    tender points, 112
        auricular distribution, 115–16
        detection in tender area, 112
        number identified, 112
        significance, 114–16
    thumb point, 111–12
    tinnitus, 143
    in treatment point selection, 232
    urinary system, 155–6
    validation, 210–14
    validation of auricular diagnosis,
        209
    vs ESRT, 178–82
pressure-probes, 115
    alternative techniques with, 115
    use on lower limbs, 117
prostate cancer, 280
protopathic sensibility, 27–8
pseudocranial nerves, 20
psychosomatic disorders, 248
Punctoscope, 143, 176
pure motor nerve, 20
pure sensorial nerve, 20

Q

qi (stasis of Blood), 93

R

'reference points' for diseases, 241
reflexes, 17

Printed in the United States
By Bookmasters